D1130472

Listening to Patients

A Phenomenological Approach to Nursing Research and Practice

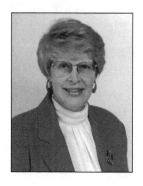

Sandra P. Thomas, PhD, RN, FAAN, is Professor and Director of the PhD Program in Nursing at the University of Tennessee in Knoxville. Her initial nursing preparation was at St. Mary's Hospital School of Nursing. She holds bachelor's, master's, and doctoral degrees in education, majoring in educational psychology. She also earned a master's degree in nursing, with clinical specialization in mental health nursing; her nursing practice and research have primarily focused on women's anger, stress, and depression. Her program of research received the Chancellor's Award for Research at the University of Tennessee. She is the editor of *Issues in Mental Health Nursing* and the author of over 80 journal articles, books, and book chapters. She is a member of the American Nurses Association, the American Psychological Association, and Sigma Theta Tau International. She is a board member of the International Council on Women's Health Issues and a charter member of the Southern Nursing Research Society. In 1996, she was named a Fellow of the American Academy of Nursing. In 1999, she became a Fellow of the Society of Behavioral Medicine.

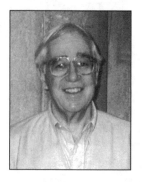

Howard R. Pollio, PhD, is Alumni Professor of Psychology at the University of Tennessee in Knoxville. He received his bachelor's and master's degrees in psychology from Brooklyn College and his PhD in experimental psychology from the University of Michigan. His areas of specialization include learning and thinking, college teaching, figurative language, humor, and existential-phenomenological approaches to psychology. He has published over 120 journal articles, book chapters, and books. He was the founding editor of the journal *Metaphor and Symbol*. He has been president of the Southeastern Psychological Association and a Phi Beta Kappa national lecturer. He is a Fellow of two divisions of the American Psychological Association and has received a number of teaching and research awards.

Listening to Patients

A Phenomenological Approach to Nursing Research and Practice

Sandra P. Thomas, PhD, RN, FAAN
Howard R. Pollio, PhD

 Springer Publishing Company

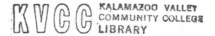

Copyright © 2002 by Springer Publishing Company, Inc.

Springer Publishing Company, Inc.
536 Broadway
New York, NY 10012–3955

Acquisition Editor: Helvi Gold
Production Editor: Jeanne Libby
Cover design by Susan Hauley

03 04 05/ 5 4 3 2

Library of Congress Cataloging-in-Publication Data

Thomas, Sandra P.
   Listening to patients : a phenomenological approach to nursing / Sandra P. Thomas, Howard R. Pollio.
     p.   cm.
   Includes bibliographical references and index.
   ISBN 0-8261-1466-0
   1. Nurse and patient. 2. Existentialism. 3. Interpersonal communication.
4. Patients—Counseling of. 5. Nursing—Philosophy. I. Pollio, Howard R.
II. Title.
   [DNLM: 1. Nurse–Patient Relations. 2. Attitude to Health.
3. Existentialism. 4. Patients—psychology. 5. Philosophy, Nursing.
WY 87 T4615L 2001]
RT42.T48 2001
610.73'06'99—dc21   2001034183

Printed in the United States of America by Sheridan Books, Inc.

This book is dedicated to the patients who shared their experiences with us. We are hopeful that nurses everywhere will hear their voices.

Contents

IV. Nursing and the Human Experience of Time

V. Nursing and the Human Experience of the World

Preface

This book began with a casual remark, a jaunty little exchange between an experimental psychologist-turned-phenomenologist (Howard) and a psychiatric nurse-turned-researcher (Sandra) who had studied phenomenology with Howard in 1981 and later developed a fuller appreciation of its relevance for the discipline of nursing. For nearly a decade, the two of us have collaborated in leading an interdisciplinary phenomenology research group on Tuesday afternoons. Sparked by discussion among the group, this book was conceived on one of those Tuesdays. Our brief exchange that afternoon went something like this: "Why don't we write a book for nurses?" "Great idea! I'll draft a prospectus." After Ursula Springer concluded that the prospectus had merit and invited us to proceed with the book, a great deal of new learning and hard thinking was required before we could complete it. The process of writing this book has deepened not only our knowledge and appreciation of existential phenomenology but also our mutual respect for each other as scholars and as people.

At times we knew what we wanted to say to nurses but struggled to find ways to say it. Writing is always a humbling experience. The philosopher Maurice Merleau-Ponty, on whom we rely heavily for inspiration, understood how writers must grope for the right words to communicate with their readers. How true we found his observation that "writers experience the excess of what is to be said beyond their ordinary capacities" (*The Prose of the World*, 1973, p. 57). At other times, we really did not know what we thought about a topic until we wrote about it. Putting words on paper, and then repeatedly revising them, eventually clarified our thoughts. Again, Merleau-Ponty was prescient: "Many writers . . . begin a book without knowing exactly what they are going to put in it" (*The Phenomenology of Perception*, 1962, p. 177). Eventually, all the words were on paper. It is our hope that readers will sense our passion for existential phenomenology and understand our conviction that it provides a basis for a new dimension of nursing science and practice.

Who are the potential readers of this book? As we wrote, we thought of graduate students and faculty, certainly, but we also meant to speak directly to clinicians, in all specialty areas of nursing, who might be interested in hearing about a humanistic philosophy and research methodology that has the potential to illuminate the deeper meanings of health crises and universal human experiences such as pain and spiritual distress.

We would be greatly pleased if teachers of undergraduates selected this book as a text. With this possibility in mind, we deliberately presented our material in a clear, jargon-free style accessible to anyone enrolled in college courses.

Every nurse hears patient stories, but not every nurse learns to *listen* to them in a way that permits *hearing* their richness and power. What this book hopes to promote is a method of hearing those stories and making meaning of the narratives within the context of nursing practice. The book is organized into five major sections. Part One introduces nurses to phenomenological thinkers, such as Merleau-Ponty, and applies insights from philosophy to the processes of engaging in dialogue with patients and interpreting what they tell us. In this introductory section, we begin the task of acquainting readers with the major contexts within which human existence is experienced (body, other people, time, and world). Thereafter, a specific section of the book is devoted to each of these contextual grounds of human life. In Part Two, for example, we examine philosophy, theory, and research about the body. In Part Three, we explore the human experience of other people. In Parts Four and Five, we address the topics of time and world, respectively. Compelling original research, conducted in a variety of health care settings by members of the research team at the University of Tennessee, is presented throughout the book. We anticipate that you will find the words of patients and their families riveting as you read these research reports.

Although we realize that some readers may be drawn by clinical interests or personal curiosity to particular chapters and not proceed in the sequence we chose for organizing our material, we urge a bit of caution. Chapters 1 and 2 provide essential information about our philosophy and approach to phenomenological research; to avoid redundancy, specific procedural details are not repeated in subsequent chapters. Thus, we strongly suggest a careful reading of these chapters before proceeding. The introductory chapters in each of the main sections of the book (Chapters 3, 6, 10, and 14) are also important in setting the stage for those chapters that immediately follow them. In anticipation of various questions that may arise, we have used the term "patient" rather than client, customer, or consumer, although no implication should be drawn that we consider the recipients of nursing services as passively dependent and unable to enter into a relationship of mutuality with caregivers. With regard to protection of the rights of human subjects, all projects were approved by the Institutional Review Boards of the university and the institutions where interviews were conducted. To preserve patient rights to confidentiality, transcriptionists and members of the phenomenology research group were asked to sign confidentiality pledges for every project. Real names of interviewees never appear on the typed interview transcripts used by the research group in our weekly thematizing sessions. While we do include verbatim quotes from patient interviews in this book, all names of institutions are removed and all names of persons appearing in the text are pseudonyms.

This is not the first book in nursing about phenomenology, but we hope it will prove to be a useful addition to the extant body of literature on this topic. This book is unique in its philosophical basis (Merleau-Ponty), its approach to clinical practice and research, and its thorough coverage of the major existential grounds described by existential-phenomenological thought. We have sought feedback about its content and readability from more than a dozen colleagues, and we are now ready for you, our readers, to enter into dialogue with us, scanning the pages we have written and critically reflecting on our ideas. We invite, and eagerly await, your response. Our hope is that we will succeed in stirring both your thoughts and your emotions. In this time of distress and turmoil produced by the corporatization of health care delivery systems, nurses are burning out and patients are feeling abandoned. It is a time for us to engage in a deepening reflection about the fundamental meanings of a practice so intimately linked to the most joyous and tragic experiences of human life. When nurses reflect deeply upon their practice, our patients will surely be the ultimate beneficiaries.

Acknowledgments

The authors gratefully acknowledge the following individuals for their contributions to this book, to our thinking, and to our richly satisfying personal and professional lives:

Stephen Krau
Dianne Briscoe
Marilyn Smith
Mitzi Davis
Johnie Mozingo
Sharon Sarvey
Becky Fields
Molly Meighan
Pat Droppleman
Janet Secrest
Karen Reesman
Carol Smucker
Mona Shattell
Kristina Plaas

I

Phenomenology and Nursing

What is phenomenology? It may seem strange that this question has still to be asked half a century after the first works of Husserl. The fact remains that it has by no means been answered. Phenomenology is the study of essences; and according to it, all problems amount to finding definitions of essences: the essence of perception, or the essence of consciousness, for example. But phenomenology is also a philosophy which puts essences back into existence, and does not expect to arrive at an understanding of man and the world from any starting point other than that of their 'facticity.' It is a transcendental philosophy which places in abeyance the assertions arising out of the natural attitude, the better to understand them; but it is also a philosophy for which the world is 'already there' before reflection begins—as an inalienable presence; and all its efforts are concentrated upon re-achieving a direct and primitive contact with the world, and endowing that contact with a philosophical status.

—Maurice Merleau-Ponty, *Phenomenology of Perception* (1945/1962), p. vii

The Patient, the Nurse, and the Philosopher: Seeing Rose through the Eyes of Merleau-Ponty

Two people are talking. One is a phenomenological nurse researcher; the other is a woman who recently suffered a stroke. The researcher, Janet, speaks first: "Can you describe for me some specific experiences you've had since your stroke that stood out for you?" Rose, the patient, replies: "Well first of all, I was just devastated that everything I had was taken away from me, you know—my jewelry, my money, everything. . . . Yeah, one day you're working and the next day you're an invalid, so you know, you think you're through."

"You think you're through?"

"You think you'll just never be a whole person again, when you realize you're paralyzed. When you can't move a finger or anything, you know."

"You didn't feel like a whole person?"

"Well, you know, I'm a person that tries to do the right thing for everyone, take care of everybody. And I just couldn't understand . . . and . . . I said if I can't get better I want to die. And if I can get better I will. . . . And like I said before, you have to want to do things. If you want to sit in a wheelchair okay. So my husband pushed me down to therapy the first day. And this big man approached me and said 'I'm here to help you. I'll teach you to walk.' He said, 'You'll stand up and I will hold you and we'll go around with the walker.' And I said, 'I can't do that.' He said, 'Well, you have the right to choice. If you don't want to, that's your right. But I've never let a person fall, and I want to help you. But you have to be willing to do it or you can sit in that wheelchair the rest of your life.' So immediately, I said [to myself] 'Well look, you know, you got to try.' And in three days I was walking . . . very slowly and very carefully, but I was walking."

From this conversation, Janet Secrest (1997) came to the conclusion that the world of the stroke survivor is one in which loss and effort are uniquely significant (see Chapter 11). In addition, each of the survivors whom she interviewed described a sense of *discontinuity* in the self: The stroke seemed to break the survivor's experience into a pre- and post-stroke person. The anxiety evoked by such an experience is clearly evident in Rose's statement, "I'll never be a whole person again." But Rose did not talk directly about who she is or was. Instead she began by describing how devastated she felt when her personal possessions—her things—were taken away. The issue of time came up next, with a clear contrast between a *before* ("One day you're working") and an *after* ("The next day you're an invalid"). There also was an ominous concern for the future: "And you think you're through." It is only at this point, however, that Rose described a bodily component of what it meant to be through ("You're paralyzed . . . can't move a finger or anything") and the personal significance of the paralysis ("[I won't be able] to do the right thing for everyone" or "take care of everybody"). This new way of being with people presents a problem for her. The narrative then comes full circle when Rose is told in physical therapy that she has the "right to choice," but if she's willing to cooperate with the therapist she won't have to sit in the wheelchair for the rest of her life. Rose's recovery requires other people, perhaps making her aware for the first time that she doesn't always have to be the one who "takes care of other people;" she can let them take care of her for a change.

This conversation is about Rose's concern over who she is both before and after a stroke. She does not talk about her "self" as a collection of habits, memories, traits, and skills encased inside her skin and separate from the world. What Rose does talk about are her absent possessions, her changed relationships to other people, her personal past and possible future, and her limited ability to negotiate space in the physical world. We might say that Rose experiences her life in terms of other people, personal objects, time, and her body's relationship to the world. *Others, time, body*, and *world*, including personal objects, comprise the *four major existential grounds of human existence*, the contexts against which human life and experience always emerge. Because nursing is interested not only in how life progresses biologically but also in how people experience their lives from their own, unique, first-person perspective, it makes sense that we should be interested in the one contemporary philosophy—existential phenomenology—explicitly concerned with these issues.

Although existential phenomenology has found its way into many nursing research textbooks, it usually receives relatively brief mention, perhaps a few pages, or at most, a single chapter. More often than not, it is presented to readers along with other inductive, qualitative research approaches that are also given a cursory overview by the authors of these texts. In conjunction with several other qualitative methods, phenomenology shares an emphasis on: (1) respect for people, (whether patients or study participants), considering them as co-researchers and not as "subjects"; (2) the use of in-depth interviewing to discover perceptions and feelings; and (3) rigorous interpretation of texts that result from such interviews. Its philosophical underpinnings, however, are unique and deserve careful examination—a task that may seem intimidating to nurses who lack a strong background in philosophy. Perhaps because of its European origins and esoteric terminology, phenomenology sounds especially mysterious to readers encountering it for the first time. Many contemporary authors continue to sprinkle their accounts of phenomenology with the German or French terms by which phenomenology was introduced, thereby creating additional difficulty for the reader who is not fluent in these languages.

Nursing needs a more comprehensive, and comprehensible, presentation of this philosophical tradition and research methodology. As a research method, it has great value for studying those aspects of our patients' experiences that are not measurable by blood pressure cuffs, rating scales, or questionnaires—such as the meaning of a stroke to a woman like Rose. Even when experiences—such as stress—have been deemed "measurable" by scientists, many questionnaires are not sensitive to cultural and/or gender differences and fail to capture what is most salient to the individuals responding to them. For example, no standard stress questionnaire measures *vicarious stress*, which proved to be the number one stressor for women in a study by our research team (Thomas & Donnellan, 1993). We had given the women a well-validated and reliable instrument, but we also asked them an open-ended question, permitting them to describe their greatest distress in their own words. By doing so, we discovered the shortcomings of the instrument and learned what was *really* causing them distress. What bothered the women most were events that were happening to their significant others, such as the impending divorce of a son, job problems of a husband, illness of a sister or friend. In these stressful circumstances the women suffered empathically along with their loved ones but had little or no control over what was happening. This type of stress has received little attention in the vast literature based on administration of standard stress questions about a person's own work, health, and finances (e.g., what is the amount of your mortgage? how many times have you been to the doctor?)

Experiences such as this to us led our research team to become dissatisfied with structured questionnaires and, eventually, drawn to phenomenological methodology for our continuing studies of anger, stress, and depression (cf. duMont, Droppleman, Droppleman, & Thomas, 1999; Fields et al., 1998; Thomas, McCoy, & Martin, 2000; Thomas, Smucker, & Droppleman, 1998; Wood, Meighan, Thomas, & Droppleman, 1997). We joined the growing number of scholars in other disciplines who had become disenchanted with the results of quantitative studies. Among the reasons for this disenchantment, Van Maanen (1982, p. 13) listed the following: (1) the relatively trivial amount of variance explained by the researcher's selection of variables; (2) the abstract nature of the key variables; (3) the lack of comparability across studies; (4) the failure to achieve much predictive validity; (5) the high level of technical sophistication, rendering many research publications incomprehensible to all but a few readers; and (6) the complexity of multivariate analysis, "which, even when understood, makes change-oriented actions difficult to contemplate."

While quantitative research is still of great value in discovering such things as precise changes in blood pressure, in millimeters of mercury, after a relaxation intervention, and we have no argument with the usefulness of many descriptive-correlational and experimental studies of nursing phenomena, such studies cannot shed light on the *meaning* of what is happening to those who are experiencing it. When our concern is the meaning of human experience, we need to use a qualitative approach. Existential phenomenology, in our view, is ideal for this purpose. A phenomenological approach also enables us to explore the experience of children (e.g., Bennett, 1991; Erickson & Henderson, 1992; Jacobson, 1994), frail elders (Porter, 1999a; Zalon, 1997), and so many others who have rich stories to tell us—but only limited ability or interest in responding to numeric rating scales. Nursing studies using a phenomenological approach have focused on the lived experience of diverse disease conditions (e.g., addiction, anorexia, cancer) and symptoms (e.g., air hunger, pain, urinary incontinence) as well as on more elusive phenomena such as empathy, courage, and caring (see Koch, 1995, or Carpenter, 1999a, for overviews of extant research).

Furthermore, we believe that phenomenology has profound relevance for our clinical practice as well as our empirics. Unfortunately, most of the extant research is "published in a language and in places that benefit researchers and not the patients and practitioners" (Miller & Crabtree, 1998, p. 295). It is the staff nurse in the rehabilitation center who could listen to Rose's story, connect with her, and explore her concerns and the deeper meanings of her health crisis. But no nurse was there for Rose. Perhaps no nurse in that facility understood how to *care* for Rose in the most elemental sense of the term *caring*.

Gergen (2000) contends that caring is not something the nurse does for the patient, but something that is co-created and negotiated in interaction with the person, a coordinated dance between two human beings in a specific relationship. The patient must teach the nurse how to care, and the nurse must listen—not only to the patient's words but to his or her unspoken bodily response. Gergen gives the example of a perfunctory back massage, delivered by a nurse who is just performing a task and whose focus is on the technical aspects of effleurage hand movements. The patient experiences himself as being pummeled and prodded but not soothed. In contrast, the nurse who is attuned to the patient's *response* continually adjusts the pressure of the touch and movements of the hands. In this latter type of encounter, tense muscles relax, pain ebbs, and the patient feels cared for.

In a profession in which the essential purpose is to *care* (cf. Bishop & Scudder, 1999; Leininger, 1991; Newman, 1994; Watson, 1985) and to provide *comfort* (cf. Kolcaba, 1995; Morse, 2000), nurses still lack an in-depth understanding of these phenomena. For too long we have considered patient complaints as problems to be solved, using a linear hypothetico-deductive thought process and specifying measurable outcomes for our interventions. And if we did not have sufficient time for the full care-planning process, a "standard" care plan could be printed by the computer and appended to the chart. Nursing research, likewise, has traditionally proceeded from defining a "problem," to operationalizing "variables," to statistical testing of the null hypothesis, hoping for a probability value of .05 or less (so that "significance" could be claimed for the results). Under this logic, nursing phenomena were reduced to a level that destroyed what the researchers had sought to explain (Robinson, 1995). In fact, isolated variables no longer seemed to represent, or even connect, to the world of everyday existence (Richardson, 1986). Sadly missing was careful scrutiny of the individual patient's experience in all of its complexity, urgency, and ambiguity. Research and clinical practice are less fulfilling endeavors when pursued within such a depersonalizing and mechanistic framework.

Unfortunately, for much of nursing's history as a profession, medicine's mechanistic lens for seeing phenomena also has been nursing's lens. It is time for nursing to change its lens (Watson, 1999). Benner (1999a) urges the profession to recover the vision articulated by Florence Nightingale. Nursing has never completely fulfilled Nightingale's vision because the service needs of hospitals and physicians "exploited the nursing vision, twisted its roots and choked potential growth" (Reed, 2000, p. 129). Reed calls for a nursing reformation based on an integrative philosophic perspective that purposely links the art and science of nursing and recognizes it as a *basic human healing process*. Jean Watson even wonders if "nursing" will still be an adequate word for the radical transformations that must take place in our healing practices.

Learning about existential phenomenology can be profoundly transformational, as our students and colleagues often report (see Post-Study Reflections at the end of each chapter). We believe that we have developed a unique approach at the University of Tennessee to the study of nursing phenomena, *an applied phenomenology for nursing*. The lens we have chosen to guide our vision is based primarily on the philosophy of Maurice Merleau-Ponty (1962). Our approach is different in several respects from Heideggerian hermeneutics (cf. Benner, 1994; Diekelmann, 1992) and other phenomenological approaches that nurses have developed (cf. Parse, 1995) or used (cf. van Kaam, 1966; van Manen, 1990). In addition to Merleau-Ponty, our thinking also has been enriched by the contributions of other existential phenomenological philosophers such as Husserl (1913/1931), Heidegger (1927/1962), Buber (1924/1970), and Gadamer (1960/1975), to name just a few, and you will see their influence in these pages. Exemplars from diverse studies conducted by nurse researchers over the past decade will illustrate the tenets of our approach, and counterintuitive findings should prove intriguing. We will take you into the familiar worlds of the hospital and the outpatient clinic, guiding you to see them freshly, from the first-person perspective of the patients. You will be dismayed, but perhaps not surprised, to learn how frequently patients perceive hospitals as inhospitable and clinics as cold and unfeeling. You will be immersed in first-person narratives of experiences such as stroke, abuse, and spiritual distress. As nurses, we often assume that we know what such experiences are like, and therefore presume that we can empathize with our patients. Phenomenology, however, demands that we initially "bracket" (that is, attempt to set aside) all that we think we know. Instead, we must enter humbly into the life world of the patient. We must listen in respectful silence as he or she describes very private experiences. Inevitably, our understanding of the other person's experience is radically altered through dialogue, and insights regarding the deeper *meaning* of an experience often have been stunning to us, even as phenomenological researchers. We have also learned that, once a nurse adopts this way of engaging patients in dialogue, routinized clinical practice is impossible: Both the nurse and the patient are irrevocably changed. The relational elements of nursing, described so beautifully by pioneers such as Peplau (1952) and Travelbee (1971) are receiving heightened attention in contemporary practice (for example, see Krauss, 2000). Why is this so? There are several reasons. The public is dissatisfied with perfunctory examinations performed in 15 minutes by monosyllabic health care providers. In fact, patients may be fortunate if they receive a 15-minute exam; one new textbook for doctors and nurses touts "expert 10-minute physical examinations!" Communication between patient and provider is often woefully one-sided, as in the following exchange between a medical student and an old man. In answer to the student's question, "what brought you to the hospital?," the patient related, "I was run down, my wife died, she had a brain tumor, and I took care of her. I got run down and got a cough." The medical student's wholly inadequate response consisted of asking, "So, you have this cough, how long have you had it?" (Shotter & Katz, 1999, p. 159).

In a recent survey, two out of three Americans said they no longer hold physicians in high regard and see health care facilities as slightly better than automotive repair shops, although less satisfactory than supermarkets and airlines (Aiken, cited in Thomas, 1998). In another survey, 79% of respondents agreed that "there is something seriously wrong with our health care system" (National Coalition on Health Care, cited in Thomas, 1998). People are being treated but not *healed*. They long for care providers who are truly interested in them and willing to sit with them and spend time listening to their concerns (Riemen, 1998).

Having such a care provider is especially important to the chronically ill patient for whom the wonders of technology proffer no cure. With the demographics of our aging population, the main focus of nursing practice now—and in the foreseeable future—is the chronically ill patient. Nurses interact for many years with their patients who have chronic conditions such as diabetes, arthritis, depression, and cardiovascular diseases—promoting optimal quality of life, rejoicing in small victories, and sharing the sadness of setbacks along the way. It is the caring relationship that facilitates patients' adaptation to the chronic condition. Having a caring "partner" motivates patients to commit to difficult medication and dietary regimens, submit to unpleasant procedures, and return month after month for appointments. Nurses, moreso than physicians, are well suited to deliver relationship-centered care to the chronically ill. Writes Peggy Chinn: "Medicine focuses on surgical and pharmacological interventions, with interpersonal interactions being an adjunct to these interventions. In contrast, technical interventions are viewed in nursing as being adjunct to the primary interpersonal interactions" (1983, p. 397). We believe that existential phenomenology, with its emphasis on deeply connecting with and understanding the human being in his or her wholeness and specificity, has much to offer nursing at this particular moment in our history.

WHAT IS EXISTENTIAL PHENOMENOLOGY AND HOW DOES IT APPLY TO NURSING?

Existential phenomenology blends the philosophy of existentialism with the methods of phenomenology to produce rigorous and richly nuanced descriptions of human life (Pollio, Henley, & Thompson, 1997; Valle & King, 1978). *Existentialism* is a philosophy about who we are and how we may come to live an authentic life. Its central concern is to prompt human beings to live with a keen awareness of both their *freedom* and their *responsibility* in shaping the situation in which they are involved (Langer, 1989). Existentialism originated with Soren Kierkegaard in nineteenth-century Denmark as a revolt against philosophy's traditional remoteness from life. As the story goes, young Kierkegaard sat in a Copenhagen cafe smoking a cigar one Sunday afternoon in 1834, musing about his failure to make a contribution to the world. His cigar burned out, and he lit another. Suddenly his mission became clear: to explore the difficulties of existence, beginning with his own inner torment, aloneness, possibilities, and limitations (Bretall, 1946). Through the years, writers such as Jaspers (1955), Sartre (1956), and Camus (1970) added their voices to the continuing discussion of basic human issues such as anxiety, despair, choice, and commitment. In the words of Sartre, upon founding a journal in 1945 with Merleau-Ponty, "We [were] hunters of meaning, we would speak the truth about the world and about our own lives" (from Sartre's *Situations*, cited in Moran, 2000, p. 397).

Lacking a systematic way to conduct their inquiries, twentieth-century existentialists turned to the methods of *phenomenology*, as developed by the German philosopher Edmund Husserl and further articulated by Martin Heidegger. Husserl first began to use the term "phenomenology" in 1900. What he meant by the term was a rigorous new science in which there could be systematic investigation of those things that we take for granted in everyday life (in what he called the "natural attitude"). His mission, like that of Kierkegaard, was to save philosophy from a "crisis" of stagnation and insignificance (Jennings, 1986). Husserl saw himself as a Moses, leading his people to a new land of transcendental subjectivity (Moran, 2000). The domain of his new science of phenomenology was consciousness, and its method was the careful description of human phenomena. He was not content with theoretical analysis but insisted upon returning to "the things themselves," in their very *essences*. Essences, by definition, were patterns of meaning that were universal, unchanging over time, and absolute (Jennings, 1986). The rigorous new science developed by Husserl called for a shift in allegiance to "a valuing of enlargement rather than reduction, generosity rather than economy, complexity rather than simplicity, the lens rather than the hammer (Psathas,1973, cited in Oiler, 1982, p. 181).

The phenomenological movement has been described as a "set of waves" (Reeder, 1987) in a vast ground swell of "anti-reductionist and anti-constructionist" thinking that had begun in the nineteenth century (Spiegelberg, 1981, p. xi). The history of the movement is fascinating, especially if we delve into the personal circumstances underlying the views of its luminaries: Husserl, who was discriminated against for being a Jew and grieved as the Nazis came to power and forbade him to teach; Sartre, who joined the French Resistance and disputed Nazi authoritarianism with his writings about the freedom of the individual; and Heidegger, who aligned himself with the Nazi regime yet deplored the societal disintegration brought about by an increasing reliance on technology. It is beyond the scope of this book to review this history, but it is helpful to know something about the disturbing context (i.e., Europe torn apart by the horror of war) in which these philosophers pondered the meaning of human existence. No wonder they were intensely seeking the meaning of *being*; it was a frightening time in which *nothingness*—which Sartre felt "lies coiled at the heart of human being like a worm"— seemed imminent.

Nurses began to find the philosophy of existentialism relevant to clinical practice in the 1960s. With its emphasis on the worth, responsibility, and potential of the unique individual, the philosophy appealed to nurse writers such as Sister Madeleine Clemence Vaillot (1966) and Anne Ferlic (1968). Both Vaillot and Ferlic viewed commitment as an intrinsic characteristic of the professional nurse. Nurses must commit to give the "whole of themselves" to individuals who are in need. Drawing from Gabriel Marcel, Vaillot urged the nurse not to be a detached "spectator" but a "witness" to human suffering, freely choosing to be fully present and engaged with suffering humans. Ferlic concluded that "existential thought seems the best philosophical foundation for the contemporary nursing profession" (1968, p. 30).

Phenomenology surfaced in the nursing literature in the 1970s. Among the first interpreters of phenomenological philosophy for scholarly inquiry in nursing were Josephine Paterson and Loretta Zderad (1976), Rosemarie Parse (1981), Carolyn Oiler (1982), and Anna Omery (1983). These scholars, and others who followed, found in phenomenology a method that enabled them to explore the chief concerns of the discipline: (a) the *wholeness or health of human beings who continuously interact with their environments*, and (b) the *patterning of human behavior* in both normal and critical life situations (Fawcett, 1995). The phenomenological approach is compatible with nursing's values and philosophical foundations. Research conducted from this perspective "becomes a caring act" (Munhall, 1994) capable of conferring therapeutic benefit to the study participants (Hector, 2000).

DESCRIPTIVE AND INTERPRETIVE PHENOMENOLOGY IN CONTEMPORARY NURSING

Most present-day nursing scholars either espouse adaptations of classical Husserlian philosophy, most commonly referred to as "descriptive" or "eidetic" phenomenology (cf. Drew, 1999; Porter, 1998), or Heideggerian hermeneutics, which is referred to as "interpretive" phenomenology (cf. Benner, 1999b; Diekelmann, 1992). Unfortunately, in written reports of their projects, some nurse researchers fail to mention the philosophical underpinnings of the approach they selected, citing only the developer of a specific set of procedures they used in their studies (for example, Colaizzi, 1978). Therefore, it may be helpful to the reader of nursing research reports to know that the approaches developed by psychologists Giorgi, Colaizzi, Fischer, and van Kaam— referred to as the "Duquesne school" because they originally worked at Duquesne University in Pittsburgh—can be classified within the Husserlian tradition of "descriptive" phenomenology (Cohen & Omery, 1994). Rosemarie Parse, a nursing scholar who studied at Duquesne, also developed a method consistent with the Husserlian tradition. A bit harder to classify are the adherents of the "Dutch school" (cf. van Manen, 1990) because their approaches combine features of both descriptive and interpretive phenomenology. Within nursing, Patricia Munhall (1994) has been a prominent proponent of van Manen's method.

Some writers contend that contemporary nurse researchers have misinterpreted European phenomenological philosophy (Crotty, 1996; Paley, 1997, 1998). Caelli (2000), however, points out that it is not nurses who have changed the way phenomenology is conducted in North America but rather that American philosophy has changed, developing new ways of applying phenomenological methods to philosophical questions. One of the changes from "traditional" European phenomenology is the focus in American phenomenological analysis on describing participants' lived experiences *within the context of culture* rather than searching for *universal* essences divorced from cultural context. This change would seem to be particularly significant to nursing scholars—and practitioners—because we must understand the frameworks within which our patients experience health problems and treatments. Caelli (2000, p. 373) advises critics of American phenomenology to consider that "changes to methodology may well have resulted from the fact that the approach is being used for research rather than for the solitary philosophical reflection of Husserl and Heidegger." This is an excellent point. The early phenomenologists might, indeed, be puzzled by the diverse ways in which their ideas have been adapted to other purposes although, of course, this is the way any genuinely novel idea progresses.

It is hard to keep track of the diverse permutations of phenomenology within contemporary nursing. At a recent conference, 18 different forms of phenomenology were identified (Caelli, 2000), indicating a high level of current interest in this approach. Striking differences may be noted in the types and amounts of data collected by phenomenological researchers. In some instances, voluminous data are collected (for example, Benner conducted 276 interviews for her dissertation in 1984). In other studies, participants may be as few as three (deKonig, 1979). While some phenomenologists obtain texts from sources such as videotapes, novels, film, and television, and others collect their data via methods such as participant observation and group interviews, in this book we present a method based on one-on-one dialogue between the researcher and the participant. Despite procedural differences among various camps or "schools" of phenomenology, all belong to a family of thinkers concerned with discovering the unexamined meanings of the phenomena of our everyday world—the world in which nurses and patients live and come to know one another.

THE PHILOSOPHY OF MERLEAU-PONTY

Fairly new to many nurses is the philosophy of Maurice Merleau-Ponty. This lack of familiarity is surprising since his philosophy is an excellent fit for nursing, encompassing holism, embodiment, and culture (duMont, 2000). *Holism* (viewing persons as irreducible wholes) is a pillar of nursing philosophy and has been a prominent concept in nursing theories since the 1970s (Levine, 1969, 1971; Rogers, 1970). More than 30 years ago, Martha Rogers (1970) introduced exotic new terms into the language of nurses to conceptualize "unitary human beings" and to describe the indivisible relation of the person to his or her environmental field. The term "embodiment" has recently assumed importance in nursing literature, replacing the well-entrenched dualistic notion of mind/body put forth by French philosopher Rene Descartes some 400 years ago. *Embodiment* is a core concept in understanding health experiences (Reed, 2000). In our view, the most eloquent descriptions of embodiment (experiencing and understanding the world by, and through, the body) is to be found in the writings of Merleau-Ponty. Perhaps that is why his work is presently attracting a new audience both within philosophy and in nursing, exemplified by scholars such as Wilde (1999). Moran (2000) speculates that Merleau-Ponty has not received the public attention accorded Sartre and other French philosophers because of his retiring personality and his sometimes difficult literary language.

Merleau-Ponty was born on the west coast of France in 1908. He was educated in the French *lycee* system and received his doctorate in philosophy from the Ecole Normale Superieure in Paris where he also conducted post-graduate research on the nature of perception. Along with Sartre, Ricoeur, Derrida, and other French philosophers, he began his philosophical career by carefully studying and critiquing the work of Husserl (Moran, 2000). He heard Husserl lecture in Paris in 1929 and later traveled to the Husserlian Archives to examine some of the philosopher's unpublished papers. Merleau-Ponty attempted to combine Husserl's descriptive approach to phenomena with an existential ground, deriving, in part, from Heidegger. But his primary interest was always in *human* being, whereas Heidegger was interested in Being as such. Merleau-Ponty offered a philosophy of meaning—the meaning that is revealed in real life—where work is done and where human beings live together and enter into dialogue (Kwant, 1963).

The outbreak of World War II disrupted Merleau-Ponty's research and profoundly influenced his views of freedom and other people. He served as a second lieutenant in a French infantry division and, as an officer, was required to call for artillery barrages or air attacks on enemy positions. He was detained and then tortured by the Germans. After the war, Merleau-Ponty wrote movingly of the changes in his values brought about by these experiences (*Sense and Non-Sense*, cited in Moran, 2000). He concluded that everyone is compromised in war. In the post-war years, he became heavily involved in radical politics, seeking answers in Marxism and communism but eventually turning away from both. In the last years of his life, prior to his death at age 53, he had begun radical revisions of his work. According to Moran (2000), he had become especially interested in the problem of relations with others (*intersubjectivity*). Unfortunately, he did not complete his analyses of intersubjectivity.

The Aim of Merleau-Ponty's Phenomenology

Merleau-Ponty's major aim was to stir us to question our "knowledge" and return to the world as we experience it, examining the immediacy of the experience before it is classified by science and rational thought: "Thinking 'operationally' has become a sort of absolute artificialism. . . . Scientific thinking, a thinking which looks on from above, and thinks of the object-in-general, must return to the 'there is' which underlies it; to the site, the soil of the sensible and opened world such as it is in our life and for our body" (from Merleau-Ponty's *Eye and Mind*, cited in Langer, 1989, p. xi). He contrasted the manipulative nature of science with the kind of truth evident in painting, with its "innocent" immediacy of vision that seizes objects in the primordial world, frequently referring in his writings to the work of Cezanne and other painters (Moran, 2000). He advised us to be astonished by the world, to make direct contact with it, and to see it with open eyes filled with awe and wonder: "In learning how to *see*, we learn how to *be*, how to be something other than what we were when we remained blind to the new way of seeing" (Macann, 1993, p. 170). Phenomenology, according to Merleau-Ponty, "tries to give a direct description of our experience as it is, without taking account of its psychological origin and the causal explanations which the scientist, the historian, or the sociologist may be able to provide" (1962, p. vii).

Because the aim of Merleau-Ponty's phenomenology is to describe human experience on its own terms and not in terms of theoretical principles, the problem is to choose a set of human activities capable of providing insight into this task. Current thought offers a number of different possibilities. If we go the way of the research laboratory, elementary movements observed under controlled conditions become a distinct possibility. If we go the way of computer analysis, conceptual activities such as thinking, remembering, and problem-solving become most significant. If we go the way of neurology, continuous monitoring of the brain, as someone goes about performing complex skills such as reading or speaking, becomes most significant. Finally, if we go the way of clinical psychiatry of the talking kind, there are symptoms and historically based personal meanings whereas, in more medically oriented psychiatry, chemical reactions and drugs are more significant. Although Merleau-Ponty may have considered such diverse possibilities, he chose *perception* as primary to the task of describing the human experience of human life. He felt that traditional philosophy had misunderstood the role of perception in the formation of awareness and experience.

The Primacy of Perception

Probably the major reason for the primacy of perception in Merleau-Ponty's phenomenology is that it provides a direct experience of the events, objects, and phenomena of the world. Unlike thinking and language, which deal with ideas and representations of the world, perception always concerns an ongoing transaction between person and world. Unlike elementary movements observed in the laboratory, the world reached by perception is not an artificial one constructed for the purposes of studying responses in isolation from one another and from the world of everyday life. Unlike computer or brain models of human activity, which make experience the outcome of intellectual acts or biological processes in the "interior" of the person, perception never wavers from directing us toward ourselves in the world. Although interior monologues, ideas, and mental images do seem to take place "away" from the world, perception invariably requires us to be securely connected to it. With perception as our reference, it is impossible to describe experience as simply mental projection from the head to the world; experience, like perception, is always a transaction between us and the world, and both aspects of the transaction are significant.

When the lessons learned from perception are applied to other aspects of human life, they are expressed in terms of the phenomenological principle of *intentionality*. Within phenomenology, intentionality emphasizes the directional nature of human experience—perception included—as it (and we) deal with objects, events, and phenomena *in the world*. Like perception, human experience is continuously oriented toward a world it never possesses but toward which it is continuously directed. At the same time that intentionality directs us toward objects of experience, it also directs us toward the person for whom these objects are present. In this case, the general maxim becomes: what I am aware of reveals what is meaningful to me. If, for example, I enter a room and notice only the furniture, I probably am a very different person from someone else who enters the room and notices only the children, the food, or the artwork. The objects that capture us, or that we seek out, reveal what is significant to us—tell me what someone notices, and I'll tell you who he or she is. In this connection, think again about Rose (as we described her at the beginning of this chapter) and her things.

For Merleau-Ponty, as for Husserl before him, intentionality captures the fundamental structure of human experience and reveals an essential interconnectedness between us and the world. One philosophical consequence to this fundamental fact is that *person and world co-construct one another*. What this means is that the alienation we sometimes feel between ourselves and our world, or between ourselves and other people, or even between ourselves and our body, is not inevitable. If intentionality describes the fundamental configuration of human existence, then connection and relationship—not alienation and distance—describe the most general properties of our being-in-the-world and of our being-with-others.

Intentionality must, however, not be confused with the ordinary English word "intention." If I say "I intend to do X," this means that I have a plan or agenda to carry out. For the phenomenologist, however, intentionality does *not* refer to plans and planning but to a general patterning of human experience which suggests that human life can only be understood as always and already in some context (as "being-in-the-world"). Intentionality, as it is used in phenomenology, describes a basic configuration of person and world that is most obvious in human perception.

Functioning Intentionality

Intentionality is also evident in other human activities, in behavior for example. Here, intentionality takes on a more directly embodied form that Merleau-Ponty and Husserl described by the term *functioning intentionality*. The embodied nature of this type of intentional relatedness to the world was well-described by philosopher David Carr:

> It [functioning intentionality] is found in the look, the reach, the walk, the mutual corroboration of the senses in the perception of an object, the general orientation of the body, which, like pure consciousness, is always . . . in relation to its world. The body is never a fully constituted object. . . . To be sure, it has limits toward which it tends, in carrying out "biological functions." [But] it is not an instrument at the disposal of a free subject; even [biological] functions link it to its environment in a way which is not purely mechanical. In sexual behavior, the body is the perfect example of 'functioning intentionality.' It is not an objective physical process, but the meaningful direction toward a definite goal. And the awareness which goes with sexual activity can never be just intellectual awareness. . . . [Sexuality] does not take place in consciousness but in the world (Carr, 1967, p. 395).

The intentionality of behavioral actions was also discussed by psychologist B.F. Skinner from a third-person perspective (something observable that an organism did in response to an environmental stimulus). For Merleau-Ponty, behavior is always about first-person significance, and any proper account of behavior would see it as "an embodied dialectic . . . a kinetic melody gifted with a meaning" (Merleau-Ponty in *Structure of Behavior*, cited in Moran, 2000, p. 414). The Skinnerian idea of "reinforcement," under this reading, becomes a behavioral way of telling us what is significant to some specific organism in some specific situation. For Skinner, there is no essential separation between meaning and action. The meaning of an action is not given by some mental plan "lying behind" the action but is the action itself. All of this takes place in the world and not in the head. What we do reveals both who we are and what is important to us. This is the case even if we, as actors, are not able to describe the meaning of our actions.

This analysis leads to several conclusions, the most important of which is that behavior exhibits many of the same properties as perceptual experience. It is intentional, it is centered on significant events, and it is always located in some context or situation. It is possible to describe an individual's first-person world on the basis of what he or she does as well as in terms of what he or she perceives or talks about. Finally, behavior and experience are not independent pieces of human life but are better thought of as reversible aspects of a single pattern or *Gestalt*. With this understanding in mind, a first-person description of human existence may be attained by emphasizing behavior and/or experience according to the possibilities of the situation, the person, the event, and/or the researcher. To the question of whether there is a significant role for behavior in a phenomenological understanding of human life, the answer must be yes, especially when behavior is considered meaningful action and not movements performed in response to contrived stimuli in research laboratories.

OTHER PHENOMENOLOGICAL CONCEPTS THAT RELATE TO ROSE'S EXPERIENCE OF STROKE

The Situational Context of Human Life

Recall that the researcher's first question to Rose was: "Can you describe some experiences since your stroke that *stood out* for you?" To achieve a phenomenological understanding of human life, we must consider the way in which human existence is related to its situational context. Heidegger suggests that we consider the meaning of the ordinary German word *Dasein*, usually translated as "being." As Heidegger notes, *Dasein* is composed of two parts, *Da* (there) and *Sein* (being), leading him to suggest that being is never "just" being but always a being in some "there"—that is, always in some place, situation, or context. Dasein is always a being-in-the-world, and the hyphens are as important as the words. This, of course, is the same conclusion Merleau-Ponty reached on the basis of analyzing how we perceive: We never just receive stimuli from the world or project our ideas onto the world. Perception is always an exchange or transaction between me and my world. In his attempt to develop this idea further, Heidegger asks us to consider the somewhat more technical term *Existenz*. In both German and English, Existenz (or Existence) is composed of two Latin roots: *ex*, meaning out, and *sistare*, to stand. Hence, the word ex-sist means "to stand out," but from what? Here the answer must be: from its context, from its "there" (*Da*, as in Dasein) or from its world (as in being-in-the-world).

Thrownness and Freedom

Two other phenomenological concepts that relate to Rose's experience of stroke are *thrownness* and *freedom*. For Heidegger, each human life comes upon itself in the midst of some situation into which it has been "thrown" beyond the person's wishes. The task of life then becomes one of dealing with our "thrownness" and "projecting" it forward to new situations in which we may realize our genuine and unique possibilities. What is important here is that each human life (or Dasein) seeks to become more and more responsible for its own being and becoming, and this can only take place if it projects itself into new situations that offer no initial guarantee of meeting personal expectations. Only by taking a chance is it possible for me (or you) to realize a life that is uniquely mine rather than one concerned with meeting the demands and expectations of convention or of other people.

To help us grasp the concept of "projected thrownness," recall Rose saying, "If I can't get better I want to die. And if I can get better I will." Thus, she accepts her "thrownness" and "projects" herself forward, concluding that if she is totally paralyzed by her stroke she would see dying as a reasonable possibility. If, however, she projects a different possibility, she will try to "get better" and accept the help of the occupational therapist who will help her learn to walk again. Armed with the therapist's support, Rose projects a new possibility: "so, immediately, I said, 'well look . . . you've got to try.' And in three days I was walking."

This fragment of Rose's interview also provides some feeling for what choice, or human freedom, might be about. If by "choice" we imagine that we are free to become anything we want, we have misunderstood the way choice operates in human life. The idea that freedom is without limits—is "situationless"—is not possible for Rose, because all being is being-in-the-world. Both the occupational therapist and Rose tell us that "choice" is not to escape from her present situation but to move toward engagement in a new situation that takes account of her original situation and projects her forward to a new one. Even in situations where no action is possible, as in the case of a prisoner in a concentration camp, we are still free, as Frankl (1959) points out, to "choose our attitude" toward the situation of unfreedom. Frankl's view does not remove the person from the situation but relates personal action to meaningful engagement in the present situation of thrownness, even if it is as confining as paralysis or imprisonment.

The Experience of Figure/Ground Phenomena

Returning, once more, to the idea that personal existence is always experienced as a type of "standing out," it is still necessary to find ways of talking about such experiences. One good way to do this is to consider the well-known perceptual demonstration of figure/ground by the Danish psychologist Edgar Rubin (1921) (see Figure 1.1). If we focus on the white area of the figure, it becomes a vase or goblet; if we focus on the dark areas at the side, it becomes two faces. What is significant is our experience of the white area when we see the faces or the vase. When we see the vase, the white area is experienced as standing out, nearer, having a definite pattern, and easier to name and describe than when we see the two faces. When we see the faces, the white area is experienced as further away, somewhat indefinite, and relatively more difficult to describe except perhaps as "behind the two faces"—in short, as *ground*. The perceived "thing," according to Merleau-Ponty, is always perceived as having a certain *figure* or form against a background (Moran, 2000).

Although this demonstration has been discussed in many different ways (see our earlier discussion of the relationship between behavior and experience as a reversible figure/ground pattern), the most important one for our present purpose is that figure and ground co-create each other in human experience. Neither the vase nor the faces can be seen without one another: Remove one, the other disappears. Although they may depend upon one another, only one figure is experienced at one time. Extending such considerations to the case of more general human experience, the ideas expressed by Heidegger in his analysis of both Dasein and Existenz lead to the same conclusion: All being can only be experienced as a being-in-the-world in which my "being" is figure and "in-the-world" is ground. There are no figures by themselves, and human experience is a patterned event constituted both by its central and contextual aspects. Also note that co-constitution does not mean *cause*: Seeing the faces does not cause the dark area to become ground; in fact, it is clear that the face and the vase cannot exist without one another and that the idea of cause seems suspect when we are talking about human perception. Cause implies two separate events; perception implies a single event.

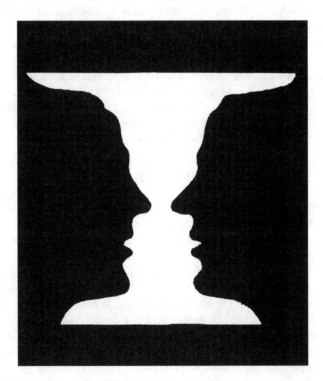

Figure 1.1. The "vase and faces" drawing.

The way Rose experiences her existence—the way it stands out to and for her—depends upon many different grounds (the world of objects and physical space, her body, time, and other people) and, although each has a seemingly clear meaning in everyday life and scientific discourse, their experiential meaning is far less clear for the person whose life is at issue. For example, we may think of the body as an object like any other object; as such, it always appears to have a clear boundary between itself and everything else (Pollio et al., 1997). This boundary is maintained if the person moves, swims, types, or watches a movie. Even in fantasies and dreams it appears as a well-defined entity. Certain individuals, such as nurses and physicians, are allowed to examine its contents and to perform procedures on it. But this understanding of the body as an object derives from a third-person perspective; that is, when you or I consider someone else's body from the outside. The body is also perceived as an object when we see our own bodies in a mirror, photograph, or videotape. Adopting a first-person perspective, however, changes the human experience of the human body dramatically. The body, which seemed so object-like from an outside, or third-person, perspective, no longer seems, from a first-person perspective, to end at the tips of my toes, nose, fingertips, and head.

Such considerations may be extended to each of the other major grounds of human existence: time, other people, and world. In each case there are two different perspectives that may be taken: that of an outside observer and/or that of the person in question. In the case of world, for example, we may talk about the geological structure of mountains or of their personal meanings to us. The same distinction may be made in regard to time defined either by the clock or calendar or by our direct experiences of it. We can experience other people as objects for our use or as centers of meaning to be encountered in moments of enriching connection. For each of the major grounds, the conclusion is the same: If we are to describe human life in terms of experience, we must begin by describing the *first-person meaning* of each of its grounds. Later in this book, we undertake this task (Chapters 3, 6, 10, and 14).

Now, however, we must turn our attention to the way in which we, as phenomenologists, do our work. How is it that we can come to know patients like Rose and feel confident interpreting what they tell us about their experiences? There is no such thing as *the* phenomenological method. We have chosen to use the lens of Merleau-Ponty to see familiar phenomena in a new light. We developed a procedure found useful in dozens of studies conducted by nurses, psychologists, and educational researchers at the University of Tennessee. Through countless discussions during the weekly meetings of our interdisciplinary interpretive group, its components have been debated and refined. In fact, a careful reader will be able to detect some modifications since publication of the 1997 text by Pollio, Henley, and Thompson. In the next chapter, we describe how our method of phenomenological inquiry works, and we present some reasons why we think it offers a useful approach to understanding the meaning of significant human phenomena as they reveal themselves in the context of nursing practice.

2

If a Lion Could Talk: Phenomenological Interviewing and Interpretation

In presenting phenomenological interviewing and interpretation to graduate students in nursing and psychology, we have sometimes used a cartoon by Gary Larson. In this cartoon, a conversation is presented between a dog named Ginger and a man with a crew cut and glasses. In the first panel of the cartoon, the phrase "What we say to dogs" appears over a drawing of the dog with these words: "Okay, Ginger! I've had it! You stay out of the garbage! Understand, Ginger? Stay out of the garbage or else!" In the second panel of the cartoon, which is entitled "What they hear," the same man is talking to the same dog, only this time the words come out as follows: "Blah, blah, Ginger, blah, blah, Ginger, blah, blah, blah . . ."

When graduate students in nursing are asked about their reactions to this cartoon, they sometimes identify the man as a physician and Ginger as a patient. Other responses, however, identify the man as a nurse and Ginger as a physician, whereas still other reactions identify the man as a nurse and Ginger as a patient. You don't have to be a philosopher of language or a communications expert to see that this cartoon applies not only to Ginger (and the man) but to any situation in which one person speaks and another tries to understand.

Misunderstandings take place not only in clinical interactions or interpersonal conversations but also when we read texts or listen to speeches. A whole discipline called *hermeneutics* has developed to deal with these and other breaks in linguistic understanding. The very name of this field, hermeneutics, provides some hint of how to think about problems of understanding and misunderstanding, especially if we keep in mind that the word "hermeneutics" derives from the name of a mythological character named Hermes whose task was to bring the word of the gods to human beings in a form they could understand—not an easy task if we are sensitive to the message of Ginger and the man. Hermes' name also recommends him as uniquely suited for this task because it derives from the Greek word *herma*, meaning a pile of stones marking a boundary between two pieces of land. The image lurking behind Hermes' name characterizes him as defining the boundary-land between people inhabiting different cultures and speaking different languages. This image also describes the discipline of hermeneutics which is best understood as the rigorous study of interpretation.

To understand what we mean by interpretation, however, it is necessary to distinguish it from a similar process, inference. Here again, the history of both words is helpful. The word "interpret" is derived from the two words *inter* (between) and *pruet* (to go), giving rise to the original meaning of "going between." A modern usage exemplifying this meaning is that of a translator who serves as a go-between capable of negotiating linguistic and cultural differences. Good translation does not *add* to what was said; it simply tries to let one person understand what another person speaking a different language has said.

The word, "infer" has a different history and meaning. It comes from the words *in* (in) and *fere* (to carry or bring). The historical meaning of infer is to carry in some idea that was *not* there in the first place. The difference between an interpretation and an inference is that one brings *out* what was there to begin with, whereas the other brings *in* something that was *not* there to begin with. Hermes was concerned with interpreting what the gods said to human beings, not with helping them infer what the gods might have had in mind.

Why is this distinction between interpretation and inference important? Because our concern while working with patients or study participants is to *interpret* what they are telling us about their experience. Consider nurses asking their patients to describe what they are aware of when they are in pain. To provide patients with as much latitude as possible in helping us to *interpret* their experience, it is necessary to allow them to tell us what *they* think we need to know. The course of the dialogue is, thus, to be jointly set by the patient and the practitioner (or researcher). An ideal conversation occurs when an interviewer's questions and/or clarifying statements provide an opening for a patient's lengthier and more detailed responses. The person to whom we are talking is the expert on his/her experience; we are there to learn about it from him or her. As Merleau-Ponty pointed out: "He is able to get across to me inasmuch as I am . . . capable of allowing myself to be led by the flow of talk toward a new state of knowledge" (1973, p. 143).

HERMENEUTICS AND HUMAN UNDERSTANDING

How is it that sometimes we understand and sometimes we do not? How do breaks in communication come about? One way this problem has been considered is in terms of ancient texts. The most important historical case, of course, involves translating the Bible from one language to another. The problem was never that the translator was not fluent in both the language being translated (Hebrew, Greek) and the language into which it was translated (Latin, English). The more subtle, and significant, problem concerned the historical period in which the Bible was written and the period into which it was to be translated. Consider a simple word like "shepherd," as in the 23rd Psalm: "The Lord is my shepherd." Since medieval times, the English word "shepherd" has been taken to imply a young person who tends sheep. In biblical Hebrew, however, there was an additional, even more primary, meaning: someone who had a large herd of sheep—hence, a wealthy and/or powerful man such as Abraham or Jacob. Both meanings are invoked in the 23rd Psalm: one who takes care of sheep (and us) as well as someone rich enough to "provide a table for me in the presence of mine enemies." If we note only the young shepherd meaning, we have missed a significant connotation of the word "shepherd" in the original Hebrew—that of wealth and power.

Part of the problem in translating the meaning of any word is that it always relates not only to some specific language but also to some specific socio-historical context. To update the problem a bit, consider the case of a welfare mother who is asked, perhaps casually, about whether or not "she had planned to have her children" (Hagan,1986). The contextual rift between the interviewer and the participant is particularly clear in this case. For the interviewer, a question is being asked about "planning;" for the participant, the question is understood as being about whether she is a "fit" mother. The meaning of a word or phrase to one person is often not the same as it is to another person, and what seems required is that both individuals explore the meaning of any and all terms before even a seemingly straightforward question can be used as a springboard for dialogue.

In the case of a text such as the Bible, the translator had to be aware not only of the two sets of words comprising each language but also the meaning of these words in the era in which they were written and in which they were translated. We never simply translate from one language to another; what seems to happen is that the unsaid—the context—must be taken into account to produce an understanding that "goes between" the two cultures, or, in the case of a phenomenological interview, between the two people speaking. We can now understand the problem facing Ginger and the man: the world of the dog and that of the man share only the name Ginger and not much else. To borrow an aphorism from the philosopher Ludwig Wittgenstein: "If a lion could talk, we could not understand him."

It was for reasons of this type that Gadamer (1960/1975) described interpretation as involving a "fusion of horizons." We must understand individual words, but we must also connect with one another in terms of past and present contexts. No interpretation is ever without its historical and personal horizons, and Gadamer is quite clear in pointing out that interpretation has to do not only with language and culture but also, in the case of written works, with different histories: that of the text and that of the interpreter. The same problem applies to human conversations that take the form of a phenomenological interview. In this situation, there are two people and two histories, and understanding takes place only when both take their ongoing life situations and histories into account.

One way in which scholars attempt to deal with the problem of misunderstanding is to develop a set of specific interpretive procedures. In the Jewish mystic tradition, for example, the Rabbis developed four rules for interpreting the meaning of obscure or complex biblical passages. The rules were formed into the acronym PaRDaS (Hebrew for garden). In this acronym, P stood for the word "Pshat," meaning literal; R stood for the word "Remez," meaning allusion; D stood for the word "Drash," meaning story; and S stood for the word "Sod," or secret. Any given word or phrase that might not have been initially clear was to be understood on the basis of one of four strategies: literally; on the basis of an allusion to a different section of the Bible; on the basis of a story created to capture its allegorical meaning; or on the basis of some esoteric secret hidden in the word or phrase itself. While these rules may seem mechanical or restrictive, it is important to remember what they were supposed to accomplish.

If we move interpretative problems to a less esoteric locale, such as contemporary quantitative nursing research, we still find that difficult problems of interpretation are solved on the basis of mechanical rules. Consider, for example, the case of $p < .05$, a rule used to judge a finding as "significant" (i.e., meaningful, important) because it could happen by chance only 5% of the time or less. The value of 5% is an arbitrary convention, and represents an agreed-upon rule by the community of researchers. Who of us has not forgotten the arbitrary nature of this value and become upset when the results of a statistical test yielded a value of $p = .10$ or even $p = .06$?

The problem with respect to ancient texts, however, was not generally solved by using fixed rules. One early technique suggested that the translator attempt to place himself or herself into the historical situation of the original text. This strategy assumes that the interpreter's present situation is an impediment to understanding. In fact, Gadamer (1966/1977) argues, it is *only* from the translator's own present situation that he or she can understand anything at all. Our personal historical situation is precisely what opens us up to past documents and other people. Understanding involves not some imaginary jumping-back in time or place but a fusion of the horizon defined by the text (or interview) with that of the interpreter's present situation. It is only because we have "prejudices" (that is, personal and historically derived judgments and knowledge) that we are able to understand; understanding is not re-entering the past but mediating between now and then as well as between you and me.

The latter understanding is crucial for conducting the kind of dialogical interviewing that we speak of in this book. We cannot "lose ourselves" and become the other person. Rather, we are who we are, just as the person being interviewed is who he or she is, and the best we can do is mediate between the two of us in the form of a meaningful conversation. One way to get to such a conversation is to recognize that dialogue works best when the conversational partners concentrate on content and not personalities. Because every conversation is "about something," our job is not to look *at* the other person as an object of concern, but *with* him or her at what is being talked about. The interpreter, like the conversational partner, must be open to the central concern of the conversation. This process of grasping the core topic allows both of us to be taken over by it and thereby to come to see the world from the developing and joint perspective of the other person and of ourselves.

SOME QUESTIONS ABOUT QUESTIONS

One way to get conversational interviews started is to ask a good question, a question that will enable respondents to talk about something they know and are willing to discuss. But questions are complex and tricky bits of language and we would do well to take a look at what they are like and how they work. Perhaps the first thing to note is that, in addition to nursing, questions are important in many different professional and academic contexts including law, teaching, survey research, linguistics, philosophy, clinical and counseling psychology, and so on. This breadth of disciplines suggests that questions are important aspects of human life and professional practice and that to learn to use them for dialogical purposes will require us to consider them for many different contexts and perspectives.

One context for thinking about questions is to consider their linguistic mechanics, that is, *how they get asked.* Questions can shape the answers obtained. In fact, major changes in research results have been noted when questions are asked in different ways. For example, whether marital satisfaction is a major or minor contributor to general life satisfaction depends on the order in which both questions are asked (Schwarz, 1999). In English, there are three ways to ask a question: (1) by a change in intonation—"You did go home?"; (2) by a series of recognizable, but complicated, transformations—"Did John go home?" (which transforms the specific statement "John went home"); and (3) by use of a *wh*-element (words such as *what, who, where, when, which, why* and an h-word having similar pronunciation, *how.*) One way of examining how questions actually work in conversation is to consider the type of answer allowed. "Do you have a pain in your leg?" allows only a response of yes or no. This type of question is commonly employed by nurses when conducting assessments. Patients often experience an extended series of such questions as an interrogation. A second type of question permits a more extensive answer and offers a better entry into a conversation: "What is the pain like? In what situations did you notice that?"

The phenomenological questioner must unlearn much of his or her previous ways of asking questions. In this context, the question is not designed to elicit a quick response or an answer already known. Likewise, the phenomenological question is not designed to elicit a theoretical explanation or statement; hence, "why questions" which lead individuals from description to theory are avoided. For purposes of description, "what questions" not only are easier to answer but also help the person describe his or her experience by directing the conversation to "what you were aware of" in some specific situation. Perhaps, most importantly, the phenomenological questioner is required to promote an air of equality with his/her partner and not assume an air of superiority because of age, position, power, or prior knowledge. In nursing practice and research, lessening the inherently hierarchical nature of the nurse-patient relationship is essential. From the stance of phenomenology, the patient is the real authority and we only are able to learn about significant human experience if this fact is continuously kept in mind.

THE PHENOMENOLOGICAL INTERVIEW

All of these concerns are extremely important in asking someone to help you understand his or her first-person world—the patient in the case of clinical practice, the participant in the case of research studies. In both cases we need some way to describe the experience of someone else (yours, for example) as it is lived. Our job as interviewer is not to tell you how to talk about your life, only to be responsive to your descriptions as they unfold in the texture of our conversation together. It is at this point that hermeneutic considerations re-enter the picture. All we ever get from you are descriptions—bits of language—and from these linguistic scraps you must help us, and we must help you, articulate your experience. Although we may not be able to understand the world of a lion or Ginger, we are able to interpret what your world is like if we are respectful enough of your language and your story, and if both of us keep working on it together. Since we are interested in understanding the meaning of your experience, we must be careful not to go beyond what we learn in our conversation.

From a phenomenological point of view, the very topic we are talking about may be uncertain at the beginning of an interview. Objective studies require the researcher to equate the topic being studied with a set of specific procedures that restrict the phenomenon to a manageable set of operations: For example, hunger may be defined by the number of hours since the patient last ate. Phenomenological research, on the other hand, is designed to explore the nature of the phenomenon as lived by the person. We have to allow for seeming imprecision and personal meanings. The very genuine first-person complexity of a phenomenon such as hunger or pain must be taken into account rather than excluded as idiosyncratic variability or "error." Individual perspectives do not confuse understanding but provide it with depth and richness.

As in any ongoing dialogue, the participant (and the interviewer) may come to learn something new about the phenomenon, themselves, or both. Within the context of a phenomenological interview, it sometimes happens that the participant shares a previously *unreflected* experience when talking with the researcher (an event in the background of an individual's life which is reflected on for the first time during the interview). With this opportunity to discuss a personal experience with another person who is equally interested in that experience, the participant may gain access to more of his or her life history. When this happens, the person being interviewed may feel understood, a rare and enriching experience.

Among the benefits of participating in phenomenological interviews are catharsis, self- awareness, healing, and empowerment: Participants often report such benefits even when their interviews explored events such as incest or the murder of a family member (Hutchinson, Wilson, & Wilson, 1994). Women with breast cancer in a study by Carpenter (1998) sent cards and letters to the investigator afterward, describing their participation in a single one- to two-hour session as therapeutic. One woman said "This was the only therapy that I ever received" (p. 63). Pennebaker's research provides extensive empirical evidence that disclosing thoughts and feelings about life-altering events is beneficial to health and well-being (Pennebaker, cited in Carpenter, 1998). These reports should serve to lessen researchers' fears that interviewing will be distressful to the patient (and, likewise, lessen the reservations of Institutional Review Boards hesitant to grant approval for dialogic studies).

During the phenomenological interview it is important to create an atmosphere in which the participant feels comfortable and safe to talk freely about significant life experiences. Unlike a structured interview with a predetermined list of questions, the flow of dialogue is set by the participant. The interviewer's role is to closely track the words of the participant, ensuring that each experience is discussed in detail and seeking clarification for any statement not fully understood. The give-and-take that characterizes a good interview is promoted by a stance of sensitivity, respect, curiosity, and openness to the participant's report. The reciprocal influence that is inevitably present, and sometimes considered a source of error in other research contexts, thus becomes an area of connection and possibility. A context for exchange is created that leads to an in-depth description of the participant's experience. Instead of being detached from the process and its outcome, the researcher fully acknowledges his or her influence and involvement in co-constituting the dialogue. For this type of research, the interviewer *is* the research tool.

Although the researcher does not control the interview or determine its content, a phenomenological interview is not to be construed as non-directive; the researcher does have a responsibility to help the participant focus on unfolding themes and details. The researcher asks for one or more examples of the phenomenon, and perhaps for comparisons or contrasts of these instances. For example, a researcher asking men about their anger may initially hear stories about anger at malfunctioning cars, boats, or computers (Thomas, McCoy, & Martin, 2000). The researcher may be wondering about men's anger in their intimate relationships. While it is inappropriate to ask a participant "What about anger at your wife?" the researcher will pose such questions as "Can you think of another situation in which you became angry?" or "What stood out to you in that situation?" or "Was your reaction in that situation similar to the incident with the auto mechanic?" The researcher seeks a complete description of each instance of the phenomenon, with full elaboration of specific details and nuances. To ensure that the participant has nothing to add, the researcher asks, "Is there anything else you would like to say about this experience?" (By the way, if the study participant *never* mentions his wife, the researcher never goes there.)

Although an effort should be made to remain at a descriptive level early in the interview, it is inevitable, and not undesirable, that some attempt at interpretation will begin during the interview itself. Because meanings are created between people, they tend to emerge in the interview. Including the participant's efforts at interpretation is important because neither the participant nor the interviewer ever returns to the original experience; rather, "the data" of phenomenological interviews are reconstructed experiences of particular situations as they emerge in ongoing dialogue. While the participant is asked to stay close to lived experience and subsequent interpretive efforts of the researcher attempt to remain close to that level of description, *reflective interpretation* is necessary to arrive at a meaningful understanding.

Kvale (1996) has offered an overview and summary of phenomenological interviewing in terms of the following 12 main points: (1) it is centered on the interviewee's life-world; (2) it seeks to understand the meaning of phenomena in that life-world; (3) it is qualitative; (4) it is descriptive; (5) it is specific; (6) it seeks to be presuppositionless; (7) it focuses on themes relating to the phenomenon under consideration; (8) it is open for ambiguities; (9) it is open for changes; (10) it depends upon the sensitivity of the interviewer; (11) it takes place in an interpersonal context; and (12) it may be a positive experience for both the participant and the interviewer. Some practical advice about interviewing, based on our experience, is offered in Table 2.1.

TABLE 2.1 Practical Advice about Interviewing

1. Arrange to conduct the interview in a quiet, private place that is mutually agreeable with the participant. Bear in mind that hospitals are extremely noisy, with doors opening and closing, carts trundling down the hallways, and a constant barrage of sounds from beepers, pagers, and telephones. If conducting interviews in the hospital setting, enlist staff cooperation in minimizing interruptions by placing a "Do not disturb" sign on the door and taking the telephone off the hook. If interviewing in the home, ask the participant to arrange for someone else to tend to small children and/or animals during the interview time.

2. Practice with your recorder and microphone prior to leaving for your appointment with the participant. Then double-check everything again once you are in the setting. Record a few minutes of chit-chat, rewind, and listen to make sure that no background noise is interfering with the taping. We have found that the loud hum of a refrigerator, sounds of traffic outside an open window, and other extraneous noises may obscure a participant's words, particularly if he or she speaks softly.

3. Take extra equipment (another recorder, plenty of tapes, extra batteries, etc.). Equipment failure is a common problem, necessitating re-scheduling of an interview.

4. If possible, place your microphone behind a potted plant so that you and your participant are not continually staring at it, ever-mindful that it is recording. An unobtrusive "pancake" mike that lies flat on the table is preferable.

5. Obtain informed consent, either via the participant's signature on a printed form or via his or her reading aloud the consent statement once the taping has begun. (Matters to be considered in advance: Is the consent form prepared at a reading level appropriate for these participants? Can your participants read? If some cannot read, how will you read the form to them in a way that preserves their dignity and self-esteem?)

TABLE 2.1 *(continued)*

6. Once you have asked your open-ended question to begin the interview, do not interrupt the participant except to ask for clarification and to make sure that you are understanding the meaning of the words. Do not inject agreement or disagreement, approval or disapproval.

7. Do not be distressed if the participant reintroduces an experience or issue several times during the interview. This indicates that the material is significant to his or her experience of the phenomenon.

8. If participants seem nervous or say, "I don't know if this is what you want," offer reassurance that you are interested in whatever they are comfortable sharing with you. Gently encourage them to continue with verbal and non-verbal prompts.

9. Do not be afraid of silence. Give participants time to formulate their answers.

10. While gender role socialization and cultural influences may forbid crying, other nonverbal cues may suggest that a participant is experiencing pain during the interview. If cues such as excessive clearing of the throat, restless fidgeting, or watery eyes indicate that the person is becoming emotionally upset, acknowledge these cues by perhaps saying, "This is difficult to talk about." Offer the person the option of stopping for a moment. From time to time, ask, "How are you doing? Do you want to go on?" Do be aware that "crying is not always a cue for the interviewer to intervene, and the absence of tears is not always reassuring" (Kavanaugh & Ayres, 1998).

11. If the participant appears to be overcome with emotion, ask if he or she wishes to terminate the interview. In our experience, no one has ever chosen to terminate, but a few minutes to gather one's composure is often appreciated. Sometimes pausing for a cup of tea is a good idea.

12. If you are not sure where to go next with a question, pick up on the last word or phrase the person said and ask for elaboration by perhaps saying, "You said you felt left out. What is it like to feel left out?"

13. If a person appears to be wandering from description of the phenomenon, do not immediately assume that the material is irrelevant. For example, in our studies of the world of the hospitalized patient, almost everyone found it necessary to relate their medical history. While we could have deemed this irrelevant, later we realized that it was not.

14. At several points during the interview, and again at the end, summarize what you have heard. For example, say, "Let me see if I can sum up what we talked about. You become angry when your husband does not listen to you and your children fail to do their chores. You are also angered when a coworker fails to do her work properly and you must do it over. It seems that the anger occurs mainly when another person is letting you down. Have I understood correctly?"

TABLE 2.1 *(continued)*

15. Do not prematurely terminate an interview. We disagree with Morse's (1991) advice regarding a nonproductive interview. Morse (p. 144) contends that "if the interview is not productive, then the interview should be terminated as soon as possible and a decision should be made concerning the inclusion of the data in the study." Based on our experience, it is not possible to determine, *in vivo*, if an interview is "productive." Often, it is not until later, when perusing the transcript, that the full richness and relevance of the narrative is evident. Terminating an interview could also suggest to the participant that the researcher found his or her story displeasing, uninteresting, or even valueless. Such a perception could intensify feelings of low self-esteem or produce other undesirable sequelae.

16. After an interview about a particularly painful experience is concluded (for example, abuse), take time to remain with the participant until composure returns. Ask participants if they need follow-up or referral. (Agreement of appropriate counselors or social service agencies to receive referrals should be obtained prior to initiating the research.)

17. The issue of subsequent interviews with a participant should be broached prior to leaving the setting. In the vast majority of our own projects, one interview has been sufficient (i.e., the participant believes that he or she has finished describing the experience). There is nothing to preclude multiple interviews, however, should both parties agree that additional conversations would be useful.

18. Make field notes of the interview immediately after you leave the setting. These can be written or audiotaped. Describe the physical setting, the nature of the verbal and nonverbal communication (especially body language) of the participant, and your own personal reactions. Note any unusual events that occurred (interruptions, technical difficulties with the taping, etc.)

19. Transcribe the interview as soon as possible, paying careful attention not only to words but also to pauses, inflections, and other paralinguistic phenomena. Make note of these in the transcript (e.g., long pause, lit cigarette, broke eye contact). Use capital letters to emphasize words that are spoken with greater volume and intensity. Change all names of persons and places to pseudonyms. After the transcript is typed, listen to the tape once again with the transcript before you, making note of any additional observations about especially meaningful segments or transition points.

20. If you use a paid transcriptionist, a confidentiality pledge must be obtained. The transcriptionist should use headphones if transcribing the interview in an office that is open to the public such as the secretarial pool in a university's departmental office. After you receive the transcript, you will need to listen to the tape, as described above, and make any necessary corrections. Bear in mind that even the best transcriptionist is likely to make several errors, especially if the participant

TABLE 2.1 *(continued)*

---

has used a lot of medical terms in describing his or her experience. (See Easton, McComish, & Greenberg [2000] for some additional points regarding careful transcription.)

21. If the content of the interview has aroused strong emotion in you (as in the case of interviewing survivors of abuse), debriefing with a colleague is strongly recommended. Journaling is also beneficial. (See Smith [1999] for an excellent article on the benefits of journaling throughout a phenomenological study.)

22. Some researchers offer to give participants verbatim copies of their transcripts and/or copies of the audiotapes. We urge careful consideration prior to making such an offer. Consider whether the participant could experience negative consequences should a family member, caregiver, or intimate partner discover what was revealed to the interviewer. Many participants (e.g., children, abuse victims) are vulnerable and privacy of their personal belongings in their homes cannot be ensured.

Space precludes extensive discussion of issues regarding interviews with children. However, phenomenology is an excellent method to discover children's experiences of illness and treatment. Most children are fascinated to hear their voices on tape and become excited about the possibility of telling stories to "the nurse with the recorder." Researchers who plan to interview children should have thorough knowledge of children's development, attention span, and ability to comprehend questions. Staying at the concrete level ("What do you do when you have an asthma attack?") is usually preferable to questions about feelings (Faux, Walsh, & Deatrick, 1988). As in all phenomenological studies, pilot testing of questions is recommended. Using drawings at the beginning of the interview can decrease anxiety (Walsh, 1983, cited in Faux et al.) A child might also be more comfortable bringing along a favorite teddy bear or doll to the interview setting. Additional suggestions regarding interviews with children and adolescents may be found in Faux et al. (1988). In the following sections, we will describe other elements of the research procedure we have developed at the University of Tennessee.

Selection of the Sample

There are two principal criteria for eligibility in a phenomenological study: (1) having experienced the phenomenon and (2) willingness to talk about that experience to an interviewer. Sample selection is *purposeful* so as to obtain participants who meet these criteria. Among the recruitment measures we have used are newspaper articles, posters and flyers, professional intermediaries (such as nurses in a particular clinic or teachers of a class), community intermediaries (such as presidents of civic clubs, leaders of support groups, or pastors of churches), and word-of-mouth (snowball sampling wherein one interviewee tells the researcher of other individuals in his or her acquaintance who have experienced the phenomenon). When seeking to recruit marginalized individuals, identifying their customary gathering places is an important first step. For a study of homeless women, Anderson (1996) found study participants through a local urban cafe that served as a safe gathering place for the women. After she described her study to women attending a support group meeting at the cafe, the researcher simply waited at a corner table for interested individuals to approach her and make an appointment to be interviewed.

Excellent suggestions for defining the eligible, accessible population for a phenomenological study and targeting intermediaries to assist with participant recruitment have been offered by Porter (1999b; Porter & Lanes, 2000). Porter's own project, examining older widows' experience of home care, required extensive effort to locate suitable participants because they had to be: (a) aged 80 or older, (b) widowed for at least one year, (c) living alone in their own homes, (d) mothers of at least one child, and (e) residing in the same community where they had lived with their spouses. Nevertheless, recruitment of an adequate sample was eventually accomplished.

Less successful sample recruitment was described by Groger, Mayberry, and Straker in their 1999 article, "What we didn't learn because of who would not talk to us." While multiple factors were involved in the researchers' difficulties accessing African-American elders and caregivers, gatekeeper bias was a prominent problem. Research textbooks seldom discuss how to deal with the resistance of "gatekeepers" for potential research participants, especially those who are patients in institutions of various kinds (nursing homes in the study by Groger et al.). Over the years, we have encountered opposition from both physicians and agency administrators to even approach "their" patients to explain a study. Despite provision of written and verbal explanations about phenomenological interviewing and assurances that (a) participation is entirely voluntary and (b) confidentiality is scrupulously protected, we have been unable to get beyond the "gate" in some settings. Planners of phenomenological studies should probably plan to allow extra time for obtaining the necessary approvals to enter a health care agency and approach patients. Being responsive to staff concerns and offering to reciprocate with staff for facilitating entree may be helpful. Anderson and Hatton (2000) recommend providing consultation or services to staff of the agency. For example, workshops on health-related matters were provided to staff of a homeless shelter by one research team (Hatton, Bennett, Gaffrey, & Berends, 1995). Agreeing to share the findings of the completed study with staff may also serve to elicit their cooperation.

An appropriate sample size for phenomenological research can range from 6 to 12 persons (Morse, 1994; Ray, 1994). Not infrequently, sample size is adjusted as the study proceeds. If redundancy is evident after hearing the narratives of six participants, the researcher may decide that it will not be necessary to interview an additional four or six. Accessing vulnerable populations such as homeless persons and abused women presents special challenges (Anderson & Hatton, 2000). It is not only difficult to locate potential study participants, but also imperative to ensure their safety from harm. The researcher must carefully consider whether the benefits of knowledge outweigh the risk to participants (Anderson & Hatton, 2000). Language of the consent form must be carefully crafted, with clear explanation of benefits and risks. Rather than obtaining written consent, leaving the participant with a piece of paper that could be discovered by an abusive husband, the researcher may choose to obtain verbal consent while audiotaping the interview. Special measures must be taken to ensure that participants are interviewed in settings where they are comfortable and safe. As in all research, "the filament of ethics that wends its way throughout qualitative research gets its tensile strength through a respect for the dignity, autonomy, and rights of the respondent" (Robley, 1995, p. 48).

The Opening Question

On arrival at the interview site, prospective participants are given a full explanation of the proposed study and provide their informed consent. As mentioned above, consent can be given either by signing a consent form or by reading the consent statement aloud during the audiotaping (The latter method of granting consent has been approved by the Institutional Review Board in situations where safety is an issue or participants have stigmatized conditions such as HIV/AIDS and wish to preserve anonymity). Some participants choose to select a pseudonym for themselves by which the interviewer will refer to them throughout the interview process.

The opening question in any phenomenological interview is worded to allow for a broad range of descriptive responses from each participant. This is no easy task given what we know about the ambiguity of questions. For this reason the researcher will usually discuss the initial formation of an opening question with members of a phenomenological research group. (If no group is available, we recommend consultation with experienced interviewers followed by at least one pilot interview.) In the case of clinical practice, a useful opening question will probably be derived from the experience of the practitioner in asking patients about particular situations or events. Hopefully, this question should be informed by many of the same considerations as apply to a research interview.

The Bracketing Interview

An essential component of the phenomenological method used at the University of Tennessee is the *bracketing interview* in which the researcher is interviewed by an experienced member of the interpretive research group about the topic of the proposed research study. Husserl (1913/1931) introduced the term *bracketing* to describe suspending the taken-for- granted "natural attitude" of daily life. Bracketing was analogous to the use of brackets in algebraic formulas. Bracketing, as we use the term today in phenomenological research, is an intellectual activity in which one tries to put aside theories, knowledge, and assumptions about a phenomenon. For example, Janet Secrest, having been a staff nurse on a neuro unit for many years, held many assumptions about the experience of stroke survivors such as Rose before she began her formal program of research. Her bracketing interview not only compelled her to become aware of her present, often implicit, understanding of the phenomenon but also provided her with some feeling for what it is like to be a participant in this type of study. The purpose of the bracketing interview is to learn about the researcher's presuppositions concerning the nature and meaning of the phenomenon and thereby to sensitize him or her to any potential demands that he or she might impose on participants either during the interview or in its subsequent interpretation. Janet realized, after she transcribed and thematized her bracketing interview, that she was expecting the lived experience of a stroke survivor to be dominated by all of the *losses* brought about by cerebral hemorrhage or ischemia. While she was being interviewed, she cried as she recalled the aphasia and immobility of some of her former stroke patients. Had she not been sensitized regarding her gloomy perception of the existence of the stroke survivor, she may have led her interviewees to focus on losses. As you will see in Chapter 11, such a picture of the stroke survivor's world would have been narrow and inaccurate.

Recently, a lively debate about the purpose and meaning of bracketing has taken place among nursing scholars. Paley (1997) pointed out that nurse researchers are not using the idea of bracketing in the way Husserl intended. But Husserl changed his ideas about bracketing a number of times over the years, making it difficult to pin down his final stance. At one point he described the concept like this: *"And the whole trick consists in this—to give free rein to the seeing eye and to bracket the references which go beyond the "seeing" and are entangled with the seeing, along with the entities which are supposedly given and thought along with the 'seeing,' and finally, to bracket what is read into them through the accompanying reflection"* (Husserl, 1907/1999, p. 257). Some nurse authors (e.g., Johnson, 2000) have pointed out the impossibility of completely setting aside one's own biases about the phenomenon being investigated. Indeed, Merleau-Ponty (1962) and Gadamer (1960/1975) long ago noted that it is not possible, or even desirable, for a researcher to be completely free of presuppositions. Bracketed material is *temporarily* suspended, not banished, repeatedly thrusting itself into awareness throughout the course of a study (Thomas, 2000). Bracketing is not a one-time event; it is a dynamic, ongoing process in which the researcher repeatedly cycles through reflection, bracketing, and intuiting (Ahern, 1999; Porter, 1998). What is essential is for the researcher to place the material "within the brackets" while engaging in dialogue with participants. Thus, the goal of the bracketing interview is to highlight to the researcher his/her individual pre- understandings about the topic of investigation. Once noted, the researcher's task is to make every effort to maintain an open, nonjudgmental attitude when conducting and interpreting interviews.

To enhance the bracketing process, we suggest that the researcher continually ask himself or herself the following interrelated questions: "Why am I involved with this phenomenon?. . . . How might my personal inclinations and predispositions as to research value influence or even bias how and what I investigate? . . . . Pursuing this line of questioning, he will discover that his approach, and all that is involved in his approach, such as personal gain and prestige, social recognition, moral, ethical, religious, political and economic features, can never be entirely eliminated. . . . Without some personal interest he could never follow through in completing or even initiating a research project" (Colaizzi, 1978, p. 55).

On the basis of this type of reflection, the researcher seeks to uncover any further beliefs, hypotheses, and attitudes that are the "necessary prejudices" (in Gadamer's terms) for any understanding to take place. Although an interviewer will attempt to "bracket" prejudices, this attempt will never work completely. What will happen, however, is that researchers (or practitioners) can place commonly held beliefs within parentheses, allowing greater openness to the specific experiences now being described by the unique human beings before them.

The Interpretive Research Group

The use of an interpretive research group also facilitates bracketing by conscientiously questioning the assumptions each member brings to the interpretation of the phenomenon under consideration. Because members of the group have analyzed the researcher's bracketing interview, it is possible for them to point out whenever his or her assumptions surface in subsequent interviews and/or analyses. These usually take the form of leading questions (questions promoting one or more of the interviewer's presuppositions). The interpretive group functions something like a jury in a legal case, although juries probably do not have as much enjoyment in their deliberations as we do! Around the table at a typical Tuesday afternoon meeting of our group are 15 to 20 researchers from a variety of human science disciplines, gathered to collaboratively thematize an interview transcript. The diverse perspectives that members bring from their disciplinary training, gender role socialization, and cultural heritage are valued. We are Christians and Jews, Appalachians and Easterners, Black and White, men and women, young and old, graduate students and faculty. All contribute their own unique and useful insights to the discussion. Group members are not expected to be experts in the phenomenon being studied; the major requirement is that they be willing to commit the time and effort needed to interpret a series of interview transcripts. Probably the most important aspect of the interpretive group is its tone: respectful but critical. Members of the group not only respect the material presented in the transcript and its evolving thematic meanings but also seek counterexamples and thematic contradictions.

All proposed thematic interpretations are continuously challenged until group members agree that an interpretation is supported by text. Interpretations that seem overly theoretical—even if they agree with the opinions of group members—are questioned and put aside until more descriptive thematic meanings are noted. Although this process may sound argumentative, such is not the case. Everyone is vitally involved in producing the most illuminating and clearly presented rendition of the themes characterizing the phenomenon in question. This communal purpose and responsibility has the effect of making every comment appear an attempt to help, not to put down, the person proposing the interpretation.

The use of an interpretive group is important for maintaining the rigor of phenomenological research methods. But there are other benefits as well. For example, 10 interviews may easily generate more than 200 pages of single-spaced, typed text. The lone researcher is likely to become overwhelmed by an interpretive task of this size and may rush the interpretation, thereby overlooking significant details and interrelations in various transcripts. The group offers a means of sharing the burden of interpretation because the ability to remember significant aspects of the transcripts is greater than that of any one individual. Finally, the group offers a means of avoiding any sense of monotony or doubt that may plague an isolated researcher. Interpretation involves going over each transcript many times. The glamour and excitement of research may fade. In addition, the isolated researcher receives no immediate feedback on the adequacy of a proposed interpretation, and several months might be spent working on an inadequate interpretation before a specific problem is noted. The interpretive group circumvents these possibilities in two ways. First, the dynamic of the group has an energizing effect on the interpretive process, bringing the transcript to "life" as it is read aloud and discussed by people who share a common interest. A second virtue is that the group serves a recognition function. If an interpretation describes a pattern in the data, other individuals should also be able to see it. Group members provide the primary researcher with immediate feedback by noting that they too are able to see the interpretation in the transcript. Master's and doctoral students consistently credit the group for stimulating their thinking and supporting them through the months or years of a phenomenological investigation.

The Interpretive Process

Existential-phenomenological interpretation is rooted in a continuous process of relating a part of some text to the whole of the text, and any and all passages are always understood in terms of their relationship to the larger whole. This part-to-whole process takes place in two distinct phases. First, the interpretive group works toward a thematic description of each interview. This consists of reading the complete transcript and then connecting specific parts that stood out as significant. These parts are sometimes referred to as "meaning units" and ultimately serve as the basis for themes. The primary researcher and the interpretive group interpret an interview transcript together, after which many of the remaining transcripts are interpreted by the researcher alone. The researcher brings preliminary idiographic findings to the group on a regular basis. To help you see how the process works, let us walk you through the complete process.

Reading the Transcript in the Interpretive Group

In the University of Tennessee Phenomenological Research Group, which meets weekly, one interview transcript is usually analyzed during a single two-hour meeting. Each group member is provided with a copy of the transcribed interview (with all identifying information removed and confidentiality pledges having been signed). The transcript is read aloud by two members of the group. Customarily, the researcher who conducted the interview takes the part of the participant to portray how he or she sounded during the interview. The transcript is read with particular sensitivity to its meaning, and an attempt is made to summarize meanings as the reading proceeds. Reading is stopped at any time a group member is struck by something in the participant's narrative, even if initially unsure exactly what about the word or phrase is striking. For example, someone might say, "I want to call the group's attention to the word 'received' in line 5." As the discussion evolves, various meanings of the word "received" are examined. It becomes clear, in this interview with a hospitalized patient, that she was using the word in a very embodied way. She had experienced admission to the psychiatric unit as being "received" in the sense of being comforted. She perceived the staff as holding her, as one might hold an infant tightly, swaddling the baby securely in a receiving blanket. Thus, her description of being "received" was a significant aspect of her hospital experience. This cluster of meaning is what we regard as a *"meaning unit."* It is not uncommon to spend 20 minutes or more discussing a particular word, phrase, or metaphor.

Mining the Data for Metaphors

We have learned to pay particular attention to the metaphors participants use. Metaphors compel attention because they occur in conversation when ordinary words fail to adequately express the intended meaning. Our understanding of experiences of anger is deepened as we listen to women using cooking metaphors such as "simmering" and "stewing" (Thomas, Smucker, & Droppleman, 1998). In anger, women are heated but not boiling over. The anger is kept inside the container. Later, we note a contrast when men describe anger as a runaway horse, flood, fire, or vortex that sweeps them along— one that captures and consumes them (Thomas, McCoy, & Martin, 2000). The words of the men vividly express their experience of the uncontainable force of anger. We have a better understanding of how it feels for men and women to be angry. And, contrary to some extant quantitative research, the experience sounds different for men and women. "Metaphor in general creeps up on you and surprises" (Janesick, 1998, p. 36). As noted by Kangas, Warren, and Byrne (1998), a metaphor gives you "two ideas for one," revealing aspects of the subject matter that otherwise might be ignored or go undiscovered if we take language literally. Other figurative and symbolic language that may prove important in our analyses can include simile, analogy, irony, and rhetoric (Lakoff & Johnson, 1980; Pollio, Barlow, Fine, & Pollio, 1977).

Deciding What is Thematic

Deciding what is thematic, in our view, is not a matter of counting the frequency of word use or "percentage of cases" in which certain elements occur, as described in a recent report by a researcher team (Butcher, Holkup, & Buckwalter, 2001) using the procedure of van Kaam (1966) for data analysis. In van Kaam's approach, an "essential structural element" must be present in narratives of 50% of the participants to be considered "essential." In the journal article by Butcher et al., tables presenting numbers and percentages documented the numeric prevalence of the essential elements (e.g., "enduring stress and frustration" was noted in 574 passages, 93% of cases). Our approach relies less on quantification and more on the researcher's reflection about recurring patterns in the data. In deciding what is thematic, the researcher ponders not only specific words but the meaning of those words in the context in which they were uttered and their relationship to the participant's narrative as a whole.

Mindful of recent criticism concerning the lack of clarity in what is meant by the term *theme* in qualitative nursing research literature (DeSantis & Ugarriza, 2000), let us be clear what we mean. At this stage of the process, the word "theme" is used to mean patterns of description that repetitively recur as important aspects of a participant's description of his/her experience. At the end of the analysis of each transcript, the group summarizes the themes that have emerged. The researcher often uses a tape recorder to capture the group's discussion and summarization of themes.

A second phase of the interpretive process takes place after all of the individual transcripts have been analyzed. At this point, the hermeneutic circle expands to include more general, or nomothetic, thematic descriptions and to seek commonalities across interviews. Once such themes are described, the interpretive group considers whether they are supported by data from individual texts and whether they offer a clear picture of human experience of the phenomenon of interest. The rationale for looking across interviews is not to produce generalizability; rather, it is to improve the researcher's interpretive vision. Themes describe *experiential patterns exhibited in diverse situations*. By looking both within and across interviews the researcher is able to consider more diverse sets of experiences and to recognize ways in which one situation bears an experiential similarity to another. *Global themes* observed across interviews must also be noted in individual transcripts. Remaining continuously mindful of each interview ensures that themes will be rendered in words taken directly from participant interviews. In contrast to some qualitative research methods, we avoid describing themes in abstract terms and attempt to present them in words and phrases that are as experience-near as possible. Usually this means that we choose specific words and phrases that were used by one or more of our participants. The development of global themes leads next to the development of an overall *thematic structure*.

Developing and Refining the Thematic Structure

The structure of a phenomenon is "the commonality running through the many diverse appearances of the phenomenon" (Valle, King, & Halling, 1989, p. 14). The thematic structure is agreed upon by the researcher and members of the interpretive group. After completion of his or her independent thematization of the data, the researcher brings a list of proposed themes to the research group with specific textual support (page numbers, line numbers, quoted words and phrases). The group then examines the proposed themes and helps the researcher to choose the most apt descriptive terms for each. The final thematic structure is sometimes (but not always) presented in the form of a diagram that depicts the themes and their interrelationships. The diagram may depict both the major grounds as well as the figural aspects of the phenomenon.

Obtaining Feedback from Participants

The analysis is not yet finished. There is a very important final step. The thematic structure is presented to each of the original study participants (or, in some cases, to a subset of them if there is a large group). Participants are asked to consider the overall findings and to judge whether the thematic structure reflects their own individual experience. Most commonly, in our experience, there is an appreciative response from the participants—"Yes, that's it!" In the case of any disagreement, participants are asked to suggest alternate wording or interpretations. In most cases, the researcher then returns to the transcripts to find textual support, and the process continues until participants agree with the thematic structure developed. However, researchers do well to remember that participants, in their intense focus on their own concrete experience, may have difficulty seeing it incorporated with other people's experiences as part of a larger abstraction (Sandelowski, 1993).

Sandelowski points out that some people even forget that they provided certain information in an interview. She gives the example of a participant who insisted that a portion of an interview transcript was incorrect. (Both the transcriptionist and the researcher had heard the woman's words on the audiotape.) The woman's failure to remember was attributed to her emotional distress during that segment of the interview. She had been crying as she spoke. How did Sandelowski resolve the practical and ethical questions posed by the discrepancy between the tape and the memory in this case? It was decided *not* to play the tape back to the woman, forcing her to listen to the distressing material again and proving her wrong about what she remembered saying. As the disputed lines were deemed "theoretically unimportant," the researcher simply thanked the participant for the correction (Sandelowski, 1993, p. 6). This way of resolving a dispute may not fit all situations. In the case of similar discrepancies, each researcher must make a decision consistent with ethical treatment of humans and good science.

ENSURING THE RIGOR OF THE ANALYSIS

The phenomenological paradigm, though divergent from ordinary social science in its methodological and conceptual bases, shares some of its standards: systematic gathering of relevant information, disciplined interpretation, and empirically derived results that are stable, consistent with the data, and open to public scrutiny. Because phenomenological research aims at meaning and understanding rather than at causality and prediction, the criteria used to evaluate quantitative research must be cast in a different light. For example, objectivity is generally understood as meaning (a) a description of reality as it "really" is and (b) an independence between a detached observer and the observed "subject." Both meanings imply that the ordinary, everyday manner of seeing and experiencing things has an intrinsic error to it and that appearances are often deceptive and require correction through experimental procedures and tests.

To the phenomenological researcher, this perspective misses the fact that everything that is observed is always *observed by someone*. Methodologically, this means that no finding is ever fully independent of the research situation. For the participant in an experiment, the researcher's presence and attitude color the meaning of the entire situation for him or her, thereby affecting what the participant does. In the realm of human phenomena, there are no facts or truths independent of experience. For this reason, objectivity from the phenomenological perspective is recast as fidelity to the phenomenon *as it is given*. Colaizzi (1978, p. 52) says:

> It is a refusal to tell the phenomenon what it is, but a respectful listening to what the phenomenon speaks of itself. To the extent that I cannot deny my own experience, I cannot deny that others have experience. Objectivity, then, requires me to recognize and affirm both my own experience and the experience of others.

Accepting the impossibility of detached observation and/or objectivity does not mean that phenomenological research is not rigorous or valid. Although existential-phenomenological researchers usually do not use statistical analyses in their work, a set of criteria for dealing with issues of validity and generalizability has been developed. These criteria guide any attempt to deal with these issues in phenomenological terms. In the discussion that follows, we have chosen to employ familiar language (reliability, validity, and generalizability), mindful that some authors have suggested abandonment of the "old" language when evaluating qualitative research (cf. Lincoln & Guba, 1987; Sandelowski, 1986, 1993).

Reliability

Reliability is most often defined in terms of the consistency of research findings. But identical replication, the hallmark of laboratory and survey research, is not possible or desirable in dialogic research. No two interviews will ever be the same. Even for a single participant, the idea of a test-retest approach to reliability will not work because human description and meanings change over time as a result of changing experiences, new insights, and ever more articulated awareness that accompanies an ongoing life event. Wertz (1983) describes reliability in phenomenological research as an understanding of the researcher's point of view. Giorgi (1975) feels that findings are reliable "if a reader, adopting the same viewpoint as articulated by the researcher, can also see what the researcher saw, whether or not he agrees with it" (p. 93).

The issue of reliability also relates to whether a specific thematic structure would replicate if a new study were done on the same phenomenon or topic. Though an exact word-for-word description of the experience is not to be expected, it is reasonable to expect that themes in any new study will be commensurate with those found in the original one. This is the same basic idea as is found in quantitative research in which statistical estimates of reliability may vary slightly but not significantly between an original study and its replications. Thus, the position of phenomenological researchers with regard to thematic consistency (or reliability) is that it is possible to identify general structures and processes of experience despite changes manifest in the unique patterns defining individuals and settings. On the other hand, because reality is ambiguous, given its dependence on multiple contexts, and because researchers are bound by the limits of their own perspectives and judgments, there may be more than one legitimate interpretation for any particular set of data. In a sense, the aim of replication is to *extend*, not to *repeat*, the themes and relations obtained in the original study. Using a different group and collecting different examples is meant to broaden the themes that have emerged but not to change their essential thematic pattern as noted during the initial analysis.

Whether across studies or within a single study, the various meanings and interpretations will not be "blind to each other nor to the data" (Wertz, 1983). Relations that can be discerned among them will serve to reveal superficial or mistaken understandings on the researcher's part and yield greater certainty and persistence of meaning. Alternative perspectives are welcomed. The attitude that one's results must be communicable and usable by others has led some phenomenological researchers to seek methods for evaluating the consistency of their categories or thematic structure. Dapkus (1985), for example, obtained 75% to 84% agreement among three raters who independently coded items using her category system. Most researchers, however, favor nonquantitative means of reaching intersubjective agreement. One crucial test of any study is its relevance and value in bringing about new insights regarding the phenomenon being studied.

Validity

Validity means whether one has investigated what one wished to investigate. In the qualitative research interview this involves the extent to which "the interviews investigate the meaning of the life-world themes of the interviewed"(Kvale, 1996). Judging validity of a phenomenological study involves both methodological and experiential criteria (Pollio et al., 1997). Methodological issues concern whether the methods used are rigorous and appropriate to the research topic; experiential issues concern whether the findings are *plausible* and *illuminating*. We should expect a reciprocal relationship between these two issues: "The more rigorous and appropriate the methodology, the more plausible and illuminating the results are likely to be. Conversely, if a study generates highly plausible and illuminating results, the more disposed the reader will be to judge the method as appropriate, and perhaps, rigorous" (Pollio et al., 1997, p. 55.) Polkinghorne (1989) observes that evaluating validity in phenomenological research is different from evaluating validity in quantitative research. Rather than asking about the relationship of findings to some external predicted or theoretical understanding, validity resides in the researcher's confidence in the meanings proposed:

> Phenomenological research approaches validity from a more general perspective —as a conclusion that inspires confidence because the argument in support of it has been persuasive. . . . The degree of validity of the findings of a phenomenological research project, then, depends on the power of its presentation to convince the reader that its findings are accurate. . . . (p. 57)

What this means is that validity is not determined by the degree of correspondence between a description and some external reality criterion but by whether convincing evidence has been brought forth in favor of the description offered.

Generalizability

As Sandelowski (1997, p. 127) notes, "the single most important factor contributing to the failure to take findings of qualitative studies seriously is the frequently cited but false charge that they are not generalizable." This false charge, aimed not only at phenomenology but also at other qualitative methodologies, can be handled in a relatively straightforward manner. In his discussion of what standard research practice would term "subject selection," Polkinghorne (1989, p. 48) notes that the "purpose of phenomenological research is to describe the structure of an experience, not to describe the characteristics of a group who have had the experience." In principle, a single individual could be studied in sufficient detail to achieve this goal, as exemplified in the work of many philosophers, novelists, and poets. Supporting this point, Sandelowski asserts that "Entire fields of knowledge, such as ethics, law, and several domains in psychology, have been constructed from case generalizations" (1997, p. 127). Likewise, in the discipline of nursing, "knowledge of particular patient populations is built up with many instances of knowing particular patients" (Tanner, Benner, Chesla, and Gordon, 1993, p. 279).

The point of inviting more than one particular patient to participate in a phenomenological study is to produce *variations*. Obtaining different narratives makes it somewhat easier to discern the essential structure of a phenomenon. Redundancies often begin to appear after a relatively small number of carefully conducted interviews. For example, in one of our recent studies, remarkable consistencies became evident after only four interviews with hospitalized psychiatric patients (Thomas, Shattell, & Martin, 2001). This experience is not unusual; thematic coherence is often provided by as few as three to five interviews. On this basis, Pollio et al. (1997), after dealing with transcripts from some 25 or 30 studies, wrote: "With this number of interviews (3–5), give or take a few, the interpreter develops a sense of descriptive patterns and relations characterizing the various interviews" (pp. 51–52). Once this point is reached—where recurrent patterns and themes are hard to overlook—the general rule of thumb is that the researcher interview two more participants. If no new patterns or themes emerge at this point, the phenomenon is thought to be well-described, and there is little or no need to seek additional exemplars or participants.

Largely because issues of generalizability have been framed by theoretically and demographically oriented researchers, the traditional proof of a study must meet the methodological requirements of disinterested observation and test. This means that the theoretical principle must be shown to occur across a wide variety of individuals and situations. Because each "subject" is essentially considered the same as any other, a large number of unknown (and randomly selected) individuals must show the predicted result for the project to prove its theoretical point or to serve as a basis for subsequent clinical intervention. The case for what might be called *phenomenological generalizability* is different. Here, "proof" does not depend solely on purity of method but also upon the *reader* of the research report. In this case, when and if a description rings true, each specific reader who derives insight from the results of a phenomenological study may be thought to extend its generalizability. Unlike other research methods where the researcher establishes generalizability on the basis of statistical and experimental procedures, phenomenological research is "validated" by its readers. As Kvale (1996) noted with regard to the clinical case study: "An example of reader generalizability . . . [involves] . . . Freud's case stories where his descriptions . . . had been so vivid and convincing that psychoanalysts still generalize [them] to current cases" (p. 234).

In like manner, we believe that clinicians reading the studies in this book about patients with chronic pain or implanted defibrillators will be able to move directly to applying our findings in practice when the findings are applicable to their "current cases." In evaluating the findings of a phenomenological study Ray advises clinicians to consider "the richness, really," [which determines] "how well somebody else can use it. . . . Does this have any relevance or validity in the context of my practice?" (1994, p. 117). *Deciding if qualitative study findings are applicable is a matter of clinical judgment.* The same type of judgment is made by a nurse in applying the findings of quantitative studies. Because research shows the "average" hysterectomy patient has gotten pain relief from 75 milligrams of meperidine, does that automatically mean that this particular patient will? The astute nurse considers the "current case" before deciding on the dose to administer. Benner (1999a, p. 316) urges nurses to reclaim the scholarly legitimacy of clinical judgment, "the reasoning about the particular patient." Perhaps *every* nursing intervention should be prefaced by something like this: "Some people with chronic pain benefit from 'X.' Therefore, I think it might be worth a try. What do *you* think?"

Recently, a more formal way of extending the findings of a qualitative study to clinical practice has been presented by Morse, Penrod, and Hupcey (2000). Drawing from previous research on hope, an assessment guide was developed to enable nurses to identify a patient's stage in the hope trajectory. Then nurses implemented strategies to modify or facilitate hope and systematically evaluated the efficacy of the strategies across cases, discarding practices that were not helpful. This approach, termed Qualitative Outcome Analysis, has great potential for bridging the often-lamented gap between qualitative nursing research and practice.

The "Unconscious"

A final issue to be dealt with in regard to interview studies is the question of so-called unconscious processes. Are participants always able to report information relevant to an understanding of the meaning of the phenomenon? What if they are repressing important material? Psychotherapists whose practice is based in existential phenomenology (cf. Yalom, 1980) locate the patient's difficulties in the present life-world and not in unconscious mechanisms (Thompson, Locander, & Pollio, 1989). Take the mechanism of *repression*, for instance. In the existential context, it is redefined as an existential choice: "The memory that is lost is lost only insofar as it belongs to a region of my life that I refuse" (Merleau-Ponty, 1962).

While many criticisms may be leveled against the psychoanalytic concept of the unconscious as a "place beneath" consciousness (see Merleau-Ponty, 1970, Chapter 6), the crucial issue for phenomenological studies is that the phenomena on which the idea of an unconscious is based (dreams, slips of the tongue, somatic symptoms) *do occur* and cannot be dismissed. Probably the best road to take is the one proposed by Van den Berg (1961) when he suggests that the interviewer (or therapist) "creates" the unconscious in his or her interaction with the person being interviewed (participant or patient). A residual sense of discontent after an interview may not be the result of "unconscious forces" but of poor questioning.

The interviewer's job is to enable participants to describe as much of their experiential world as possible. By carefully asking "what" questions ("what did you notice?") rather than "why" questions concerning an analysis of causal factors, the interviewer helps the participant describe personal experience as it is lived. Sometimes, there are seeming contradictions in what the participant tells the interviewer. When this happens, what is required is not a switch to "why" questions but an attempt to enable the participant to describe the phenomenon more fully. When this happens, both participant and researcher will come to discern the experience as it now is for the participant, even if the experience is described in terms of contradictory aspects. (See the discussion of a syzygy of feelings in Chapter 4). By focusing on "what" questions, the interview proceeds to a deeper and richer description of first-person experience. This does not mean that all ambiguity is cleared up, especially since some experiences are ambiguous and confusing by their very nature. Contradiction and/or ambiguity do not necessarily imply either the operation of "unconscious factors" or poor experiential description. Each participant reports what he or she reports, and it is the interviewer's responsibility to interpret such descriptions without recourse to theoretical mechanisms that may be significant to the interviewer but not to the participant. As Peplau noted, when two people are in the midst of developing a common understanding, not all experiences can be shared or understood (1952).

A Final Word About Rigor

Striving for rigor in phenomenological research does not have to result in "quasi-militaristic zeal to neutralize bias and to defend our projects against threats to validity" (Sandelowski, 1993, p. 1). In many published accounts of studies, a defensive posture is assumed by the researcher. An excessive number of pages is devoted to raw data (for example, lists of statements from which themes were extracted) and detailed description of the rigid and laborious steps that were taken to ensure rigor in arriving at the "findings." The reader is worn out before ever *finding* the findings in such a report. We agree with Sandelowski's admonition to "soften our notion of rigor to include the playfulness, soulfulness, imagination, and technique we associate with more artistic endeavors (1993, p. 8).

SUMMARY AND CONCLUSIONS

As one way of bringing together many of the concerns and procedures we have described, Pollio et al. (1997) offered the following flow chart (see Figure 2.1) to describe the sequencing of procedures and practices in an existential-phenomenological study based on dialogical interviewing procedures and thematic interpretation. Although the original flow chart was developed as a somewhat tongue-in-cheek invocation of cognitive psychology, we have since learned that researchers have found it to be helpful. As long as the researcher/practitioner does not take this sequence of steps as the final word, it seems appropriate to use as an organizational mnemonic.

As previously discussed (and reiterated in the chart), the original focus for any specific piece of dialogical research is the investigator. For this reason, the researcher is asked to consider two different questions: (1) what about the topic was important enough for me to make it the major concern of an investigation? and (2) in what ways and situations have I experienced the phenomenon? The purpose here is not to make the researcher "objective" but rather to enhance awareness of the personal perspective he or she necessarily will take in dealing openly with participants and patients. Prior to embarking on the study, the researcher also thoughtfully considers its ethical aspects

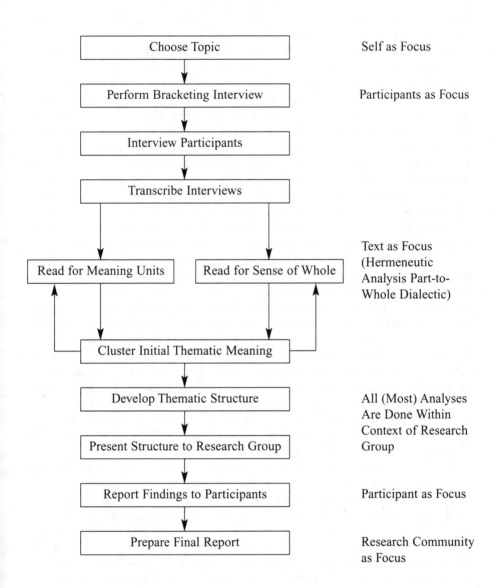

Figure 2.1 Summary of Steps in Conducting an Existential-Phenomenological Study. From Pollio, H. R., Henley, T., & Thompson, C. B. (1997). *The Phenomenology of Everyday Life*. New York: Cambridge University Press. Reprinted by permission.

and the steps that must be taken to protect participants. (We suggest a review of the American Nurses' Association's "Ethical Principles in the Conduct, Dissemination, and Implementation of Nursing Research" [Silva, 1995].)

We need to make one more comment here about the researcher's preparatory phase. In some accounts of phenomenology in the nursing literature, it is stated that "the review of literature follows data analysis" (Carpenter, 1999b, p. 61). We disagree with this position. Prior to undertaking any research project, one needs to survey what is already known, and not yet known, about a phenomenon. Although the phenomenological researcher does not choose a theoretical framework to guide the study, he or she should be familiar with the theoretical lenses used by previous scholars to view the phenomenon. A critical analysis and synthesis of previous research findings is also essential in evaluating the potential contribution of this particular project to the ongoing stream of discoveries about the phenomenon. Having a sophisticated command of the pertinent literature does *not* imply that "biases will influence the research" (Carpenter, p. 61)—provided that the researcher initially brackets, and continually re-brackets, prior knowledge while interacting with participants and analyzing data.

The second focus depicted in Figure 2.1 is the interview itself. Enough has been said about the interview process, but perhaps once again we should remind the reader of the humility with which the interviewer approaches the participant who is considered the expert on his or her experience. The next stages of the process involve the text and the care that must be taken in its initial transcription as well as in its subsequent interpretation. If a major concern during interviewing is not to lead the participant or the dialogue on the basis of personal or theoretical pre-conceptions, a similar injunction must be raised during the interpretation phase. In our view, the major task of interpretation takes place within the context of the research group. Researchers with no access to a group are encouraged to avail themselves of the technology permitting conference calls, online Internet dialogues, round-robin e-mails, and overnight mail delivery of transcripts or portions of transcripts to colleagues and consultants. Journaling is another helpful adjunct in this as well as other stages of the process.

To avoid giving priority of interpretive place to the researcher's intuitions, all meanings and themes must be located in the text. Although some investigators (cf. Giorgi, 1975) argue that it is necessary to transform the language of the participant into that of the researcher and/or the discipline, our view is more compatible with that of Husserl (1913/1931) who advised that phenomena can be characterized in language that may be "derived from common speech." We have found that the specific words of the participant invariably are powerful enough in their evocative and experiential meanings to capture the "essence" of the phenomenon. (Consider the difference between labeling a hospitalized psychiatric patient's experience as "regression" versus using his own words describing hospitalization as mercifully allowing him to "cool his head and mind.") For this reason, we prefer to describe the structure of meanings in the simple and powerful personal language of participants whenever possible.

Such reliance on the participant as a research collaborator also extends to the next phase of a phenomenological study. During this phase, participants' individual descriptions are presented to them, along with a summary of the overall findings, for comments and reactions. The purpose of doing this is not to have them "validate" the results but to engage them, once again, in a dialogue about possible points of disagreement. Participants do not have the final say about "correctness" of the description any more than we do; instead, the purpose is to seek a fusion of horizons between two different, but complementary, perspectives on a topic of interest to both. Neither the researcher nor the participant is afforded interpretive priority: All results are co-constructed on the basis of open and continuing dialogue.

The final step in any research is the writing of a public report. Here, a shift in focus takes place from the participant and the researcher to the larger disciplinary community. It goes without saying that the same attention to detail that prevailed during the interview and its interpretation must also be observed at this stage. In our view, the researcher is obligated to share the themes identified in analysis of his or her bracketing interview (Thomas, 2000). Extensive disclosure of painful private experiences such as sexual abuse is not necessary; the reader does, however, have a right to know where the researcher is "coming from." As noted by Polkinghorne (1989, p. 58), "It is important to include in the phenomenological research report an implication section where the significance of the findings for practice and policy is spelled out." Throughout the written report, the researcher must follow the ordinary amenities of clear writing and compelling example. We use participants' words liberally in our reports because we believe their words are far more vivid and compelling than our paraphrases of them.

In a phenomenological journal article or book, consideration also must be given to the fact that not everyone who reads the results will understand or approve of this type of research. For this reason, some effort must be made to describe the rationale behind the procedures used and to situate present findings within recognizable horizons of meaning for the reader. The researcher must clearly specify the *methodology* (the "branch" of phenomenology, whether descriptive, hermeneutic, or a hybrid) and the *method* (systematic sequence of procedures, e.g., Thomas & Pollio, Colaizzi, Newman, or another). Janesick (1998), however, warns against *methodolatry* (devoting too many pages of the report to extensive defense of one's method rather than the substance of the research findings): "In the final stage of writing up the project, it is probably wise to avoid being overly preoccupied with method" (p. 48). Here, perhaps, the best hope is to say something of such significance to the reader that he or she will be able to see beyond the method to new insight about the phenomenon.

One additional point remains. Although these steps have been described for the specific case of research interviews, it seems clear that various aspects of this process are also useful to nurses in the clinical area. Perhaps the major implication is that our patients are able to tell us what is significant about their experience when in our care. Nursing practice is never just an analytic assemblage of numbers and charts designed to make the patient into a package of biological functions. As we know, and as our practice tells us every day of our professional lives, people come to our clinics and hospitals having significant information to provide if only we will listen. The problem, however, is how to hear and use what they tell us. The lessons taught by Ginger,

Hermes, and Wittgenstein's lion seem particularly apt—every understanding requires a negotiation on our part and on the part of our conversational partners. Only if we make the effort to understand does it become possible for language to connect rather than separate us from our patients. This would seem a particularly relevant consequence for nursing practice as well as for nursing research.

Here is an example of using phenomenological concepts in practice. Suzanne Beddoe, a nurse practitioner, seeks to attain what she calls the "reachable moment" in her everyday work with patients. She tells the following story. A middle-aged man with chronic back pain was talking at length about his previous ability to provide for his family, often holding two jobs. At first, Beddoe was annoyed and failed to understand what he was trying to communicate. Gradually, she understood that this man was "in mourning for a life that he would never know again," so she said to him: "The world you knew, and thrived in, and were successful in is gone. You are wondering how to cope with a situation you never imagined. Before your injuries, you were a successful provider for your family and now you don't know where you fit" (Beddoe, 1999, p. 248). He was astonished, tears welling in his eyes as he replied, "I've seen dozens of physicians and nurses, but no one has ever talked to me this way. . . . I have never cried in front of anyone" (p. 248). In their dialogue in this "reachable moment," Beddoe and her patient forged a bond. She did not cure him of his back pain, but that was not what he was seeking from her.

Dialogical procedures imply a philosophy of what is crucial in, and about, human life. Using dialogue as a point of reference, communication and conversation become the overriding issues in what it means to be a human being. Our lives are lived neither in fusion with other people or social institutions, nor in isolation from them, but in connection with the interpersonal, social and natural worlds of everyday life. The human world is a network of interconnections whose complexity and significance are given voice both in the language of the artist and in conversation. As Martin Buber (1924/1970) pointed out a number of years ago, all human life is lived in the in-between. Who we are and how we are depends as much on our situation, our history, and our relationships as upon our self-reflections and our body. We are always and already in relationship to something beyond us, and this existential fact defines both the method and philosophy motivating an existential-phenomenological approach to nursing.

II

Nursing and the Human Experience of the Human Body

Keeping Things Whole

In a field
I am the absence
of field.
This is
always the case.
Wherever I am
I am what is missing.

When I walk
I part the air
and always
the air moves in
to fill the spaces
where my body's been.

We all have reasons
for moving.
I move
to keep things whole.

—Mark Strand
Copyright 1964 by Mark Strand. Reprinted
with permission of the Wylie Agency.

3

The Human Experience of the Human Body

Anursing assessment often involves a collection of numbers—simple ones such as height, weight, temperature, and heart rate and more complicated ones such as cholesterol levels and red and white blood cell counts. Patient numbers are then compared to standard values, with "health" being defined, in part, by the outcome of these comparisons. The nurse also performs a physical examination of the patient's corporeal body in which the body is scanned for any obvious abnormalities or wounds. The picture of the body that underlies the traditional physical examination is one in which the body is conceptualized as a self-contained machine that can be assessed and diagnosed by relatively straightforward physiochemical and observational procedures. But what we know about the body from a nursing or medical point of view will be incomplete until we also take a first-person view into account. The human body is never experienced by the person as a machine, object, or thing.

Consider the simple task of trying to feel your left hand with your right. As Merleau-Ponty (1962) pointed out, the left hand is also able to feel the right hand as the right hand attempts to feel the left one. Although the left hand may "let itself be felt" by the right, at any given instant the situation may be reversed. A similar state of affairs describes the adult experience of examining his or her body for lumps or a child's experience of sucking his or her thumb. While we are often able to experience physical objects from many different perspectives, the human body is always experienced *from the same perspective*. Unlike physical objects, we are never able to move away from our bodies nor can they be moved away from us. Merleau-Ponty (1962) writes: "[An object's] presence is such that it entails a possible absence. . . . The permanence of [the human body] is not of a permanent object in the world but of a permanence of my point of view."

For Merleau-Ponty (1962) the body is the fundamental category of human existence. In fact, the world is said to exist only in and through the body. It is the body that first grasps the world and moves with intention in it (Leonard, 1999). The body is the focal point of living meanings, the carrier of our mortality, and the origin of all spatial relationships. The place the individual occupies within the world, his bodily "here," is the beginning point from which he takes a bearing in space and makes intelligible ideas such as far, near, beside, above, and below. With the growth of the body over time, the meaning of space changes; what is high for a child is no longer high for an adult. Even the perceptual qualities of objects require the body's participation—"There is no 'weight' without lifting, no 'smoothness' without a caress, no 'circle' without a curving glance, no 'depth' without reach, and no 'distance' without gait'" (Merleau- Ponty, cited in Wertz, 1989, p. 86).

The lived body is regarded by phenomenologists such as Merleau-Ponty as worthy of serious philosophical and empirical investigation. This stance contrasts sharply with many of the disembodied philosophies that have dominated Western thought for centuries. Within Cartesian thought, for example, the mind was more significant than the body which belonged to the lesser realm of things. Only recently have some philosophers, most notably Lakoff and Johnson (1999), concluded that even intellectual meaning is grounded in and through our bodies. Consider the meaning of "losing" one's voice. Merleau-Ponty (1962) tells the story of a girl, forbidden to see her lover, who "loses" her voice. The body is the place where life hides away, its movement toward the future arrested. The girl recovers her voice not by intellectual effort or an act of will, but through a conversion in which the whole of her body reopens itself to others.

THE "BODY OBJECT" AND THE "BODY SUBJECT"

Merleau-Ponty distinguished between the "body object," the body of medicine, and the "body subject," the body of subjective experience. The orientation of medicine—body as material object—has "allowed us to have body parts repaired and replaced, becoming interchangeable, at the external level, without consideration of the inner world of the body-as-self, as experience" (Watson, 1999, p. 135). It is not surprising that medical students come to perceive the body as "object," given the fact that they begin their study of the body by dissecting lifeless cadavers. One well-known medical school professor actually introduced his students to the human body by writing "dead mammal" on the blackboard the first day of class (Watson, 1999). In contrast to the professor's stance, Merleau-Ponty reminds us of the sacredness of the body. If we keep this sacredness in mind, "it [is] impossible for us to treat a face or a body, even a dead body, like a thing. They are sacred entities" (from *Structure of Behavior*, cited in Moran, 2000, p. 415)

A number of activities can be undertaken to demonstrate that the human body is not an object. Consider the way in which we attempt to see our own body using mirrors. Here, we are struck by certain effects that would not be possible if our body were truly an object. Von Fiandt (1952/1966) points out that, when he shaves his face in the mirror, it is his mirror face and not his corporeal face that he experiences himself shaving. This event may become even more ambiguous. The person shaving may experience his face both *here* (on this side of the mirror) and *there* (in the mirror) and be able to move back and forth between the two perspectives. Young children behave quite differently with respect to their image in the mirror, often treating it as if it were another person. The experience that I am both the "see-er" and the "seen" takes a while to develop: very early in life, the infant seems able to experience himself or herself as a locus of seeing but not as the continuing perspective from which seeing takes place.

Mirrors allow us to see reflections, and it seems apt that the same word, "re-flect," also describes a different human ability to bend back on itself, that of thinking. If we choose thinking as the most significant way that we have of being a human—as philosophers such as Descartes have suggested—then the reflected body becomes more important (and "real") than the body doing the reflecting. The problem arising from these concerns was summed up quite neatly in the words of Helmuth Plessner (1961/1970): "The human being both is a body and has a body." Although the second body derives from reflection—and Descartes would say it is the only one worthy of concern—the first body captures the experience of our human body in everyday life, and, as Merleau-Ponty (1962) would say, it is the more basic one.

Although medicine has struggled long and hard with the role of psychological factors in illness, the idea that a human being both is a body and has a body is explicitly agreed to whenever the word *psychosomatic* is used. Can such illness be understood by considering the body as an object or machine, or must we recognize a different way of understanding the body of psychosomatic illness? To help think about this question, consider two very different phenomena that fall in the category of psychosomatic: the relatively esoteric and elusive phenomenon of voodoo death and the well-researched, everyday phenomenon of hardiness or resiliency. In the case of voodoo death, the eminent physiologist Walter B. Cannon (1942) long ago specified three conditions as necessary for a voodoo curse to work: (1) the person had to believe it, (2) the culture had to believe it, and (3) the cursed person had to be expelled from the social life of the community. In the case of resiliency, research by Kobasa (1984) has shown that hardy, resilient people tend to: (1) view change as a challenge; (2) trust in personal efficacy rather than luck or powerful others; and (3) be strongly connected to some social or religious community. Taken side by side, these results suggest that both resiliency and voodoo death depend upon the person's specific experiences of time (as challenging or closed), personal efficacy (as under my control or not under my control), and relationships to other people (as alienated or connected). Viability is as much a question of the person's present situation of being-in-the-world as of the objective status of the corporeal body.

THE EXPERIENCE AND CONCEPT OF BODY IMAGE

Many of these ideas come together in a particularly clear way in terms of the experience and concept of *body image*. Even a casual examination of research on this topic reveals that body image means one of two different things: (1) the body as a system of biological parts that work together as an overall pattern, and (2) the body that I think about when considering myself in terms of social attitudes and evaluations. The first of these meanings originated in response to issues raised by the experience of phantom limbs as well as by medical observations of patients having undergone certain types of brain damage. The second meaning arose in attempts to think systematically about personal attitudes and values concerning the appearance of the human body to oneself and to other people.

Phantom Limbs

The first-person facts concerning phantom limbs are well known, having been reported long ago by Admiral Horatio Nelson who lost his right arm in July 1797 and viewed his phantom limb experience a "direct proof of existence of the soul." He came to this conclusion by assuming that, if an arm could survive physical destruction, so too could his soul (Riddoch, 1941). Nelson was among the first to describe pain in the phantom arm, including the experience of absent fingers digging into an absent palm. Such experiences are well-established medical phenomena, as are the following:

1. Over 90% of all patients experience a phantom after the loss of a limb. In some 65% of cases, the phantom appears within 24 hours of the amputation or at most within a few days or weeks.
2. In some cases, the phantom fades from awareness in a few weeks. In other cases, it seems to have an extraordinary persistence of years and even decades (Sunderland, 1978).
3. Although, as the name suggests, phantoms most often involve arms and legs, they have also been reported for almost all body parts (Ramacharandan & Hirstein, 1998). In the case of arms and legs, the phantom usually assumes a habitual position—for example, flexed at the elbow. Ramacharandan and Hirstein (1998) note that "we have seen a patient [preoperatively] where the arm was in a vertical wooden splint . . . with fingers hooked over the end of the splint. . . . Several weeks later, his phantom was in exactly the same position . . . with the finger hooked over an imaginary splint."
4. For some individuals, telescoping of the phantom occurs. In some 50% of cases the patient may be left with a phantom hand "attached" to the stump of the arm. Such telescoping can be re-extended—for example, in situations in which it would have been appropriate to "shake hands," to protect oneself from a blow, or to pick up a cup.
5. The phantom often evokes personal memories; some patients experience a wedding ring or watch on the phantom hand or arm. Ramacharandan and Hirstein (1998) even report that one of their patients experienced arthritic pain in her phantom fingers whenever the weather was cold and damp.

What do all of these clinical phenomena tell us about the human body? Merleau-Ponty (1962) suggests that in order to derive some implications for our understanding of the body from these findings, we must simultaneously consider a different phenomenon of abnormal bodily experience termed *anosognosia*, a phenomenon recent texts refer to as neglect. Following right parietal lobe damage, either part or all of the left side of the body "ceases to exist" for the patient. Not only are things and sounds on the left not responded to, the patient frequently does not groom that side of the body. When asked, "What is that?" (referring to the left arm) the patient will report that he or she does not know; some early reports indicated that patients described their left arm as a "rope" or a "long cold snake" (Merleau-Ponty, 1962, pp. 76, 148).

Considering the phenomena of phantom limbs together with those of anosognosia produces a peculiar paradox. In one case, a body part that is absent to clinical observation is present to personal experience; in the other case, a body part that is present to clinical observation is absent to personal experience. To deal with these phenomena Merleau-Ponty suggests that we must not think of the body and the world as separate but as always in communion with one another. We must not think of the body as simply a bit of biological machinery. Instead, we must think in different terms, terms that do not view the body as a thing separate from the world or our intentions toward the world. The ordinary split of mind from body and body from world leaves all of us with a set of uncomfortable barriers: between "me" and "my body" and between "my body" and "the world."

It is precisely this sort of conceptual disconnection that is meant to be overcome by existential phenomenology's seeming fascination with the hyphen, as in the phrase, being-in-the- world. What hyphens do is remind us that "I am not a mind, in a body, in the world" but that personal existence is the nexus between personal intentions and the world. Existence is never a simple summation of mind plus body plus world but rather an integrated system in which the three terms define a total pattern constantly responsive to changes in any one or all of them. In the present context, this implies that the human body is not an assemblage of components but a system committing us to the world. Perhaps this is why the infant looks toward the world and not toward its own hand when it first attempts to grasp an object.

Phantom limbs and contralateral neglect (anosognosia) both concern issues of presence, absence, and possibilities. Body parts that are absent to objective (third-person) observation retain experiences of possible movement, whereas body parts present to objective observation do not afford possibilities of movement and are experienced as absent. What this synopsis of facts suggested to Merleau-Ponty was that, somewhere between "objective" movement and "subjective" intention, threads of possibility continue to connect person to world. When nothing directly calls the impossibility of movement to the person's attention, the person-world connection remains alive and vital. Thus, the presence or absence of movement possibilities (i.e., *functioning intentionality* in philosophical terms) defines the relationship between body and world, not the presence or absence of body parts. The first-person experience of the lived body is not to be found in the subjective phenomena of mental life or in the objective phenomenon of physical movement but in a third realm that does not fit the ordinary categories of mind and body.

Body Image as Appearance

The term "body image" is meant to capture first-person thoughts, values, and attitudes toward the human body. As the word "image" suggests, the experience we have of our body may be likened to that of "a picture." Under this reading, my picture should be similar to someone else's picture of my body (say, that of a nurse) and both "pictures" should correspond to what that person or I might see in the mirror or in life. This view, however, does not accord with what we know from a first-person point of view. First of all, there is the case of looking at my body in the mirror: "Think . . . about the last time you looked in the mirror and consider what highly selective details you saw—a misplaced hair, a slight paunch . . . or a pimple. An extreme example would be a young woman with anorexia nervosa, who stares into the mirror and selectively focuses on a fold of fat on her thigh" (Moss, 1989, p. 66). We do not look at our mirror body in an objective way, like a nurse or physician. Rather, we are extremely selective in what we notice and look for. What we notice and look for tells a good deal about what is important to us about our body.

A different way to study body image is in terms of figure drawing. If we consider the picture actually drawn as providing information as to how the person "sees" or thinks about his or her body, a number of interesting facts emerge. First of all, there is the developmental context. Research indicates that children of four or younger draw pictures in which few details are correct and that children of eight or older draw pictures in which almost all details are correct. These differences are so clear and orderly that it is possible to use the number of correct details a child draws to predict his or her IQ score.

If we combine these observations with those of Simmel (1962) concerning the ages at which children develop a phantom limb (greater than eight years of age) or do not develop a phantom limb (less than four years of age), it is possible to propose that the body system characteristic of adult being-in-the-world develops during the period between four and eight years of age. Other data supporting this possibility may be derived from an infant's reaction to his or her own image in the mirror. Here, results indicate that an infant does not invariably recognize itself in the mirror until approximately two years of age and that during earlier periods the infant may smile at its mother's mirror reflection but not at its own. During the period from 6 months to 24 months, not only does the infant attempt to touch or talk to the mirror child, but it also may attempt to wipe off the mirror image, paint placed on its own nose or cheek. These observations all suggest that the infant does not come to its own body image on the basis of mirror reflection but on the basis of first-person experiences associated with prior actions in the world. The mirror only lets the infant, and later the child or adult, recognize from a different point of view what he or she was already aware of but had not yet explicitly claimed. Results from both mirror reactions and (somewhat later) from figure drawings suggest that the initial aspects of body image come together between two and four years of age and are only completed, in the sense of providing a useable body system, by eight years of age.

Drawing a picture of the human body also tells us about the person's pre-reflected attitudes toward his or her body. In the case of child figure drawings, issues of gender hardly ever appear in early drawings (less than six years of age) but only appear as the child grows older. By adolescence, absence of gender differentiation is potentially significant. By the time we come to the adult, sociopersonal attitudes toward the body are quite apparent in figure drawings. Moss (1989), for example, presents figure drawings by clinically obese adult women. In these drawings there is a characteristic head/body split: the head is drawn in great detail whereas the rest of the body is drawn in little or no detail. On the basis of many conversations with these women, it is also possible "to hear" a similar head/body split: "From here up I am valuable and competent; from here down, I am simply this thing, and I can't do very much with it." In summarizing these and other observations, Moss returns us to the idea of existence as being-in- the-world:

> To this division in her body image corresponds a split in her world . . . when a part of the world has become a region of futility, incapacity or shame . . . it is relinquished and the related parts of the body . . . described as "not me" or as the "thing I am helplessly encased in." With this loss . . . comes mourning, grieving and tears, (and we) discover that intimate bonding of body and world. (pp. 77–78)

Obesity is not the only condition wherein appearance-based aspects of body image exact a price. Two other significant domains concern cosmetic surgery and the clinical conditions of anorexia and bulimia. Take the case of surgical breast augmentation. Despite an FDA ban on gel implants and widespread publicity about adverse consequences of other types of implants (e.g., silicone), the number of operations continues to run to over 120,000 per year (Thompson, Heinberg, Altabe, & Tartleff-Dunn, 1999). The average cost of breast augmentation surgery is anywhere from $2500 to $5000 and up. Such cosmetic surgical procedures, and their associated personal and economic costs, make sense only if we consider them in terms of results produced by three large scale surveys done by the popular magazine *Psychology Today*. Although their specific numbers may not be representative of the total population, they do indicate that in 1972 15% of male respondents and 23% of female respondents were dissatisfied with their appearance; comparable values in 1985 were 34% for men and 38% for women. In 1996, these values rose to 43% for males and 56% for females (cited by Thompson et al., 1999). These results suggest that, when asked directly, between one-third and one-half of all adult respondents are dissatisfied with their appearance. When a partial list of things we do not like about our appearance is tabulated, the following often come up as needing "repair": weight, specific facial features, hair loss, level of muscularity, wrinkles, chest/breast size, etc.

The case of anorexia and other eating disorders such as bulimia also reveal that dissatisfaction with one's appearance is a significant predictive risk factor. Rosen (1992, 1996) has gone so far as to propose that body-image distortions are at the base of these disorders (perceiving oneself as too fat overall or in some specific body area, then controlling weight by fasting, starving, or purging.) The relationship between body image and anorexia was first described by Bruch (1985) who noted a clear gap between a patient's self-perception of her body and her appearance to a parent or nurse. Rosen (1992) later described it in the following terms: "In essence, patients with eating disorders tend to perceive themselves as unrealistically big or fat and as being grossly out of proportion or protruding at certain body regions. . . . No matter what feedback the patient may receive she relies on her own perceptions and feelings of being too big" (p. 193).

Despite clinical agreement on these perceptual distortions, "hard" medical evidence has been difficult to come by. The nub of one early controversy concerned the finding that control (non-eating-disordered) subjects frequently overestimated body size by about the same amount as was true for anorectic subjects. As a partial answer, Cash and Brown (1987) tallied all existing studies at the time, noting significantly greater overestimation in patients than in controls, especially in the case of bulimia. The fact that non-eating-disordered women overestimate their size suggests that there is a ubiquitous concern for being thin in Western culture. This assumption was tested in a series of prospective studies performed on many different groups of women in the 1990s and summarized by Thompson et al. in their book *Exacting Beauty* (1999). When girls and young women were followed for a period of time, ranging from 9 months to 8 years, "body dissatisfaction" predicted a wide variety of eating problems and disorders. More sophisticated statistical modeling procedures indicated that "eating disorder symptoms were affected by the interaction of social pressure for thinness, negative self-appraisals, and negative affect, but *body dissatisfaction mediated the relationship* between most risk factors and eating disorders" (Thompson et al., 1999, p. 36).

THEMES IN THE HUMAN EXPERIENCE OF THE BODY: FINDINGS FROM PHENOMENOLOGICAL RESEARCH

These considerations, all of which derive from research concerning the body, indicate that, although we know a great about the physical body, we know considerably less about the human experience and *meaning* of the body, what Merleau-Ponty (1962) would call the "lived body" or "body subject." To learn more about these topics, MacGillivray (1995) asked 16 healthy adult men and women to "please tell me about some times when you are aware of your body, and then tell me what you are or were aware of in that situation." The first request was designed to discover the specific situations in which an awareness of one's body is figural, the second request to learn about the specific meanings the human body holds for adults. When MacGillivray analyzed participant responses, three major thematic categories emerged.

The first thematic category, **Engagement**, concerned situations in which the person experienced his or her body in terms of full participation in some project. The focus was primarily on the world of the project, and the person either reported no particular experience of the body or a "curious absence" of specific experiences. Sartre (1956) spoke of this mode of experiencing the body as "passed-over-in-silence." Sometimes these situations concerned experiences of **Vitality** (feeling totally alive and absorbed in the world) and at other times they concerned experiences of **Activity** (focusing on the concrete movements in which the person was engaged). Specific examples of both of these subthemes of engagement are as follows: **Vitality**—"And I guess [I'm aware of] the feeling of well-being; you go outside and take a deep breath and feel good all over;" **Activity**—"In running I enjoy the feeling of the muscles burning, the tightness of the skin with the wind on it;" **Vitality and activity**—"[When walking] . . . I'm aware of the good feelings of stretching the legs . . . of taking in breaths . . . of walking in the cold rain and having it hit my face."

The second major thematic category, **Corporeality**, had to do with experiences of the body- as-physical. In these settings, the body was experienced as an object in a world of objects or as a mechanism or instrument capable of attaining goals. Examplars from the interviews included: **Instrument**—"In the early stages of learning how to dance, you have to think about the process, all those pieces;" **Object**—"I'm most aware of my body after I eat, aware and self-conscious of my belly;" **Instrument and object**—"I think a lot of my awareness of my body has to do with maintenance, going to the bathroom, eating . . . my body is like a car . . . making sure it is oiled and gassed up."

The third major thematic category, **Interpersonal Meaning**, concerned experiences in which the body was described in regard to its social and symbolic meanings. These meanings were described either as open and public (Appearance) or closed and private (Expression). Examples of both subthemes follow: **Appearance**—"I'm aware of my body just before meeting people . . . the immediate thing that comes to mind is . . . the face, facial features, my eyes . . . ;" **Expression of self**—"I often feel I am fighting to be the way I am in a world that tries to tell me what to look like, what clothes to buy, etc.;" **Appearance and expression of self**—"I've always been hard on myself, seeing room for improvement. I guess I've fallen into the trap of the modern American male always trying to look like the model in *Esquire*."

The first-person meaning of the human body, as revealed in these conversations, is that our bodies are experienced in terms of what they look like to other people and how they and we see them as expressions of ourselves. We also experience our bodies as objects that allow us to accomplish projects in the world, sometimes impinging upon us in both pleasure and pain. Finally, our bodies provide us with experiences of personal vitality and enjoyable activity. In short, our bodies may be experienced as objects for ourselves (or others) as well as a mode of experience by which we accomplish projects and experience the vitality of our lives.

Results of MacGillivray's phenomenological study thus agree with, and extend, previous conclusions drawn from medical and psychological research. They confirm the idea that the lived body relates both to instrumental activity and to issues of appearance and self-expression. What they add is a concern for experiences of vitality and activity, those human experiences serving to define feelings of health and well-being.

Such feelings, often missed by non- phenomenological studies of the body, serve not only to make the other aspects of the body possible and worthwhile but also to enable each of us to endure and overcome the pain, deterioration, and damage of the object body usually considered the sole or primary focus of medical practice.

IMPLICATIONS FOR NURSING PRACTICE

What does all of this have to do with nursing practice? All of these considerations lead to some powerful implications for the practice of nursing. Probably the major implication is that the human body is never experienced by our patients as one object among many. Serious illness confronts patients with bodies that are recalcitrant and baffling, but they still want to be acknowledged in their wholeness as unique human beings. Patients want the hands that probe and poke their bodies to do so with sensitivity. They do not want to think of health care providers joking about their bodies while they are in surgery. As you will see in Chapter 16, patients feel great resentment when they are being treated by care providers as mere limbs and parts on a conveyer belt, moving through a factory-like assembly line. Recently, Max van Manen (1998) expressed concern about patients' feelings when their caregivers don protective gloves before touching their bodies—a standard practice of doctors and nurses taking "universal precautions" against HIV/AIDS and other communicable diseases. Patients may wonder if their gloved caregivers find their bodies repulsive or offensive. The gloves may serve as a barrier in more than one sense.

How can nurses prevent their patients' feelings of being objectified? When caring for individuals who are ill, Gadow (1980) urges nurses to affirm "the value of the lived body through the intimacy of physical care and comforting" (pp. 96–97). Gadow (1990) further reminds nurses to take into account their *own* embodiment, so that they can avoid bodily objectification of their patients. If nurses cut off their own sense of embodiment when inflicting pain during care, patients not only experience more discomfort but also become mistrustful and alienated (Schroeder, 1992). Although during an illness a major thematic focus may be on the body as a mechanism (and restoring it to good working order), we must always keep in mind the correlated thematic issues of bodily experience: how our patients appear and express themselves in their own eyes and in the eyes of other people, and how (and whether) they are still able to experience activity and vitality in their lives. "Getting well" means recovering the social and vital body as well as the corporeal body. When a patient's relation with his body has been "broken, disrupted, or disturbed," Max van Manen (1998, p. 9) suggests that "the healing relation of the nurse consists precisely in the ability to *reunite the patient with his body*" (emphasis added). The job of nurses and other health professionals is to make it possible for the bodies of our patients to resume their multifaceted roles in contextualizing everyday experiences and activities.

In the following two chapters, the human body is the context for a set of unique and complex phenomena, which, until now, were poorly understood by nurses and other health care providers. We explore what it is like to have one's body altered by the implantation of something foreign: a device that aborts a heart's wild dysrhythmias. We will also examine experiences of living with what our study participants referred to as the "monster" of chronic, debilitating pain.

4*

"It's Like Getting Kicked by a Mule": Living With an Implanted Defibrillator

> "It's like getting kicked by a mule, but there's no point of impact for it to hurt. . . . You don't yell because you don't know it's coming. It just knocks the sound out of you."
>
> —words of an AICD recipient interviewed for the present study

In 75% of patients who experience sudden cardiac death, the precipitant is ventricular tachycardia or ventricular fibrillation (DeLuna, Coumel, & Ledercar, 1989). To reverse such potentially fatal dysrhythmias, a device called the automatic implantable cardioverter-defibrillator (AICD) was invented and approved by the United States Department of the Food and Drug Administration in 1985. This device senses ventricular tachycardia and ventricular fibrillation and aborts these dysrhythmias with countershocks of between 25 and 30 joules delivered through electrodes having direct contact with the heart. Through an operative procedure, the AICD is implanted in patients who meet strict selection criteria (for example, having had a previous cardiac arrest). Although the effectiveness of the device in preserving life has been amply demonstrated, its impact on the subsequent life of the recipients is not well understood. Despite the fact that thousands of patients have had these devices implanted, there has been no systematic attempt to study their lived experience. What does it mean to live with something in your body that sets off metal detectors and "kicks like a mule"? It stands to reason that more than cardiac function changes as a result of an implanted AICD.

---

* This chapter is based on an unpublished doctoral dissertation, "An Existential-Phenomenological Study of Living with an AICD (Automatic Implantable Cardioverter Defibrillator)," by Stephen D. Krau, the University of Tennessee, Knoxville, 1995.

RELATED LITERATURE

Much of the literature outside the discipline of nursing discusses indications for the implanted defibrillator, its efficacy, and the operative procedure by which it is implanted (cf. Bigger, 1991; Cannom, 1992; Horowitz, 1992). The nursing literature, however, is concerned with helping AICD recipients manage and maintain their AICDs. For example, Nichols and Wolverton (1991) focus on teaching persons with AICDs what they are likely to experience after implantation of the device before they leave the hospital. Articles regarding nursing outcomes and goals for persons with AICDs abound (cf. Bower, 1994; Davidson, VanRiper, Harper, & Wenk, 1994). Ethical issues surrounding the removal or discontinuance of the device when death is imminent are provoking comment in the literature (Quill, Barold, & Sussman, 1994). Fabiszewski and Volosin (1992) discuss the nurse's role when an AICD patient refuses to have the device's generator replaced. A comprehensive presentation of indications for implantation, operative conditions, and nursing care of AICD patients may be found in Moser, Crawford, and Thomas (1993). In all cases, however, the focus tends to be on the device and not on the response of the patient receiving it.

Research concerned with psychological reactions to AICD implantation is limited and tends to examine selected aspects of living with the device rather than the recipient's lived experience in its totality. Studies illustrative of this particularistic line of investigation have examined patients' anxiety and depression (Keren, Aarons, & Velti, 1991), anxiety and anger (Vlay, Olson, Fricchione, & Friedman, 1989), and quality of life (Cooper, Luceri, Thurer, & Myerburg, 1986). In the first two studies, questionnaires were used to measure the selected emotion variables, while in the latter study a structured interview protocol was followed. Taken together, findings of the studies suggest that having an implant is not a benign, innocuous process. Researchers discovered considerable psychosocial distress and difficulty in adapting to life with the device. In the study by Cooper et al. (1986), for example, patients reported decreased social and sexual activity, sleep disturbances, concerns regarding body image, and fear of the shocks administered by the device. Additional concerns expressed by AICD recipients in nurse-led support groups included premature battery replacement and device failure, fear of driving and other travel-related issues, and concern over a potential loss of consciousness in public (Teplitz, Egenes, & Brask, 1990). In one study, only 3 of 12 AICD recipients felt that their general sense of well-being had improved as a result of the device (Keren et al., 1991). In summary, a variety of post-implant reactions, concerns, and emotions have been examined. Missing from extant literature on AICD recipients, however, are studies undertaken from a holistic perspective. Knowledge of this unique patient population remains fragmented and incomplete.

THE PRESENT PROGRAM OF RESEARCH

This study aimed at uncovering the meaning that living with an implanted defibrillator has for its recipients. Twelve participants were obtained through two AICD support groups. All persons who were interviewed had the device more than six months, and all had received at least one post-hospital shock prior to the interview. Eight of the participants were men, four were women. Six were retired or unemployed, while the others still worked. Eleven participants were Caucasian; one was African-American. None had been patients of the investigator. Audiotaped interviews took place either in participants' homes, or at their workplace after hours. The interview focused directly on the experience of living with an AICD. Prior to conducting any interviews, the researcher (Krau) submitted to a bracketing interview which produced the following insights.

Bracketing Interview

The persons with AICDs whom I knew on a professional basis from my clinical practice in critical care were in life and death situations of cardiac crisis, and the importance of the device to their subsequent day-to-day existence seemed quite removed. The need for my study emerged from an interaction with a patient who had been presented with the possibility of AICD implantation to control ventricular arrhythmias. This particular patient had been on antiarrythmics that were either non-effective or induced side effects that so diminished his quality of life that he considered terminating the medication and "taking his chances." At one point he asked me, "How will the AICD affect my life?" To answer his question, I located several studies that measured the psychosocial impact of the device and the efficacy of the device in preventing dysrhythmias and maintaining life. Very proud of my findings, I reviewed them with the patient who, at the end of my delivery looked at me and said, "No. I want to know how the device is going to affect my life." I had no answer and could find none in the literature. The naivete of my understanding of the AICD's impact on a recipient's day-to-day existence was clear and served as an impetus to the study.

The bracketing interview revealed my bias with regard to the evolution of technology used on humans. It was my belief that technology was evolving at a rate much faster than people were able to adapt. Advances were being made, but the general populace who uses the technology does not have a firm understanding of it.

FINDINGS

Narratives of the experience of living with an AICD usually began with a contextual history of cardiac events leading up to the implantation. The men and women in the

Tag	Ind 1	Ind 2	Field Data
000			00934nam__2200301_a_45x0
003			OCoLC
005			20031111161858.0
008			010507s2002____nyu_____b____001_0_eng_c
010			‡a 20103418
035			‡a (OCoLC)ocm52264529
040			‡a YUS ‡c YUS ‡d R2A
020			‡a 0826114660 ‡c $41.95
042			‡a pcc
050	0	0	‡a RT42 ‡b .T48 2001
049			‡a R2AA ‡l m-04108 10/03
100	1		‡a Thomas, Sandra P.
245	1	0	‡a Listening to patients : ‡b a phenomenological approach to nursing / ‡c Sandra P. Thomas, Howard R. Pollio.
260			‡a New York : ‡b Springer Pub. Co., ‡c c2002.
300			‡a xiii, 294 p. ; ‡c 24 cm.
504			‡a Includes bibliographical references and index.
590			‡a NURS 210 NURS 230 NURS 240
650		0	‡a Nurse and patient.
650		0	‡a Existentialism.
650		0	‡a Interpersonal communication.
650		0	‡a Patients ‡x Counseling of.
650		0	‡a Nursing ‡x Philosophy.
700	1		‡a Pollio, Howard R.
994			‡a X0 ‡b R2A

study spoke of their myocardial infarctions, aneurysms, balloon and bypass surgeries, valve replacements, and cardiac arrests, a saga of life-threatening events taking place over 20 years or more for some of them. The significance of receiving an AICD could not be separated from the history of cardiac experience and the profound meanings of the heart in human existence. Each participant related a unique **story of assimilating** the device into his or her body and overall being. In each story, there was a clear trajectory over time; the progression was not uniform but rather an ongoing, dynamic process. This process of assimilation was mediated by understanding and by specific experiences with the device, primarily the initial shock.

All study participants had experienced at least one shock from the defibrillator at the time of the interview. One individual had experienced 35 shocks in the three years since his implant. Participants' descriptions of the shock sensation appear in Table 4.1. Accounts of these experiences included a mixture of discomfort from the shock, apprehension in waiting for the next shock, and relief that the device was functioning properly. Prior to the first experience of the shock, participants reported being fearful, not knowing what to expect. There was relief once the shock had occurred with comments such as: "Once it finally fired, after 18 months, and we saw that it didn't do anything to me, you know, then it was a whole lot better. If we could have made it fire earlier, it would have been a lot easier to live with."

TABLE 4.1 Description of the Shock Sensation by Each Participant

Abe:	Well, it's kind of like, I guess you'd say, a young mule kicking you in the chest.
Bob:	Felt like you stuck two fingers in a socket at the same time.
Carl:	I had first thought the table had shocked me. It shocks hard enough to let you know it's there, but it wasn't that bad.
Don:	We were having sex and I felt this "WHACK!" Sudden jerk like that.
Eve:	It's like getting kicked by a mule. . . . You don't yell because you don't know it's coming.
Fred:	Just like getting shocked. If you grabbed a couple of open wires, you know.
Gail:	I thought I was going to faint. . . . Everything started to turn black, and it shocked me. . . . If I hadn't been sitting down it would have knocked me over.
Helen:	It had like needles, thousands of needles in my arm and like somebody had hit me in the chest . . . with their fist in my chest.
Ian:	It just kind of lifts you up, it sounds like a bomb went off in your head.
Jill:	A like thing would be when you have static electricity and you touch something and it shocks you. . . . Multiply that several times, and it hurts.
Ken:	Just like picking up two loose electrical wires and getting a real jolt. I mean it shakes your whole body, down to your feet.
Lee:	The first time, it's . . . probably no more than getting a hold of a spark plug or something. Second time is a little stronger, and that third and fourth is probably like standing in water and getting 110 volts.

The meaning of the shock varied across participants; in some cases it was perceived as restoring order ("bringing it [the heart] back in line"), while in other cases it served as a kind of alarm or wake-up call, reminding patients that they had violated certain regulations on their activities. One man actually used his AICD to regulate his activities, saying, "My wife gets on me a lot. She says, 'You're doing too much.' I say, 'Well it's not going off. . . . As long as I'm not getting shocked, I'll just keep on doing whatever I'm doing. Now if it starts shocking me, I'll just do something else.'"

Study participants frequently spoke of the "bulk" of the boxy AICD and its impedance of their customary body positions and movements. It protruded from their bodies to the extent that it could be seen by others unless well-camouflaged by loose clothing. Participants reported being acutely aware of the device when sitting, turning, bending over, or bumping into things. Vivid metaphors were used to describe attributes of the AICD. Participants' words usually concerned the symbolic meaning of incorporating the mechanical device into their bodies (e.g., "filling in my tooth"). Through analogy and metaphor, an intimate alliance with the device was conveyed, and it was often personalized as a companion (guardian angel or doctor). This perception of companionship was evident in one person's statement that "I'm not alone with it." The AICD represented security for most of the individuals in this study. To them it provided the miraculous means of restoring equilibrium to a body that had become turbulent; sometimes its action was compared to a "good laxative," leaving the body cleansed and refreshed. In addition, it was seen to stave off death, especially for those individuals who had faced death previously (e.g., "I dodged three bullets. Three times I would have been dead"). Table 4.2 presents various participants' descriptors of the device.

THEMATIC MEANING OF LIVING WITH AN AICD

The meaning of living with an implanted AICD was captured in terms of six different themes: **choice/no choice, understanding, support, trust/absence of trust, syzygy of feelings,** and **special actions. Choice/no choice**, the first theme, defines the actual starting point for the story of assimilation. It is the device itself that provides a choice,

TABLE 4.2 Symbols Used to Describe the Device

The box	Doctor with me	A sack
Guardian angel	Lifesaver	The silly thing
Insurance policy	Safeguard	Not alone with it
Security blanket	Protector	Piece of machinery
Filling in my tooth	Works like a good laxative	to do miracles

and choosing to have an AICD is an affirmation of life in the presence and awareness of death. The topic of death continually emerged in the interview data, as exemplified in Lee's description of the terrifying sensation of ventricular tachycardia prior to having the AICD: "You'd just get dizzy and feel like all of the life is draining out of you." Because these people chose life, they had no option to refuse the AICD. One participant had initially refused AICD implantation, having overheard a conversation among physicians about a patient who had died because her AICD did not work. But after she elected to have her arrhythmia treated medically, her quality of life was greatly diminished, "They gave me medication and I was on that for 18 months and it just about killed me. Literally, I mean that was the worst experience because I felt terrible all the time. I had . . . muscle spasms. I couldn't think." Ultimately, the medication regimen was unacceptable to this patient. Choosing the AICD enabled her to "flush them [the pills] down the toilet."

Choosing to have the implant was sometimes an affirmation of concern for family members. For example, Eve related, "My husband and I decided that I didn't want it, that I would rather take my chances. . . . But then, looking at my mother, I thought if I don't have this done, she will never forgive my husband. Once I'm gone, she will turn on him and say, 'If you had made her have that device put in, this would not have happened.' And my mother was the basis for me deciding to have it. . . . Because of what I thought it would do to her. . . . Losing one of your children is the worst that can happen to you. I didn't think she could take it. I couldn't get her ready for it. So we had it put in."

Understanding, the second theme, was acquired through education or experiences, and was seen to facilitate the process of assimilation. In some instances, considerable time was required for participants to comprehend what the AICD was or did. For example, Ian did not understand the purpose and function of the device for over three years after having it implanted, although he had seen videos and received counseling prior to the operative procedure. Understanding is sometimes blocked or postponed as each individual interprets experiences and understands the meanings of those experiences somewhat differently. Understanding offered by other people (or their lack of understanding) affected the assimilation process as well. Many participants expended considerable effort in explaining the device so that other people would understand and not be afraid. The following remarks are illustrative.

". . . I went to see Dr. ____. . . . And he explained to me what the defibrillator is and why I have a defibrillator, and that was the first time it really got through to me about irregular heart rate or cardiac arrest. . . . And that made me feel a lot better since then. . . . I've improved steadily and that was probably one of the turning points in making me feel better because I began to understand, you know, what I had and that I had no reason to be overly concerned about it."

"Now the pastor of our church has been supportive. He understands about the AICD. Most people still don't understand about it."

"I say [to others], 'You've seen 'em take paddles and hit people to start their hearts back? That's what it does.' And they'll say, 'Oh, okay, I understand.'"

Support is a common thread described by persons with AICDs. Support was reported as coming from assorted individuals and groups. The experience of living with an AICD, or living with someone who has an AICD, creates an important bond, although formal organized support groups were not perceived as helpful by everyone. Some participants viewed support groups as a reminder of their illness and possible death.

Support came in many different forms. In the case of Lee, his 13-year-old son's non-special treatment was perceived as supportive. Descriptions of support from participants follow:

"Lucky I have a supportive wife. She's stuck through it all."

"I have a friend who calls every day, sometimes more than once or twice a day, just to shoot the breeze and see how I am."

"Family support is the best support, and those support groups, the meetings we go to every month. . . . You get together with everybody who's got these things, you know, and you get to talking about your experiences and they'll tell theirs. . . . You find out that you're not the only one having the problems. . . . It makes you feel good to know that there's just beaucoups of people who have these devices and have learned to live with them."

Trust/absence of trust was another common theme in living with an AICD. Trust was seen to depend upon: (a) the reliable functioning of the device, (b) health care personnel knowledgeable about the device, and (c) being related to a spiritual being, often identified as "the Lord." There were times when an absence of trust existed, or when both trust and an absence of trust existed at the same time, as shown in the following quotes.

"I don't take any pills now. I just rely on this." (trust in the device)

"I am not out to sue anybody, I just want some answers and it seems nobody wants to tell anybody anything." (mistrust in the medical community after a frightening malfunction of the device)

"I knew it was there and I knew it would do the job, but what if my heart gets so bad that a shock won't bring it back in line?" (trust/absence of trust)

Syzygy of feelings, the AICD patient's simultaneous experience of opposite feelings, is also thematic. As the term is used in astronomy, syzygy describes the conjunction and opposition of two celestial bodies. Applying the term to non-celestial events, Kainz (1988) suggests that a syzygy occurs when various opposites enter into a "dynamic unity-in-distinction in which there is simultaneous conjunction of ideas which would not be permitted to cohabitate if the rules of ordinary logic and usage were followed" (p. 42). Conjunction and an appearance of opposition occur simultaneously and are a part of the whole. It soon became evident that the feelings conveyed by persons with an AICD could be viewed as syzygies. Whereas the emotions described were not necessarily opposite, they did appear incongruous to participants. Seemingly antithetical pairs of feelings included depression and gratitude, freedom and restriction, security and doubt, fear and safety, comfort and annoyance, and feelings of similarity and difference. Inherent in a syzygy is movement and change, both of which are aspects of the story of assimilation. The sides of a syzygy fluctuate in time and patterns, and there is usually no final resolution to the syzygy.

Special actions created by the presence of the device is a final thematic element in the general structure of living with an AICD. Such actions included: (1) attempts to make the physical presence of the device more comfortable to the recipient's daily being, (2) actions specific to preventing the device from delivering a shock, and (3) actions employed to bring resolution to conflicts (such as those surrounding driving). The latter two actions could be condensed into a single category of self-regulation. Actions that make the physical presence of the device more comfortable include positioning for comfort while working or sleeping, wearing non-restrictive clothing, and avoiding objects that may bump the device. These actions emerge from the recipient's experiences and personal understanding of the device. Actions to prevent the AICD from delivering a shock include stress reduction, diet changes, taking deep breaths at the recognition of preshock symptoms, and monitoring the types and amount of physical movement. Resolution of conflicts regarding driving include seeking assistance from others for transportation, explaining and justifying continued driving to self and others, and driving more carefully than before the AICD implant.

The trajectory of accommodation to an AICD is individual and gradual. Fear recedes as recipients embrace the mechanical regulator of their compromised hearts and trust its dependable functioning. Several patients spoke of a particular point in time when they abandoned a cautious stance toward existence and resolved to "go on with things." For example, Eve noted that, "You cannot live on a knife edge. You've got to go on with things." Participants expressed gratitude for their prolonged lives and the "amazing" technology making it possible for them to "go on."

DISCUSSION AND CONCLUSIONS

Existential phenomenology was used to formulate a description of the lived meaning of having an implanted defibrillator. Symbolic meanings of the device and its attributes were vividly depicted by the men and women who took part in this study. The complex and multidimensional aspects of their experiences were revealed in their narratives of assimilation and tend to raise concerns about the usefulness of the some of unidimensional studies discussed earlier. Tools used to study anxiety or depression in persons with AICDs are limited in scope and do not seem to adequately capture the

gamut of conflicting emotions reported by participants. By identifying both components of the syzygy, a more realistic picture of the experience was derived. Fear and
anxiety were described by the AICD recipients in this study but did not seem as prevalent as in the cases discussed by Cooper et al. (1986). This difference may be due to
the more widespread use of the AICD since the mid-1980s, thereby lessening its nov-
elty and fearfulness.

Although the study was not based on any pre-selected theoretical framework, the
value of the findings is enhanced when related to a nursing perspective. Parse's theory
of human becoming (1981, 1992, 1995) is a human science theory that provides a har-
monious structure from which to consider the findings of this study. The theory, drawn
from the work of Martha Rogers and from existential-phenomenological thought,
involves three major principles:

1. Structuring meaning multidimensionally is co-creating reality through the lan-
   guaging of values and imaging.
2. Co-creating rhythmical patterns of relating is living the paradoxical unity of
   revealing-concealing and enabling-limiting while connecting-separating.
3. Co-transcending with the possibles is powering unique ways of originating in the
   process of transforming. (Parse, 1981, p. 69)

Aspects of the present thematic structure of the AICD experience can be discussed
in relation to each of these principles. In regard to the first principle, the experience
of living with an AICD is endowed with meaning, and the structure of that meaning is
linked to valuing and imaging. Values such as the affirmation of life and concern for
one's family that went into the choice to have an implanted defibrillator were unique
for each person, as were the metaphors used to depict their unique experiences of this
device and its action. The identification of the syzygy is consistent with Parse's (1992)
notion of paradox: "These rhythmical patterns are not opposites; they are two sides of
the same rhythm that coexist all at once" (p. 38). Parse's paradox of *revealing-concealing* pertains to the very human tendency of revealing one aspect of oneself while
concealing another. In the present study, this was typified by Lee's dread of having his
battery changed in two years. In his dread there was concealed hope, hope that he would
be around for two more years to have the battery changed.

Lee's case also seems to illustrate Parse's paradox of *enabling-limiting* (i.e., that as
people move in one direction, they are presented with opportunities that limit movement in other directions). As Lee chooses not to think about his device, he is limiting
his understanding of the device and his ability to deal with it. Because he did not know
what to do when he received his initial shock, he allowed ambulance attendants to intervene, thereby causing him to experience additional shocks.

Connecting-separating in Parse's second principle can also be observed in Lee, as
he separates himself from other people who have the device and moves toward situations where he is with people who do not have the device, thus creating both distance

and opportunities for interactions. With regard to the third principle, Parse holds that powering and originating propel *transforming*: "The shifting of views of the familiar as different light is shed on what is known" (1992, p. 39). Transforming is evident in the trajectory of assimilation described by recipients of the AICD, and understanding and experience served to transform the recipients further.

IMPLICATIONS OF THE STUDY FINDINGS FOR NURSING PRACTICE

Care provided by nurses to AICD recipients can be augmented by a thorough understanding of the experience of living with an AICD as described from the perspective of the patient. This knowledge can be of value to nurses as they prepare candidates for the operative procedure, present information essential for obtaining truly informed consent, convey an accurate scenario of the postoperative course, and provide empathic support throughout the processes of assimilation and healing. Education should be ongoing, as consent to have the device placed does not assure the person will understand what it is like to live with the device on a day-to-day basis. Not everyone is ready to receive and incorporate information at the same rate or at the same time in the process. Nurses need to identify key experiences in the recipients' postoperative trajectory of assimilating the device and to help them comprehend and interpret the meaning of these experiences.

POST-STUDY REFLECTIONS FROM STEPHEN KRAU

As a critical care nurse and nursing professor, I am very aware of the continual advances in medical technology. Beyond knowing or understanding the mechanisms of the technological device and its impact on physiological processes in the human, I have always been concerned with the human responses to technology. The AICD is a prime example of a technological advance that prevents mortality; its utilization, however, is accompanied by multiple issues that surpass physiological knowledge and understanding. The nurse is obligated to consider not only the physiological effects of the technology but also the patient's response and the family members' responses to the device. The technology invariably changes something about the patient. The presence of the technology always has meaning.

The study on living with an AICD was the beginning of my endeavors to understand the meaning that technology holds for the recipients of such technology. As a nursing professor, I encourage my students to explore the meanings that machines have for their patients. I continually seek research to broaden student understanding of the complex moral and ethical issues involved in increasing technology use. As a practitioner, I actively seek the patient's or family member's perspective. Currently, I am exploring family decision-making as it relates to withdrawing technological life support. Through a careful understanding of this experience, health care providers will be able to support family members both at the time of the decision and in the months and years following the decision.

5

"Now It's Me and This Pain": Living With Chronic Pain

"Pain . . . teaches us how unfree, transitory, and helpless we really are, and how life is essentially capable of becoming an enemy to itself" (Buytendijk, 1962, p. 27).

Human beings fear and dread the helplessness of pain more than any other element of illness. In fact, it has been said that "most people fear death less than they fear continuing pain" (Seitz, 1993). St. Augustine called pain "the greatest evil." Pain stuns us, stops us, humbles us. We wonder what we could have done to deserve its cruelty. Consistent with its origin in the Latin *poena*, meaning penalty or punishment, the word pain suggests retribution for sin.

Since the time of Florence Nightingale, whose vision for nursing was created amid the anguished groans of thousands of wounded and dying British soldiers at Scutari, patients have looked to nurses for analgesia and comfort. "Nurse, I need something for pain" is repeated countless times per day in health care facilities everywhere. Injections are given, backs are massaged, pillows are plumped. With short-term pain, such as the pain of childbirth or minor surgeries, relief is promptly received. A grateful patient tells the nurse, "Oh, it's much better now. Thanks."

Long-term pain presents a different picture. The fantasy of prompt relief has been shattered. By the time patients earn the diagnostic label of "chronic pain," these individuals have tried to get relief from a variety of medical interventions. They have been

* This chapter is based on a study conducted by Sandra Thomas and an unpublished doctoral dissertation, "The Experience of Coping with Chronic Pain: A Phenomenological Investigation," by Dianne Briscoe, the University of Tennessee, Knoxville, 1999. Contributions of the following members of Thomas's research team are gratefully acknowledged: Vicki Slater, Linda Hafley, Karen Heeks, Tracey Martin, Rebecca Ledbetter, Lisa Fleming, and Pam Watson. Portions of Thomas's study were previously reported in an article in "Western Journal of Nursing Research" (Vol.22, No.6, pp. 683–705) and are used with permission of Sage Publications.

poked, prodded, x-rayed, and scanned. Many of them have also dabbled in "alternative medicine" and sampled a variety of psychological interventions. Although a number of individuals with chronic pain respond to cognitive and behavioral treatment protocols, some patients show little or no response (Keefe & Lefebvre, 1997). Both patients and caregivers are frustrated with one another when treatments are ineffective and suffering is prolonged. Very often, they come to an impasse. As Wolf (1977, p. 54) relates, "The pain person wistfully clings to an inadequate, but heartfelt, conviction that all pain should be short-term. Our word choices, then, betray the terrible truth that we simply do not know what to do about persistent pain. . . . The prospect of there being no end to the experience is so devastating that all but the most determined personality can be reduced to a whine and a whimper." The cryptic advice of "learn to live with it" is often the final salvo of the health care provider to the departing chronic pain patient. But the biomedical approach, with its focus on pathophysiology, does not address the complexity of chronic pain nor does it provide guidance for successfully living with it.

Some chronic pain patients reach a point when they no longer wish to live. A survey of patients who were members of a national pain self-help organization revealed that 50% of them had considered suicide—a particularly disturbing finding, given that this was a select group of well-educated and financially secure individuals who had actively sought out a group to help them manage chronic pain (Hitchcock, Ferrell, & McCaffery, 1994). Data indicate that the longer the duration of pain, the greater the likelihood of suicidal ideation (Hinkley & Jaremko, 1994).

From the perspective of nursing's holistic philosophy, the existing literature on chronic pain has significant limitations, including the tendency to focus on discrete aspects of the chronic pain experience ("the parts") rather than on its interrelated wholeness. Researchers have seldom invited patients to describe their lived experience. In this chapter, we present the findings of two phenomenological studies designed to "give a voice to the voiceless" (Hutchinson, et al.,1994)—the men and women who endure pain daily. Conducted independently, both Thomas's and Briscoe's studies explored the *experience* of chronic pain, although only the study by Briscoe also plumbed the phenomenon of *coping* with the pain. When the findings of both studies were integrated, a remarkable convergence of themes suggested that the essence of the experience of chronic pain was accurately captured.

RELATED LITERATURE

Qualitative Studies of Chronic Pain

There is little scrutiny of chronic pain in the phenomenological research literature. Three unpublished dissertations were located (Cademenos, 1981; Erdmann, 1987; Newshan, 1996), one book chapter (O'Loughlin, 1999), and one journal article

(Bowman, 1991). The O'Loughlin study (1999) involved only one participant whose lifetime of chronic pain was inextricably intertwined with sexual and physical abuse beginning in early childhood. Cademenos (1981) investigated the social/psychological implications of the divergences between medical definitions of chronic pain and patients' reports of their experiences. Unfortunate misunderstandings and distrust resulted from these divergent perspectives. Newshan's (1996) study of chronic pain in hospitalized AIDS patients corroborated the miscommunication created by the different experiential worlds of doctors and patients. Erdmann (1987) used an existential-phenomenological approach to describe emotional concomitants of chronic low back pain and some of its long-term effects. Participants described situations in which they were cut off from other people, resulting in feelings of depression and self-pity. Bowman (1991) also studied individuals with chronic low back pain, recruited from two pain management centers. However, her data were not plumbed deeply; typical themes were "varied psychological reactions" and "related physical symptoms." Although her interpretations were plausible, they were not highly illuminating.

Two other pertinent qualitative studies were located. A British interview study of 75 chronic pain patients (Seers & Friedli, 1996) had several significant limitations. The interviews were not audiotaped, and there is a possibility that the researchers' field notes may have been subject to selection bias (the tendency to record what the researchers were interested in or wanted to hear). At best, field notes must be regarded as incomplete accounts of participants' subjective experiences. Furthermore, the data coding scheme was superficial (e.g., "psychological state," "social activities"), and some themes such as "desperation of doctors" were not well-supported by quotations from study participants. Semi-structured interviews by Henriksson (1995) with 40 fibromyalgia patients (half Swedish, half American) yielded a useful typology of strategies for managing activities of daily living, although the researcher did not attempt to explore the deeper meaning of having continuous muscular pain.

OTHER STUDIES OF CHRONIC PAIN

Most research on chronic pain has been conducted using quantitative methods. Studies have examined the epidemiology and socioeconomic impact of chronic pain as well as its association with a plethora of psychological variables such as anxiety, depression, fatigue, helplessness, and locus of control (Ackerman & Stevens, 1989; Bates & Rankin-Hill, 1994; Covington, 1991; Elton, Hanna, & Treasure, 1994; Latham & Davis, 1994; Skevington, 1983). One popular line of inquiry focuses on the effect of psychosocial variables on the pain experience, but this body of research has been criticized for failure to consider indirect effects (Keefe & Lefebvre, 1997). A number of studies have been undertaken with the presupposition that pain patients must have psychopathology. Physiologic mechanisms in chronic pain have been explored by Markenson (1996) and others. Physiological explanations, however, have not been sufficient to account for discrepancies in identified physical pathology and the severity of reported pain and disability. As Morris (1998) points out, ongoing tissue damage is not required for chronic pain.

Studies which illuminate the nature of interactions between pain patients and their caregivers are particularly relevant to nursing. This literature documents: (1) paternalistic staff stoicism (Edwards, 1989), (2) labeling of pain patients as "difficult," "demanding," "manipulators," and "addicts" (Faberhaugh & Strauss, 1977), and (3) adversarial relationships between patients and their care providers (McCaffery & Thorpe, 1989). Physical and occupational therapists have reported poor alliances with chronic pain patients, especially those who were depressed, angry, and irritable (Burns, Higdon, Mullen, Lansky, & Wei, 1999). Physicians tend to discount chronic pain patients' reported levels of pain (Tait & Chibnall, 1997), especially when pathology is ambiguous or inconclusive (Chibnall, Tait, & Ross, 1997). Nurse estimations of patients' pain intensity are often erroneous, especially when assessing the chronic pain patient. For example, in a study of 268 registered nurses, the chronic pain sufferer was negatively stereotyped and judged to have less intense suffering than an individual with acute pain (Taylor, Skelton, & Butcher, 1984). Particularly pejorative views of the chronic low back pain patient were noted, perpetuating the stereotype of "low back loser."

Nurses admit that they are more sympathetic with "teeth-gritters" than with patients who express distress more overtly (Faberhaugh & Strauss, 1977). In fact, one research team found that stoicism was even expected of *infants* (Seymour, Fuller, Pederson-Gallegos, & Schwaninger, 1997). In an ethnographic study of pediatric nurses, there was disapproval of babies who were crying when there was no observable source for pain. Moreover, nurses were unsympathetic if the babies were thought to have caused their pain by moving excessively (Seymour et al., 1997). And despite research showing that drug addiction occurs in less than 0.1% of patients in pain, nurses consistently undertreat pain because of their irrational fear of promoting addiction (Henkelman, 1994).

This review of the literature reveals notable gaps in our understanding of chronic pain. Methodological problems lessen reader confidence in some of the conclusions that have been drawn. It is notoriously difficult to measure pain, and many of the commonly used instruments fail to exhibit adequate psychometric properties. Researcher bias is evident in the use of labels such as "immature defense style," and no study has sought to discover strengths on the part of the chronic pain patient.

THE PRESENT PROGRAM OF RESEARCH

Given the gaps in our understanding of chronic pain, both researchers sought to illuminate its deeper meaning. A total of 25 participants were interviewed for the two studies, 12 by Briscoe. and 13 by Thomas and her research assistants. All participants met the criteria of willingness to talk about their lived experience, age 18 or older, and the presence of nonmalignant chronic pain consistent with the North American Nursing

Diagnosis Association (NANDA) definition: "Chronic pain is an unpleasant sensory and emotional experience arising from actual or potential tissue damage or described in terms of such damage . . . without a predictable end and a duration greater than six months" (NANDA, 1996, p. 76). Individuals were recruited for the study in a variety of ways, including a newspaper article, a flyer posted on a university campus, and network sampling. Additionally, five participants were recruited from a pain clinic. No attempt was made to locate patients with a particular diagnosis or disease trajectory. As noted by Dworkin, Von Korff, & LeResche (1992, p. 7), "chronic pain conditions at different anatomical sites . . . may share common mechanisms of pain perception and appraisal, pain behavior, and social adaptation to chronic pain." Moreover, variation in experience is considered desirable for phenomenological research because it "enhances the opportunity for the thematic structure of the phenomenon to reveal itself" (Hawthorne, 1988, p. 111).

Table 5.1 presents the sociodemographic characteristics of the combined sample. Ages of participants ranged from 27 to 79 years. Most were white. There were slightly more women ($n = 14$) than men ($n = 11$). Duration of pain ranged from 7 months to 41 years. Back pain was the most common type; pain was present at multiple sites for many participants.

In-depth individual interviews, lasting one to two hours, were conducted according to the procedure described in Chapter 2. Informed consent was given prior to initiating data collection. Both of the researchers thoughtfully reflected on, and thematized, their own bracketing interviews before interviewing the study participants.

Bracketing Interviews

The two researchers who probed the chronic pain experience began their work from vastly different perspectives. Thomas needed to bracket the "provider" stance, based on years of nursing clinical experience, while Briscoe had to thoughtfully reflect upon, and then temporarily set aside, the "patient" perspective, based on her own experience with chronic pain. Each describes insights gained from her bracketing interview:

Thomas: Like Nightingale roaming the vast halls of the Scutari barracks hospital with her lamp, I used to make nightly rounds on the orthopedic unit with my flashlight. Squirming, grimacing patients welcomed me. Patients in traction and body casts, patients whose bones had been pinned and nailed. They hurt, and they could not sleep. I was nifty with a needle, and soon dispensed their morphine and meperidine. They liked me because I was more generous with the medicines than the 3 to 11 nurse, who had an irrational fear of facilitating drug addiction. And so I was Lady Bountiful, the bringer of the opiates and sleeping pills. I ministered, they rested.

What came up in my bracketing interview was a lot of anger at nurses who were not enlightened about analgesia, nurses who were rigid about times and doses in violation of their moral obligation. What I expected to hear when I interviewed pain patients was anger at these uncompassionate nurses. After all, these were *chronic* pain patients. They had been denied comfort repeatedly. Of course they would be outraged!

TABLE 5.1 Characteristics of the Sample

Participant	Gender	Age	Race	Occupation	Type of Pain	Duration of pain
#1	Female	45	Black	Former Military/ Unemployed	Lower back & sciatic nerve pain	6 years
2	Male	79	White	Retired	Back and leg pain	7 years
3	Female	48	White	Counselor	Neck, jaw, back, & shoulder pain	12 years
4	Male	65	White	Retired Accountant	Shoulder, arm & neck pain	41 years
5	Male	33	White	Construction Worker	Back pain	7 months
6	Female	27	White	RN	Back pain	1 ½ years
7	Female	50	White	Master's Student	Joint pain, headaches assoc. with lupus	15 years
8	Male	52	White	Counselor	Back, hip and leg pain	15 years
9	Female	44	White	RN	Shoulder pain	4 years
10	Female	62	White	Retired	Ear pain	1 year
11	Female	45	White	Housewife	Joint pain, rheumatoid arthritis	8 years
12	Female	42	White	Teacher, now unemployed	Hip, sciatic nerve pain	20 years
13	Female	39	White	Cable Splicer	Low back and shoulder pain	2 years
14	Female	42	White	Office Manager, now unemployed	Neck & Back	8 years

TABLE 5.1 *(continued)*

Participant	Gender	Age	Race	Occupation	Type of Pain	Duration of pain
15	Female	44	White	Housewife	Neck, Shoulder, Jaw	5 years
16	Male	50	White	Retired Army Colonel	Legs, Back, Lungs	20 years
17	Male	51	White	District Manager	Back, Hip, Feet, Chest	10 years
18	Male	47	White	Graduate Student	Back & Hip	3 years
19	Female	43	White	Counselor	Neck & Back	8 years
20	Male	43	White	Mail Carrier, now unemployed	Neck & Back	6 years
21	Male	45	White	Psychologist	Shoulder & Back	7 years
22	Male	34	White	Machinist, now unemployed	Back & Legs	5 years
23	Male	43	White	Business Owner	Back, Neck, Leg	8 years
24	Female	37	White	Route Carrier	Neck & Back	6 years
25	Female	34	White	Factory Worker, now unemployed	Back, Hip, Leg	4 years

But, as you will see, anger, although episodic, was neither focal nor prominent in the narratives of these individuals; in fact, nurses were barely mentioned.

Surfacing from an even deeper level of my psyche was old anger, anger from childhood at the suffering of my mother when cancer swept through her body like a ravenous beast. Even medications such as Dilaudid, given whenever her moaning resumed, failed to alleviate the pain once the cancer had spread from breast to bone. All night long her cries of distress permeated the house, reverberating in the walls. The analgesics, and I, were powerless. It is easy to understand why I found my work on the orthopedic unit so gratifying a decade later.

Briscoe: I became interested in how people cope with chronic pain both from the personal experience of chronic pain following an automobile accident, and from the experience of working in a pain clinic. I noticed that some patients adapted to limitations and continued their involvement with the tasks of daily living while others progressed toward withdrawal and disability. I became interested in the nature of coping, the structure and process of coping with chronic pain on a daily basis. What made the difference between adaptation and hopelessness?

From my bracketing interview and the research group's interpretation, I learned that I was prone to withdrawal from others during pain flare-ups. My coping style left out other people. Therefore, I could have been unduly attuned to independence and aloneness with pain when listening to my study participants.

FINDINGS

The analysis of participant interviews revealed a two-part thematic structure : one describing the *experience* of chronic pain and the other describing the experience of *coping* with chronic pain. Chronic pain patients described their experience as an individualized interactive process between themselves and their painful condition. Their life-world was shrunken, their way of life irrevocably changed, their freedom greatly constricted. The pain set up a wall or barrier that separated them from other people. Pain dominated their consciousness, as shown in these remarks from the transcripts: "You can't think about anything else, really;" "Pain is king. Pain rules;" "The pain just rides on your nerves;""Pain dominates what you can do;" "Pain is a monster. All I can say is that it's tormenting."

Pain was a formidable opponent with whom they fought daily: "I'm battling it. And I think if I give up the battle, I'll give up more than—I'll just give up completely and turn into a couch potato. I don't want to do that. I need to battle it." The dyadic nature of the relationship was succinctly captured as follows: "Now it's me and this pain. It's a thing. And you've just got to fight it continuously."

Descriptors of the pain included "devastating," "excruciating," "debilitating," "grating," "nerve-wracking," "incapacitating," and "tiring." Gradations and levels of pain were detailed with extreme precision. For example, one participant contrasted the ubiquitous flu-like feeling of "achy all over, just yucky all over" with the more episodic "excruciating pain [in a] particular place like my shoulder or back." Pain was described in vivid metaphorical language: "The nerve in my leg is like a toothache when a filling has fallen out, and there is an open nerve root;" "I can feel my leg cramping, just like a steel rod was embedded, anchored in my toe and up around my leg, up to my groin, and somebody's drawing on the steel wire;" "It's like an old movie I was watching the other night about torture, a drop of water dropping on your forehead in the same place."

In the following sections, we turn to elucidation of the figural themes, i.e., those that stood out most prominently in participants' accounts. There were four interrelated themes in the description of the chronic pain experience: *limitations, out of control, invisibility*, and *separation from others*. Five coping themes were identified: *hiding/revealing; accepting/denying; enduring/managing; connecting/withdrawing*; and *monitoring/evaluating/deciding*. In subsequent sections of the chapter, all themes will be illustrated with richly descriptive verbatim quotations from the interview transcripts. Participants' words show how the themes interrelate.

FIGURAL THEMES IN THE EXPERIENCE OF LIVING WITH CHRONIC PAIN

Limitations

In most accounts of healthy individuals, the body is "silent," quietly performing its functions without compelling moment-to-moment awareness. Only when a foot falls asleep does it attract attention, only when hunger gnaws are we reminded that there is an internal organ called the stomach. Only occasionally do incidents of ill health or injury interrupt a general confidence in our bodies' sturdiness and reliability. The lived experience of the chronic pain patient presents a dramatic contrast: he or she is exquisitely and perpetually aware of the body. Within the body is housed the pain which has become the most salient aspect of daily existence. For most study participants, every movement of the body produces twinges, aches, spasms, or other unpleasant consequences. They do not have the healthy person's luxury of moving spontaneously and thoughtlessly, nor can the body be ordered to perform desired movements. Even when simple activities such as brushing teeth are carefully planned and calibrated, sharp reminders of disability capriciously occur. In describing a routine trip to her mailbox, one woman reported being "stunned with the pain" as she was halfway across the grass.

The chronic pain experience profoundly altered participants' perceptions of their bodies. Once familiar and predictable, their bodies were now baffling. Moreover, the body had become a barrier or obstacle rather than an enabler. Gone was "the possibility of cooperation between the person and his body" (Plessner, 1961/1970, p. 33). The body was seen as recalcitrant, damaged, inert, or useless in contrast to the body that was previously active and productive. Trying to force the body to perform an action could be costly: "If you do this, you will pay for it for quite a while . . . for a couple of weeks."

Participants described numerous limitations. One woman who had ridden horses competitively and played "a lot of tennis" in the past spoke with nostalgia of her slim body and athletic ability. Greater immobility had brought about considerable weight gain, which she deplored. The simple joy of cutting firewood was no longer available to a 33-year-old man: "I've done it since I was 15 years old every year. . . . This year, my wife had to get some of her friends and my brother to go cut it. It's hard to sit there and just watch." A woman who had experienced a fulfilling military career compared herself to a useless inanimate object: "It's like being a vase on a table, you're not doing anything. You're just there. You don't see any self-worth." An excellent summary of the theme of limitations was provided by this participant:

> It's just limiting in various areas of life. You know lots of things I can't do. . . . There are things that I would like to do, but I probably shouldn't. I'm aware that one of my worst back spasms comes from reaching up to move the rear view mirror and so I'm aware and cautious of things like that. Anything that has a twist to it or a kind of twist and a forward motion at the same time, I'm very aware of. . . . It's not only physically painful, but it's mentally painful to know that at a point through your life you were always strong and you were healthy. Nothing could stop you. You could do anything. You could lift anything, go anywhere, do anything. All of a sudden you're not able to do that anymore. You can't even sit at a picnic table and get comfortable.

Clearly, the limitations described by participants profoundly changed the nature and meaning of their existence. Strangeness and unpredictability replaced an easy enactment of daily routines. Participants' narratives call to mind Heidegger's (1962) description of existential dread, "a relation to the world that encompasses being in all its aspects but without the familiar feeling of being at home in the world."

Out of Control

All participants talked about feeling out of control. Part of feeling out of control was the unpredictability of the pain. It was not possible to know what it would be like from moment to moment. There also was no assurance that the agony of the moment would end; the future was unfathomable. Participants described good days and bad days. Interestingly, a "good day" was described in terms of what was achieved (productive "doing"), not by how well the person felt. A "bad day" was when the pain was unpredictably worse and the participant was unable to "do" or was completely incapacitated: "I can't plan for when it's going to happen." Not knowing what was happening, as the painful condition progressively worsened, led to the strongest sense of being out of control: "Everything starts falling apart and that's scary. That really is. At the same time, I started to have other things that I didn't understand. What was happening to me? I didn't know what was wrong with me. I just knew that I was hurt. I kept trying to ignore it and then just go on about my daily routine and I couldn't do that and so I felt very out of control."

Sharp distinctions were drawn between mind and body, in Cartesian fashion. Participants spoke of the incongruity between their thoughts of productive activity and the physical inability to enact their intentions. Pain sometimes obliterated the mind, expanding to fill the body completely. Efforts to control the body through cognitive strategies such as distraction were seldom efficacious, leaving the patients once more at the mercy of the recalcitrant body: "I'll try to get involved with something that's going to take my mind off the pain. But then when I start to move around, there's the pain again."

A humiliating incident of feeling out of control and making attempts to regain control was described by a male participant. He reported being with his wife and children in a department store when he lost control of both his legs and his bowels due to the unpredictable flare-up of a previous spinal injury. He described lying helplessly on the floor trying to explain his situation to store personnel and asking for help to get to the door. Not only did members of management refuse to help him, but also they intimated that he had staged a "slip and fall" scam in order to file a lawsuit. He tearfully related this story, insisting that all he had wanted was for someone to help his wife get him to his car. Being out of control left him, and other participants, feeling helpless and degraded.

Invisibility to Others

Despite profound changes in their bodies, study participants ruefully acknowledged that the chronic pain was not readily apparent to other people. Chronic pain was invisible, a "secret disorder" with no outward manifestation. Because their bodies looked healthy in the eyes of others, they were accustomed to hostile glances when they disembarked from vehicles parked in spaces for the handicapped. Some longed for external manifestations of disability that could provide greater societal legitimacy: "You can't look at me and say, 'I guess she has rheumatoid arthritis.' You can't tell by looking;" "It's so hard for people to understand if I say I'm in pain because they don't see it; I'm not in a wheelchair or walking with a cane." Ironically, a woman whose arm was in a sling—who conceivably might have welcomed the device as a badge of legitimacy—actually resented the attention it garnered: "I just want to wear a sign that says 'Please don't ask.'"

A particularly unfortunate aspect of the invisibility of pain is that it is also invisible to the medical profession. Participants experienced frustration when their pain was not acknowledged: "If they can't find anything right away or if it's marginal what's wrong, then they're going to say, are you sure this isn't some sort of emotional problem that you're dealing with as opposed to a physical problem?" When a diagnosis was given, participants experienced relief at having a concrete label to refute doctors' assumptions that they were "crazy" or "lazy."

Separation from Other People

Even though the experience of pain is created in the body, it is also constituted in the person's relationships to society. Participants perceived society to have pejorative views of "pain patients." Thus, they generally kept "the secret" of having a chronically painful condition because they anticipated adverse outcomes if it were revealed. They expected skepticism and disinterest rather than sympathy and support. One elderly man explained that he tried not to limp in public because of anticipated negative reactions, and even at home (although he could limp there) his freedom to discuss his condition was constrained: "I don't even tell my wife about it, because I have a feeling [that] she doesn't have much sympathy for me." A professional woman, who continued to work despite her condition, felt it important to laugh and make jokes to maintain a normal facade for coworkers. Statements such as the following were common: "Only as a last resort did I ever let anyone know;" "People don't really want to hear about your pain."

Isolation was evident in all interviews. Dialogue took place between the study participants and their nonhuman tormentor, the pain, more so than with other human beings. Participants described their pain as imprisoning them. For example, they used terms such as locked off, roped off, and caged off. Pain had somehow reset their interpersonal parameters, creating separation and distance from the world and other people, even family members. They felt that they no longer had much in common with others and no longer "fit in." Relationships in which they could be honest and authentic were few or nonexistent. Comments from the transcripts illustrate the isolation: "Pain separates you. It's really hard to be involved with people when you're in pain;" "I feel like I'm on this little island all by myself;" "My life is pulled in to where I have very little contact with anybody;" "I am absolutely alone."

Study results also indicated that when pain patients do leave their solitary "island" to have contacts with others, they are most likely keeping an appointment with a physician. Clearly, the most significant "others" in narratives of pain patients, more significant than family members or friends, were physicians. Despite repeated experiences with "bad" doctors who were impersonal, unkind, or even cruel, participants could not abandon their search for a "good" caring doctor out there somewhere who could provide relief for them. Therefore, they were willing to entrust their bodies to MRI machines and scalpels again and again. But their fragile trust of physicians fluctuated, with considerable disillusionment and mistrust evident in some narratives: "He didn't even want to listen to what I said. He just wrote out a prescription;" "You wonder—are they really trying to help or are they just trying to take the money?" "Some of them think females are just a bunch of walking complaints." One participant said that a physician made him feel "like something on the bottom of his shoe."

Nurses were virtually invisible in the narratives, a curious omission given the numerous contacts patients had with both acute care facilities and doctors' offices. One individual spoke briefly about hospital nurses and their poor management of acute pain. Another made a vague statement of admiration for nurses and doctors but described no specific incidents or interactions. No participants mentioned nurses as part of their support system, and none of them were involved in nurse-led support groups.

FIGURAL THEMES IN THE EXPERIENCE OF COPING WITH CHRONIC PAIN

Hiding/Revealing

Participants said they began the coping process by deciding when to hide their pain from others and when to reveal it. Because they did not expect compassion, empathy, or nurturance from others, usually they did not risk asking. Making the pain visible could have negative consequences such as jeopardizing continued employment or preventing them from getting a job: "Absolutely nothing was going to keep me from interviewing for that job. The fact is, I think he [the prospective employer] felt that was going to be a continuing problem and that's one of the reasons why I didn't get the job . . . perhaps that's the reason why you do conceal pain . . ." On the other hand, it was critical to reveal the pain and extent of disability in order to receive disability income: "I'm afraid that sometimes I'm overly defensive about convincing somebody that I really do feel bad, and that probably stems from having to go through getting disability income and proving it and them making sure I'm not faking it or malingering or anything."

There was a catch-22 quality to revealing chronic pain to intimates. Realistically, help is needed on many occasions. Revealing the pain to family and friends is necessary in order to get assistance with tasks such as tying shoes or getting out of bed. But the patient fears that others will get tired of helping and become impatient. Participants did not want to appear weak, dependent, or whiny. So they stoically hid the pain and declined to ask for help. Thus, there were negative consequences of asking for help and negative consequences of not asking for help.

Accepting/Denying

Coming to terms with the reality of a chronic condition involved tension between the polarities of accepting and denying. The meaning of life itself was called into question by some participants. Life's normal rhythms had been disrupted. Participants had been confronted with events that had radically revised their expectations: "I was just 25 years old when it happened. I didn't think anything like that could happen to me . . . I'll probably never be able to carry a child;" "What happened to me was quite existential. It made me aware of my age, very aware of becoming less able, in the process of growing old. Becoming aware and accepting age and dying in all things."

Most denial centered on the issue of chronicity or the fact that the pain could not be "cured," mandating acceptance of the permanence of limitations. But an eternity of suffering was inconceivable, and patients tended to go from doctor to doctor, hoping an error had been made in their tests and looking for a cure. Some put their lives "on hold" waiting for a return to their old selves and normalcy. However, exacerbations of the painful condition often shattered tenuous hopes, and attempts at denial were ultimately ineffective because the reality of the pain could not be denied. As one individual explained: "I believed that there was going to be a cure for what was wrong with me. After about three to nine months, it began to seep in that there might possibly be no end to this. That's when I became aware of *chronic* and *pain*. Prior to that, I think I just viewed it as pain from the accident." Participants discussed coming to an acceptance of their limitations through grieving their losses and dealing with their fear:

"I think to say that you deny it would be to try to then do something that you know you can't do. If you accept it and you acknowledge it and you live within the constraints imposed by it, then you live with it and I think there is a fundamental difference. That's the way I see it."

"There is some grieving at not being able to do some things . . . It's like grieving anything else. . . . That whole piece of my life is gone."

"You know, fear to do things. Fear to experience it. Fear of what it means. When the pain is no longer connected to danger or uncertainty, it's not as bad."

Making the decision to accept a changed way of life was an important part of coping with limitations. But acceptance was an ongoing process as new limitations surfaced. An example is provided by a participant with headaches and dizziness following a head injury. She had accepted that, at times, she was unable to walk unassisted, so she began to use a walker. Then she discovered that the world had new barriers; for example, going to the mall or another place that was crowded increased her difficulties with balance and dizziness because of the constant movement of others. She discovered that it was more difficult to use her walker in such crowded areas and that others became impatient with her because she had to move slowly to keep her balance. Some of her friends no longer wanted to go places with her because she couldn't keep up with them.

Understandably, some participants expressed bitterness about the lack of a definitive solution to their distress. In a world of highly touted medical miracles and dramatic organ transplantations, where was the remedy that eluded them? One participant lamented: "After six surgeries, I am probably no better off than I was to start with." Another wryly observed, "We can go to the moon, but nobody can find something to change this."

Enduring/Managing

Choosing to live with the pain or choosing to die appeared to be the ultimate solution to the issue of lack of control. Thoughts of death as liberating were described in some interviews. One participant expressed the feelings of many: "Really don't fear death because one day I won't hurt. . . . On a day where you feel like things are hopeless, you wonder whether you want to go on . . . and whether the quality of your life is enough to keep plugging away." In a particularly poignant segment of an interview, one participant described an occasion of desperation in which he grabbed his pistol and sat "out back on a brick," contemplating "blowing my brains out for relief." Another participant admitted trying to imagine how his suicide could be made to look like an accident or a natural death. Another was acutely aware that a means of liberation from suffering was already available to him: "These pills are very tempting to take more than you're supposed to."

Participants in this investigation, despite recurrent thoughts of suicide, had made a decision to endure. They appeared to confront the possibility of death and through this confrontation made the decision to live within the limitations on life associated with chronic pain. With this decision came a redefinition of the self, the me-with-pain, which was the cornerstone of enduring. Enduring was described as an active choice to be inactive, to let time pass, and live through the worst of times. Enduring involved simply *being* rather than *doing*. One participant related: "Probably the primary thing is to stop, stop whatever you're doing. You can't do anything anymore. You have to lie down, sit down, lay down, whatever. It's this humongous giant stop sign that says 'stop functioning in the normal way.'" Another said, "It [is] something you endure alone. You survive it alone . . . you survive the pain. There's an achievement in surviving."

Managing involved active manipulation of feelings, attitudes, and thoughts. Participants described self-talk such as "Take it day by day" and "Don't ever give up." They gave themselves permission for necessary self-care: "I have to be very tender and caring toward my body—give myself permission to lie down, withdraw from activities that the rest of the family is involved in or permission to withdraw from a chore I'm involved in. Give myself permission to do it without guilt and without beating up on myself, and that's not easy." Managing also included information-seeking and developing "rules to live by." For example, one participant reported: "I do not do things that I know make me hurt. I no longer jog or run. I simply walk. During the day, I may change shoes several times, changing the height of the heel, changing the composition of the material in it. I might change shoes three times in a day." Other individuals listed prohibited movements such as jumping, lifting, running, or bounding up steps. Unable to rely on others, self-protective actions were undertaken:

> "I still go to the library and check up on something a doctor has told me. Because I had lost a lot of trust [during the years before lupus was diagnosed]"

> "In every state we have moved to, I try to get a book telling me those doctors who have had some type of disciplinary action."

Medication did not assume prominence in participant narratives of enduring/managing. In fact, there was considerable aversion to analgesics. Many participants were adamant that they took little or no pain medication, waiting until the pain was intolerable before seeking relief through chemicals. One participant denied any use of medication, no matter how severe the pain, after being accused of drug-seeking behavior when visiting a physician. A number of individuals, while working with a psychologist or psychiatrist, had learned relaxation techniques they continued to use after termination of therapy.

Coping was a continual process of reevaluation and redefinition, of learning to live as me-in-pain, finding meaning in the pain, and transcending it. Participants identified a need to make some kind of sense out of their pain or wrest some benefit from it. One woman speculated that, "Maybe there's a reason, maybe it's to slow me down [to] look around to see other people are in pain. I'm more and more interested and want to be involved with helping battered women." If the pain resulted from an activity judged by society as meritorious—such as in the case of an Army pilot with three purple hearts—the self could be seen as valuable and heroic and the pain as meaningful. On the other hand, pain resulting from a senseless accident led to a different type of self-evaluation. One participant who was injured in such an accident saw his pain as retribution for past sins: "I must have done something wrong." Not all participants had found meaning in their suffering at the time they were interviewed for the study.

Connecting/Withdrawing

Some participants chose to connect with others through providing education about chronic pain. One wrote articles for a newsletter; another became active in giving public lectures. Another participant uses his experiences to work therapeutically with people in pain: "Being a therapist who, in part, deals with people in chronic pain, I have had to stop and analyze what that means to me in a way that I don't think most people have. I think you only focus on your own experience of pain for the most part, and to explain it to somebody else over the years and to talk to people about their pain is to bring some form and structure to it. . . . The issue becomes fundamentally: does pain become your life or do you live your life?"

No matter how open participants were with other people regarding their pain, they often chose to withdraw and be alone, especially at times of extreme distress. In some respects, this withdrawal was self-protective; it also lessened the likelihood of "tiring" family members. Participants said they did not want to dampen others' moods or cause relatives to worry.

"When I ruptured that disk, I didn't want anybody near me—anybody. I didn't want anybody to touch me. I didn't want anybody to talk to me"

"It's almost like you have to go deep within a hole or something in order to block out everybody's everything whether it's their thought, their opinion, their need, even their conversation. I desperately want to be left alone at a time like that. I think that is because I need every single resource that I have in order to cope and I can't share those resources at all at that point."

"I was trying to curl up inside myself because I hate to keep making an issue. It's got to be horrible for someone who is healthy to live with someone who isn't. As tired as I get of having bad days, can you imagine how tiring it must be from the other person's point of view? At any rate, I didn't even want him to look at me. I just wanted the whole world to go away and leave me alone."

Monitoring/Evaluating/Deciding

Participants described daily existence in terms of a continual monitoring of their bodies, their environment, and the reactions of others to them. They evaluated this information and decided how to respond to their world. These three activities were a constant in their lives, determining how they would react and how they would choose to cope with other aspects of their experience. The theme of monitoring/evaluating/deciding moved back and forth across all of the other themes of coping.

DISCUSSION AND CONCLUSIONS

Findings of this study contribute to a phenomenological understanding of the human body and its symbolic meanings. In contrast to the healthy individual's relative lack of body consciousness, the body becomes the main focus of a chronic pain patient's existence: "bodily events become the events of the day" (Merleau-Ponty, 1962, p. 85). In addition, the life-world is virtually restricted to the patient's body, as described by Plugge (1967). Bodily performance is experienced as capricious and unpredictable, rendering planning fruitless. One cannot know from day to day, or even from hour to hour, what the state of the body will be. Neither commanding nor cajoling will result in compliance of recalcitrant bones, joints, and muscles. Vigilant monitoring of the body and avoidance of sudden motions like twisting or bending are necessary to prevent even greater discomfort. But vigilance does not prevent flare-ups of pain. Pain invariably intrudes and imposes its will.

Themes found in the present study sharply contrast with MacGillivray's (1986) phenomenological study of healthy adults (discussed in Chapter 3). One of the three figural themes of the lived body in that study was engagement in the world (i.e., the body as vital and active). Vitality involved feeling highly energetic and fully in control of the body while engaging in an absorbing project. For example, a runner spoke of the good feelings of stretching his legs and taking in breaths as he ran. Perhaps because volitional control over the body was largely absent in the present sample of pain patients, there were no similar anecdotes of body as an instrument of mastery over the world. Participants' perceptions of their bodies were discrepant from the "socially engaged, skilled bodies" described by Benner (1994, p. xvii) but consistent with MacGillivray's (1986) theme of "body as object": "The body 'owns' the person, demands attention, and calls the person back from the world and projects" (cited in Pollio et al., 1997, p. 79). The chronic pain patient dwells in the world of "I cannot" instead of the world of "I can," much like the cancer patients who were studied by Kesselring (1990).

Most notably expressed in the powerful metaphors used by study participants, the essence of the chronic pain experience is unremitting torment by a force or monster that cannot be tamed. Accepting the chronicity of their limitations changed the nature and meaning of personal existence. Recall that Heidegger (1962) referred to "being thrown" as the way one finds oneself in the world. Participants' conscious decision to accept their "thrownness" involved redefining the self as a self-living-with-pain and grieving for the more active "old self" that was gone forever. Although the battle with the monster dominated patients' consciousness and imposed severe limitations, there were no external indications. Pain is invisible. The theme of invisibility revealed in this study is similar to one described by Fernandez (1992) in his study of women with lupus. The women were thought to be malingering, or lazy, because the complex symptom pattern made the disease difficult to diagnose. Patients expressed relief at finally having a diagnosis and becoming validated in their social context as having a "real" disease. According to Braden (1991), the issue of "secondary gain" is an important factor in the diagnosis and treatment of chronic pain and a major concern of health care professionals. The invisibility of chronic pain further complicates this issue. Others cannot know with certainty when a patient is suffering or malingering. The importance of validating the reality of chronic pain was discussed by Howell (1994); the women in her study did not make a transition to an effective coping pattern until their pain had been diagnosed and thereby made legitimate and visible.

As described in this study, patients walk a tightrope between hiding and revealing their pain. Revealing it is necessary to get help from family, but asking for the help is done only with great reluctance and misgiving. In contrast to Friedemann and Smith's (1997) report of intense family involvement in the lives of chronic pain patients, such intense involvement was not evident in the present study. Friedemann and Smith's interviews, however, were conducted for the specific purpose of obtaining descriptions of family functioning, and their interviews took place after participants had completed a questionnaire about their family's stability and growth. In phenomenological interviewing, if the respondent does not volunteer information, the researcher does not probe. Participants in the present study seldom mentioned family members except to deplore their lack of understanding. They were more likely to conceal their discomfort from family, even from spouses, rather than seek sympathy or assistance. These findings call into question the prevalent notion of the "secondary gain" (cf. Braden, 1991) chronic pain patients allegedly receive from significant others.

The need to hide pain, a prominent element of participants' narratives, has been noted by other researchers (e.g., Hitchcock et al., 1994). The culture does not offer a "natural home" for these patients, leaving them on the "amorphous frontier of nonmembership" in society (Hilbert, 1984, p. 375). Existential philosopher Albert Camus once referred to illness as a convent. If his metaphor is taken to mean closed off from the world and deprived of worldly pleasures, it seems relevant to the chronic pain patient. The concept of internalized stigma, which Phillips (1994) examined in AIDS patients, is perhaps germane to chronic pain patients as well. Society's pejorative aspersions are incorporated into the psyche, reinforcing a desire to hide from others and conceal a shameful condition. Participants' narratives of pain are consistent with its portrayal by Hannah Arendt as "a borderline experience between life . . . and death" (cited in Engelbart & Vrancken, 1984). If there is no one who understands and no place where one fits, is this not a kind of living death?

The grim, ongoing struggle with pain is a very individual one ("Now it's me and the pain"), although the sufferer longs for a rescuer. Physicians are both trusted and mistrusted, with the pendulum swinging toward greater mistrust and alienation after repeated experiences of being unheard and unhealed. Not being listened to by doctors is a well-documented complaint of many patients but may be particularly galling to the pain patient. No electrocardiogram can reveal the pattern of the pain; only by talking is the patient able to describe his or her subjective sensations. But physicians studied by Tait and Chibnall (1997) relied heavily on physical findings and tended to rate both pain and disability lower when physical damage was not readily visible. And patients interviewed by Miller, Yanoshik, Crabtree, and Reymond (1994) all claimed that their physicians didn't listen to them when they tried to describe pain and its impact on their daily lives. When these researchers interviewed the physicians, a different understanding of "listening" was discovered. To the doctors, it meant hearing patients' words as diagnostic cues, not placing the words into the context of the patients' life-world. This gap in communication between physician and patient was the strongest theme in Miller et al.'s study and was frequently alluded to by participants in the present study as well.

It logically follows that chronic pain patients begin to doubt that health professionals can help them. In one recent report, 78% of patients with chronic neuropathic pain resulting from breast cancer treatment declined an offer of free treatment in a pain center because they did not believe the treatment would alleviate the pain. Despite an average of 29 months of living with the pain and a significant decrease in quality of life, the women remained unconvinced that pain center therapies were efficacious (Carpenter, Sloan, & Andrykowski, 1999).

IMPLICATIONS OF THE STUDY FINDINGS FOR NURSING PRACTICE

Approximately 75–80 million Americans currently suffer handicapping chronic pain (Matas, 1997), and chronic pain is estimated to be the third largest health problem in the world (Latham & Davis, 1994). The problem will continue to grow as people continue to live longer and as more people become ill or injured each year. Every practicing nurse, therefore, will undoubtedly encounter patients struggling to cope with this cruel condition. As more nurses obtain graduate preparation and move into advanced practice roles, they will be expected to assume more prominent roles in pain management and pain modulation (Davis, 1998). Although hospital accrediting bodies are mandating the use of pain rating scales, the foremost mandate, in our view, is to listen to these patients. The most frequently voiced complaint of participants was that no one wanted to listen to them talk about their pain. Their isolation can be lessened when nurses engage them in dialogue. The psychological pain of being disbelieved and stigmatized is surely as devastating as their bodily pain, perhaps moreso. Therapeutic benefit was obtained by some participants in the present set of studies simply by talking to a respectful listener. As one put it, "I believe there has been a release here." Nurse-led support groups would address this need to tell their stories.

Nurses can help promote greater trust and fewer misunderstandings between patients and physicians by facilitating communication between them. Physicians need to know that chronic pain patients consider listening more important than "fixing." Indeed, most of them cannot be fixed. Patients can be helped to articulate their symptoms, making the pain visible, in a way that may serve to establish a positive relationship with their physicians. Fortunately, the zeitgeist in medicine is rapidly changing, with increased acknowledgment of postmodern models of illness that grant legitimacy to a patient's subjective experiences as well as to his or her biological functioning (Morris, 1998).

Given the plethora of coping strategies developed by participants, nurses must share this information with other chronic pain patients. Awareness of the power to choose one's stance toward pain is the core of coping and the key to regaining a sense of control. In designing interventions for patients involved in senseless accidents, it may be important to help them reframe their experience. Indeed, they were "dealt a bad hand," to use a card-playing analogy, but they need not concede defeat. In the words of an expert duplicate bridge player, "winning is how you play your bad hand." Because chronic pain patients place such a great emphasis on "doing" and feel useless when pain limits their activities, they must be helped to reframe what doing means. For example, doing could mean not only developing a sensible self-care regimen with workable "rules to live by," but also allowing oneself to simply "be" when the body requires rest. Taylor and Epstein (1999) recommend cultivation of a loving attitude toward the body despite its inability to function as it once did.

Psychoeducational nursing interventions, such as the Chronic Pain Self-Management Program (CPSMP) described by LeFort (2000), have achieved outcomes such as decreased pain and dependency, increased sense of efficacy and resourcefulness, more involvement in valued roles and activities, and greater life satisfaction. This program is not prescriptive but facilitates individual exploration of problem-solving approaches so that chronic pain patients can find what works best for them. Learning new self-management skills takes place within a supportive group environment.

Lastly, nurses and other health care professionals should facilitate the grieving process, which is a necessary component of learning to endure/manage as a redefined self. Jacob, Kerns, Rosenberg, and Haythornthwaite (1993) introduced a construct called "pain accommodation" which shows similarity to the redefinition of self as "me-in-pain" described by some of our participants. Pain accommodation does not imply passive resignation. In fact, it is significantly correlated with greater self-control, fewer depressive symptoms, and viewing oneself as a problem-solver (Jacob et al., 1993). It seems that winning the battle with the monster of pain involves incorporating the pain into oneself. It is possible to live a full, rewarding life even with a chronic condition, as shown by 15 years of studies reviewed by Thorne and Paterson (1998). Positive images of normality, courage, and transcendence were evident in these studies of chronic illness. Patients were depicted by researchers as strong, powerful, and competent. It seems that the dread of nonbeing allows a person to confront the patterns of his or her life, subsequently continuing life in a more authentic way.

> *"In the depth of winter I finally learned that within me there lay an invincible summer."*

> —Camus

POST-STUDY REFLECTIONS FROM DIANNE BRISCOE AND SANDRA THOMAS

Previous research has shown that nurses who have personally experienced intense pain are more sympathetic to the patient in pain (Holm, Cohen, Dudas, Medema, & Allen, 1989). Perhaps readers of this chapter will prove to be more sympathetic as well. Polkinghorne (1989, p. 46) asserts that the reader of a phenomenologic research report should come away with the feeling that "I understand better what it is like for someone to experience that." Munhall (1994) emphasizes that the reader of a phenomenological study should feel compelled to *act* as well. It is our hope that our readers will find ways to act, and interact, on behalf of this isolated and stigmatized patient population.

III

Nursing and the Human Experience of Other People

Home is where one starts from. As we grow older
The world becomes stranger, the pattern more complicated
Of dead and living. Not the intense moment
Isolated, with no before and after,
But a lifetime burning in every moment.

—T.S. Eliot, "East Coker," *Four Quartets*
Reprinted by permission of Harcourt, Inc.

6

The Human Experience of the World of Others

"Man is but a network of relationships, and these alone matter to him."

—A. De Saint-Exupery, cited by Merleau-Ponty (1962, p. 456)

There is a very powerful exercise sometimes done in group therapy. In this exercise, each person is asked to "list as many people as you wish who are or were important to you. These individuals may be alive or dead, fictional or real." Few participants take this task lightly, and most produce a list of people truly significant to them. Once this list is complete, a number of questions can be asked, the most straightforward of which concerns the number of people on the list. While the specific number is not usually significant—it may be if the person can think of no one or lists a hundred or so individuals—what is more important is when in life the person first encountered each of his or her significant others. The usual result here is that the two largest groups derive from early periods in the individual's life (roughly, family members) and from more contemporary ones (roughly, one's present family or friends). To be sure, significant individuals appear on the list who are from the individual's "middle period"; these, however, are usually fewer in number.

Once these issues have been considered, every one in the group is given a sheet of paper containing five concentric circles. Each person is then asked to place each of their people in various circles, with the most significant ones in the center and somewhat less significant ones in the outer circles. At this point, some people object and say, "They all belong in the center" although, if asked again, they are able to locate specific individuals in specific circles. At this point, the facilitator may ask one or both of the following questions: (1) What would happen if you were to learn that you were not on the list of the people you listed? (2) When do you experience the people on your list and what is that experience like for you?

The use of concentric circles to help people think about significant relationships operates on the basis of an obvious spatial metaphor: We are closer to, or more distant from, some people than others; some people form our "inner circle" while others do not. We use distance metaphors for changes in relationships, such as "we grew apart" or "he became distant from me." Nurses often hear patients speak of such changes after a diagnosis such as cancer. Relationships with old friends, even family members, may become awkward and strained and visits less frequent. If we take the metaphor of interpersonal closeness seriously, it is possible to see why the loss of a significant relationship often leaves us feeling as if a part of us had been removed or destroyed.

THE LEGACY OF EARLY LIFE RELATIONSHIPS

Our significant others often serve as a context for experiencing relationships outside the family circle. Sometimes this circumstance brings about a positive feeling toward an individual, perhaps because she is similar to a much-loved grandmother. By the same token, sometimes we may experience a strong negative feeling toward an individual because he or she conflicts powerfully with one of our significant others. While such reactions are fairly common, there are times when they may be problematic. From the time of Freud on, we have termed the unsuspected effects of prior relationships on present ones as *transference*. Technically, transference as defined by Freud referred to the tendency of patients, while in therapy, to behave in terms of prior ways of behaving with their parents or other people prominent earlier in their lives.

In addition to transference, Freud called attention to behavior on the part of the therapist in which responses to the patient were made in a manner appropriate to the patients' past relationships but *not* to the present context of therapy (*counter-transference*). Thomas (1998) and others have urged nurses to be alert to transference phenomena in clinical practice. Is a certain patient reacting to the nurse in the same way as he once reacted to his critical mother or punitive father? Is the nurse responding accordingly? Such reactions may interfere with the effective collaboration of nurse and patient in managing a chronic illness such as diabetes. Many psychotherapists regard the working through of transference relationships as a crucial aspect of therapy. The patient must come to experience present relationships as *grounded* by earlier ones but not *determined* by them.

SOCIAL ASPECTS OF RELATING

We learn and relearn who we are throughout life on the basis of our encounters with other people. Merleau-Ponty reminds us that newborn infants are oriented first toward their mother's face, not towards objects in the world; the first "objects" an infant sees are smiles (Moran, 2000). As the infant grows and comes to experience a variety of other people beyond the family of origin, he or she discovers a certain consistency in what infants, and later, children are allowed to do and not do. Children absorb the social norms regarding appropriate behaviors for their age, gender, race, and geographic area. For example, white girls growing up in the southern region of the United States may learn that overt expression of anger is not consistent with the ideal of the genteel "southern lady" that their mothers are trying to inculcate. Black southern girls, in contrast, may be told by their mothers that the world is a tough place and they will need their anger to defend their boundaries and their rights (Fields et al., 1998).

When learning social norms, sociologists Berger and Luckmann (1966) point out that there is a progression from "Mommy is angry with me now" to "Mommy is angry with me whenever I spill the soup." When other individuals also show the same attitude, the child learns that it is "wrong" to spill soup. The most decisive step, sociologically considered, takes place when the child learns that no one is allowed to spill soup. As part of this new learning, the child realizes he or she is included in this social injunction. Such learning leads to the idea of a *generalized other*. Once a child identifies with the "generalized other," he or she has learned social norms in a specific and powerful way. When this happens, other people may be experienced in a number of different ways: as significant others who are extremely important, as generalized others who capture social rules, or as "other others" who simply are present in the ongoing social world.

SELF-OTHER RELATIONSHIP AS PERCEPTUAL-COGNITIVE EVENTS

Many actions we engage in as adults are designed to conceal from others a too-clear expression of our intentions or feelings. At the same time, there are many things we don't see or know about our own social actions. Taking both possibilities into account suggests not only that we sometimes "hide" a bit of knowledge we have of ourselves from other people but also that sometimes we are "blind" to the reasons for our actions. Building on these two possibilities, Joseph Luft and Harry Ingram developed the diagram shown in Figure 6.1 (cited in Luft, 1970). They named their diagram the Johari window (a combination of their names, Joe and Harry).

The Johari window consists of four different quadrants, each representing a different class of information which I am either aware or unaware of and which you are either aware or unaware of. For example, the upper left quadrant, the "open quadrant," concerns things that both you and I know about me. This information, along with the corresponding information you and I have about you, forms the basis for our usual dealings with each other. Quadrant 3 concerns information about myself that I hide from you. In interactions between you and me, the relative sizes of these quadrants vary. If our relationship is close and intimate, the open quadrant predominates; if we are acquaintances rather than friends, the hidden quadrant is larger.

	Known to self	Not known to self
Known to others	1 Open	2 Blind
Not known to others	Hidden 3	Not known 4

Figure 6.1 The Johari window. Adapted from J. Luft (1970). *Group processes: An introduction to group dynamics*. Reprinted by permission of Mayfield Publishing Company.

Although you and I may try to deal openly with each other, this is sometimes impossible. Often I do not know why I do what I do. In quadrant 2, the "blind quadrant," you know some things about me that I do not. You then have a decision to make: whether to tell me what you know or to keep it to yourself. In some relationships, as between a patient and therapist, I may expect (but not always be ready for) you to tell me; at other times I may not want to know. The final quadrant (4) is not there just to complete the diagram: It emphasizes that some things about me are unknown to both of us. We may come to understand something about our relationship only after the fact— after something happens that neither of us expected. Luft (1970) feels that this quadrant contains "untapped resources" for the person, and each person only reaches his or her fullest scope dealing with others.

SOCIAL INTERACTION AS DRAMA

A different way of talking about social interaction was offered by Erving Goffman (1959), who described human relationships as similar to staged performances. For Goffman, social interaction represents an attempt to manage the impression that we make by treating the other as an audience. Many different actions are "performed," including the use of a personally useful "line" to promote the interests of the "actor." Metaphors such as these provide testimony to Goffman's view that social interactions are similar to theatrical performances and terms like "on-stage," "off-stage" and "playing a part" are essential aspects of social life. Goffman also likes to point out that the word *persona* derives from the Greek word for an actor's mask.

In the case of playing one's role, consider the "bedside manner" of health professionals, a brisk, falsely cheerful way of acting while making patient rounds. The people in white coats, stethoscopes draped around their necks, whisk in, and out of the patient's room after conducting a few rituals (rustling the pages of the chart, listening to the patient's heart for a moment). The people in white coats do not sit down in the patient's room (indicating their intention to keep the visit brief) but stand above the recumbent patient in the bed while speaking (reinforcing the hierarchical nature of the provider-patient relationship). Such role performances are not unkind, just detached.

Making rounds in this way does afford nurses and doctors a certain distance from the horrors of metastasizing cancers and infected wounds. Professional detachment also conceals embarrassment when handling the bodies of others in ways that customarily are defined as taboo (Wolf, 1988). When well-armored in their roles, caregivers are able to hide their disgust, fright, and vulnerability. Although Sidney Jourard (1971) understood the need for professionals' "armor," he also deplored its dehumanizing effect on patients. He called the impersonal bedside manner displayed by many nurses "a peculiar kind of inauthentic behavior. . . . Some nurses smile, others always hum, and still others answer all patients' questions about medications with the automatic phrase, 'This will make you feel better'" (pp. 179–180). Dryly, Jourard commented that this performance sometimes functions as an emetic.

SOCIAL ROLE ENACTMENTS

Nurses nonetheless do learn "bedside manner" and other aspects of their professional role during the intense period of role socialization conducted by their instructors. Social roles represent the way in which a social institution such as medicine becomes experientially real to us. As sociologists point out, social roles usually occur in pairs: nurse/patient; teacher/student, etc., and partners in role-related interactions are usually aware of what each role requires. This means that, should one partner say or do something (as Goffman might put it) "out of character," the other will attempt to restore order to the situation. In routine interactions, role behaviors are accepted and recreated without change; in nonroutine cases, negotiation modifies role performances. At any one moment, however, social actions and meanings are known and followed, and participants assume present actions express their usual meanings.

Although role is a well-known concept in the sociological and medical literature, few if any studies have been concerned with the ways in which we experience ourselves when enacting a role. In one attempt to deal with this topic, Beier and Pollio

(1994) asked individuals to report what they were aware of when in a role of one sort of another. When responses were analyzed, the researchers discovered that enacting a role was described in terms of three interrelated themes: (1) an ideal form for the role as understood by the person, (2) an experience of how well or poorly the role fit the person's body, the present situation, and the person's sense of "who I am," and (3) an experience of being "hyperaware."

The experience of *form* in role performance, to return now to the first theme, concerns what the person experiences as expected in carrying out the role. Such expectations one described as "oughts" of the role and include an understanding of what the role entails, although some perceived obligations may be idiosyncratic. The second theme pertained to the person's experience of how well the form of a specific role "*fit*" the person with regard to three domains: (1) fit to situation (appropriate/inappropriate)—whether present actions were felt to be appropriate to the expectations of others and/or to one's own self-expectations; (2) fit to one's self (real/fake)—how "real" or "fake" the person felt when performing the role; and (3) fit to one's body (comfortable/uncomfortable)—how the person felt moving the body to enact the role and how "natural" it felt compared to other actions. The final theme, *hyperawareness*, describes a heightened sense of self, body, other persons, and/or the social situation in which the person performs the role. Occasionally this hyperawareness was not experienced until the person made a misstep.

In discussing their experiences in different roles, participants reported using "different aspects of themselves" in different roles. Roles usually became figural when something was not completely settled about the role, as, for example, when student nurses described their first day at the hospital. Sometimes participants felt "untrue" to themselves when enacting a specific role: "I didn't really feel like a nurse." As discussed by Berger and Luckmann (1966), roles also may become figural when we reflect on some role that was enacted earlier. When a role fits the person's body, the present situation, and one's experience of self, there is little or no experience of role and a more powerful experience of the ongoing activity itself.

Returning now to the specific performance situations defining the practice of nursing, it seems clear that patients hope for a certain kind of professional role behavior from their nurses (attentive, caring, competent) and that nurses expect a certain type of role behavior from patients (cooperative, not too demanding, and willing to "help themselves") (Thomas, 1998). Learning to be a "good patient" while feeling sick and helpless is no easy task (Viney, 1989): Think for a moment about the indignity of having to ask a complete stranger to lift you onto a bedpan or hold a basin while you vomit. Studies show that nurses become angry at "difficult" patients who "whine" or "cling." Even stronger reactions are provoked by patients who do not comply with the prescribed treatment regimen (Brooks, Thomas, & Droppleman, 1996; Smith, Droppleman, & Thomas, 1996). In some instances, the nurse's impulse is to abandon the "bad" noncompliant patient.

Mike, a nurse interviewed by a member of our research team, related the following incident: "The patient had chronic obstructive pulmonary disease and then developed laryngeal cancer, had a laryngectomy, had a tracheostomy, and was still smoking. He would smoke through his tracheostomy. The first time I walked in and saw him smoking, I just had to walk out in disgust. I couldn't take care of him" (Brooks et al., cited in Thomas, 1998, p. 146). Unfortunately, by walking out, Mike lost an opportunity to learn about himself as well as his "self-destructive" patient. When we shut out a patient such as this, we are closing off access to an important part of ourselves (Stein, cited in L. Dossey, 1984). We also are making a judgment that such a patient is not worthy of our care. Taking a phenomenological stance, the patient would be viewed differently: "No matter how dysfunctional . . . the person is, the phenomenologist believes that the client . . . is living as best as she or he can" (Becker, 1992, p. 224). What if a deep, enriching connection had been established with this patient, going beyond the "patientness" of the person, opening up new possibilities for him? Such relationships may be transformative for patients, as shown in a study by Pieranunzi (1997). What if Mike had engaged his patient in *dialogue*, gently exploring the meaning of his nicotine addiction within the context of a therapeutic relationship?

INSIGHTS FROM EXISTENTIAL PHILOSOPHERS ABOUT DIALOGUE

The origin of the word "dialogue" is "meaning flowing through" (Newman, 1994, p. 130). Dialogue is at the heart of many different philosophical analyses of human relationships. For example, Heidegger takes this perspective in his analysis of the role language plays in allowing us to experience and know one other. For Heidegger, the language of *Dasein* (a being-in-the-world) is neither the "idle chatter" or "gossip" of everyday life nor the super-precise language of science and technology; rather, it is the language of poetry and metaphor, both of which abound in Heidegger's own writings and provide a way for human beings to dwell meaningfully in the world. Unfortunately, contemporary human life does not dwell poetically and seems determined to alienate itself from other people, and even from itself. The impersonal nature of modern urban living serves to alienate us from what Heidegger proposes as the essential task of human life: to make contact with the authentic nature of existence. Although each person achieves authentic existence alone by confronting non-being ("I will die")—and other people may become distractors from this pursuit of authenticity—Heidegger acknowledges the importance of significant relationships. One of the reasons that confronting death is so difficult is because significant relationships with other people are lost.

Many of the existential philosophers seem to have a rather dark view of humanity, espousing individualism and writing disparagingly of the "crowd, the herd, the mass" (MacQuarrie, 1973, p. 122). In contrast, Merleau-Ponty (1962) sees the benefits of connecting with other people: When I am connected to others, not only do I transcend my isolation but also "experience myself as something more than I am given to be by myself" (Macann, 1993, p. 192). For true connection to take place between human beings, however, Merleau-Ponty (1962, p. 354) asserts that there must be *reciprocity*. He explains:

> *"In the experience of dialogue, there is constituted between the other person and myself a common ground; my thought and his are interwoven into a single fabric. . . . We have here a dual being, where the other is for me no longer a mere bit of behavior in my transcendental field, nor I in his; we are collaborators for each other in consummate reciprocity. Our perspectives merge into each other, and we co-exist through a common world."*

Martin Buber's work (1924/1970) sheds additional light on such reciprocity. Buber calls authentic connection between humans "I-Thou encounters" and begins his analysis with the idea that we experience the world in two different modes: I-It and I-Thou. Every person takes one of two relational stands in regard to the social and natural world, and it is only in this stand that the specific nature of the I exists. Because the pattern of this relationship defines what sort of person I am at the moment, the I of an I-Thou relationship is different from the I of an I-It relationship. In the case of I-It, the I relates to everything in the world as an object to be sensed, used, or categorized. Extreme instances of the I-It relation are prostitution and slavery, but less extreme examples are observed wherever there is discrimination (MacQuarrie, 1973).

The world that Buber calls Thou is not set in time and space as we usually understand them: It is a domain that Buber calls "meeting." To "meet" another human being as Thou, the I has to stop being an "it" both for himself or herself and for others. When this happens, the other person becomes Thou, the I becomes I, and both I and Thou live in the meeting of I-Thou. Buber suggests that we think about I-Thou relationships in terms of a "true" conversation, that is, where the participants do not know how it will progress and in which they find themselves saying and experiencing things they had no idea they were going to say, do, or experience. Such deep and meaningful conversations often take place between phenomenological researchers and their interviewees, as demonstrated in the interview excerpts cited throughout this book. Despite the hectic pace of the work in most health care settings, the possibility of I-Thou is also present when clinicians are genuinely open to, and accepting of, the "otherness" of their patients. Benner (2001, p. 68) shares this example of a psychiatric nurse who, in our view, met her patient as Thou; the nurse engaged in dialogue despite the patient's initial belligerence toward her:

> *"I was making my rounds. And I walked in and I said, 'Hi, I'm Sue. You must be Ann.' And she said 'What the hell is it to you? I'm so goddamned mad.' I . . . said, 'Well, why don't you tell me about it?' I knew from the beginning that there was such pain under her vile language—such intensity, almost agony. And I didn't even know her history. I didn't know anything about her . . . and over the next month I found out about the agony and the pain."*

THE SOCIAL ORDER—MAKING FIGURAL WHAT IS NORMALLY INVISIBLE

In addition to experiences of other people, the world of others concerns experiences of the social order in which we live and in which our interactions must take place. But the social order is difficult to experience directly and requires us to perform the social equivalent of a figure-ground reversal—to make figural the normally invisible ground of social structure. To help do this, consider a trip to work. Where, in this trip, is it possible to discern aspects of the social forces that ground everyday life? First, before we can even take the car out of its garage we must have up-to-date license plates, a state-issued driver's license, and current automobile insurance. Once the car is started, we must drive on a specific side of the road—on the right in the United States, on the left in England. Lanes separate the two sides of the pavement. A dotted line means passing is possible; a double line means it is not. Then there is the issue of red, yellow and green lights as well as stop, yield, and construction signs, all of which direct or constrain our possible actions and movements. Should we need gasoline, we note that the price includes two parts—tax and the cost of the gas itself. Once moving again, there are speed limits, school and hospital signs, and curb markings that tell us where we can park. Should we find a parking spot, there are meters that cost different amounts in different parts of the city. Finally, meters tell us the number of hours we may park for a given amount of money.

The major conclusion that arises in regard to the social order, once it is made figural, is that it is designed to direct, or prevent outright, what we may or may not do. We are enmeshed in power relations that operate on us. Foucault (1991) writes persuasively of "power grids," the intersecting influences in a society that affect each of us according to our race, sex, economic status, and other factors. The social order is defined by more or less explicit rules instituted to regulate human behavior. Sometimes these rules and norms are collected together into a single entity called a social institution. The total order of any society consists of many different social institutions, each with its own rules of conduct, accreditation, and concern.

Since any particular social institution, say medicine, may run into objections raised by a competing institution, say business (in the form of HMOs), some attempt must be made to explain the significance and necessity of both institutions. In sociological terms, there must be a body of thought to legitimize both institutions, even if they remain in partial conflict with one another. No society has ever been able to successfully adjudicate competing claims, and in complex societies such as our own we regularly have to live in the tension generated by rival claims to legitimacy.

Most nurses spend their working lives in large bureaucratic, often patriarchal, institutions such as hospitals and health departments. They often experience themselves as oppressed, having little control over their own practice (Roberts, 2000; Thomas, 1998). What is most important to the present discussion is that these institutions are experienced as legitimate and immutable objective reality. We hardly ever notice that many parts of our work world are socially constructed. We forget that we (or our ancestors) produced this world. We tend to experience it as beyond our present control. The social order strikes us as natural and eternal, as the mountains or the sea. But man-made institutions, policies, and rules can be *deconstructed*. Sartre reminds us that people are more free than they realize. Rodgers (1991), among others, urges nurses to begin deconstructing the dogma promulgated in nursing procedure manuals and standardized practice guides, and she asks them to question the institutional mandates that stifle nurses' curiosity and creativity. Instead of socializing nursing students to be obedient to authority, Bevis (1993) challenges nursing faculty to foster students' ability to think through, and resist, the hidden cultural conditioning that has inhibited nurses' personal and professional growth.

An additional consequence to the view that social reality is constructed (and may be deconstructed) is that our views as to what it means to be human have been quite different at different points in history. The human being is always a product, as well as an originator, of historical process, and how we look at one or another aspect of culture changes in different historical eras. According to Dutch psychiatrist J.H. Van den Berg, it is even possible to conclude that what it means to be human changes from generation to generation; a caveman is not a simple historical variant on a Renaissance man, nor is a Renaissance man simply a variation of contemporary man. The human being is not static, and each historical period gives rise to its own unique type of person.

For this reason we ought to place the whole of human life within the proper time frame of its own century and culture. Any understanding of human life at the end of the nineteenth century must be somewhat less correct today than it was years ago when it was written. Any description of human life is correct only for the "us" who live here and now. We must never expect any description to pierce, once and for all, the mystery of what it means to be human. We must be satisfied with the idea that even sensitive thinkers of the stature of Heidegger, Buber, and Merleau-Ponty will probably be "right" only for the time being.

THEMES OF THE HUMAN EXPERIENCE OF OTHER PEOPLE: FINDINGS FROM PHENOMENOLOGICAL RESEARCH

Bringing this discussion back from sociocultural institutions to people, there is still the question of how we experience other people in everyday life. In an attempt to explore this question, Pollio, Henley, and Thompson (1997) interviewed 20 adult participants, asking them to talk about what they were "aware of when they were aware of other people." Participants ranged in age from 22 to 45 years; 11 were women, 9 were men. All participants described at least five, and usually more, situations in which other people were figural to them. Interpretive analysis of these interviews revealed that three major themes describe the human experiences of other people: **Relationship, Comparison,** and **Benefit.**

The first of these themes, **Relationship,** refers to an awareness of relational patterns in our day-to-day dealings with people. Included here are feelings of closeness and synchrony as well as those of distance and asynchrony. This theme has great relevance to the experience of the hospitalized patient who is dislocated from his established social network. At a time when closeness and emotional support are greatly needed, significant others may not know how to respond and cope. In one study, disturbances in relationships with family or friends were observed in over 25% of hospitalized patients (Plutchik et al., cited in Viney, 1989).

The second theme, **Comparison,** refers to our tendency to categorize other people as similar to and different from ourselves, each other, and/or social norms. For example, we may make judgments on the basis of a person's sex, class, nationality, or race.

The third theme, **Benefit,** refers to the fact that we experience people in terms of their ability to meet our needs. The theme of Benefit also includes our judgment of people as good or bad for us and/or for others; this is exemplified in nurses' judgments of "good" and "bad" patients.

The three themes are not mutually exclusive; each defines one aspect of the experience of other people at different times and in different situations. Which aspect is figural depends on the situation as well as upon the individual describing the experience. In many interviews, all three themes appeared in a single description.

In this connection, consider the case of one young man who described changes in his experience of connectedness to family members after the death of his grandfather. He described becoming aware of how much he valued present relationships among family members as a result of his loss:

> Just like, everyone was together . . . that changed my awareness of people to this day about that group of people, my aunts and uncles . . . like we all have something in common now. . . . It might be about death, and it might be about family, I guess, or life, maybe. About how we are all, like, still living and are all together, maybe, and we all realize that life has a high quality. It's like precious to all of us, maybe, and when we're together, it's like we live pretty good, I guess, like everyone's together.

This quote returns us to our starting point: We are always affected by people who are significant to us, and they shape our experiences and actions in many and varied ways. While not everyone in the world is a significant other, our experiences of ourselves and of others, our patients included, are always affected by prior relationships, our modes of interacting with one another, our social roles, and our perception of the present social order as stable and unchanging. Although the ground provided by other people and the social order is a complex one, it is not incomprehensible, and all of our experiences are subtly, and not so subtly, affected by the usually quiet meanings this world holds for us and to us.

In the following three chapters, we explore the meaning of postpartum depression, eating disorders, and diabetes to the significant others who live with individuals who have these conditions. The voices of these husbands, mothers, brothers, and sisters have seldom, if ever, been heard by nurses. As you will see, their relationships with the ill member of the family were profoundly disrupted and forever altered.

7

"We All Became Diabetics": The Experience of Living with a Diabetic Sibling

"When M became a diabetic, we all became diabetics. . . . We all ended up having to wear shoes outside. . . . We couldn't do a lot of things because of having a diabetic in the family."

—excerpt from an interview with a healthy sibling

T he chronic illness of a child can create many changes for the entire family, including the healthy siblings. Decreased family satisfaction (Gayton, Friedman, Tavormina, & Tucker, 1977), severe financial strain (McCollum, 1971), communication difficulties (McKeever, 1983), and disorganization of family routine (Boyce et al., 1977) have all been reported in the literature for several decades. A study involving parents of chronically ill children revealed that the majority did not talk about their own feelings nor did they encourage their well children to talk about feelings. Reasons given for not talking to the well children included: (a) it did not occur to them to do so and (b) they did not want to make the child feel worse. In this way, parents believed they were protecting their well children from pain (Canam, 1987).

Relationships among siblings are beginning to receive attention in the literature on families with a chronically ill child. Given that sibling relationships are conflicted and competitive in the best of circumstances, this attention seems long overdue. Sibling relationships have a major impact on any child's development (Powell & Gallagher,

---

* This chapter is based on a doctoral dissertation, "Protective Shield: A Thematic Analysis of the Experience of Having an Adult Sibling with Insulin Dependent Diabetes Mellitus," by Marilyn E. Smith, the University of Tennessee, Knoxville, 1996. An earlier version of this paper appeared in *Issues in Mental Health Nursing* (Vol. 19, No.4, pages 317–335). Reprinted by permission of Taylor and Francis Publishing Company.

1993). Clearly, a more complete understanding of the sibling subsystem in families with a chronically ill child is needed. Information obtained directly from siblings about their experiences will presumably be more reliable than information obtained from parents, teachers, or health care providers.

RELATED LITERATURE

For the well sibling of a chronically ill child, a unique set of stressors has been recognized. Some of these stressors include social isolation (Taylor, 1980), emotional deprivation (Kramer, 1984), increasing responsibility (Gallo, Breitmayer, Knafl, & Zoeller, 1991), and fear regarding one's own health or death (Menke, 1987; Walker, 1988). When well siblings participate in giving care to an ill brother or sister, Chesler, Allswede, and Barbarin (1992, p. 28) warn that the "unique and separate development of their own identity" may be hampered. Gallo (1988, p. 32) cautions that the well siblings may view parental expectations for increased participation in household and caregiving chores as "an indication that the parents are not concerned with them as individuals but only as persons meeting the needs of others." Despite the similarity of stressors resulting from chronic illness in the family, well siblings have reported experiences that are both positive and negative. Positive outcomes identified in the literature are increased nurturing, compassion, personal maturation, and family cohesion (Ferrari, 1984; Kramer, 1984; Taylor, 1980).

Does the experience of having grown up with a chronically ill sibling yield any long-term effects on well siblings when they enter adulthood? Definitive answers to this question are not available in extant literature because adult siblings were selected as the source of information about a sibling's chronic illness in just five studies. Each of these will be briefly reviewed.

One retrospective study of well siblings of childhood cancer survivors showed that the illness was seldom talked about in the family (Gogan, Koocher, Foster, & O'Malley, 1977). Because of a lack of communication between parents and children, some of the well siblings harbored guilt feelings for many years. Intensified sibling rivalry and jealousy also were acknowledged by study participants. Using a semi-structured interview, Gerace, Camilleri, and Ayres (1993) interviewed adult siblings of schizophrenia patients. Some were experiencing guilt about wanting to get away as well as "unreasonable" feelings of both responsibility and powerlessness. A limitation of this study is that it was not clear how many of the participants were living with the ill sibling at the time of diagnosis. The impact of a sibling's illness is likely to be different if well siblings still live in the parental household.

Using existing data from the above-cited study, Main, Gerace, and Camilleri (1993) examined descriptions of the siblings' experiences of information-sharing as it occurred presently and while growing up with the schizophrenic brother or sister. In families where denial and information withholding prevailed, children grew up feeling embarrassed about their sibling's illness and withheld information about it from others. Even as adults, because of the stigma of mental illness, some of these individuals continued to withhold information about their sibling's illness.

To determine the impact schizophrenia has on siblings, Lively, Friedrich, and Buckwalter (1995) interviewed 30 adults, and content analysis was used to generate theme categories. Growing up with a sibling ill with schizophrenia created conflict and distancing in all family relationships, although the relationship most affected was the one with the ill sibling. Well siblings expressed a distancing from the ill sibling as well as sadness and grief over their sibling's change in personality. The ill sibling was the central focus of the family, depriving other members of time and attention. Well siblings as adults experienced conflict between giving attention to the ill individual and to their own spouse.

Martinson and Campos (1991), using a semi-structured questionnaire, interviewed 21 siblings of children who had died from cancer 7 to 9 years earlier; the surviving siblings were between 17 and 28 years old. Interviews were coded using the Ethnograph qualitative software program. Sixteen percent of these young adults reported that the death of their sibling still had a negative impact on them. Aspects of this negative impact included dissatisfaction with the relationship with the dying sibling, avoidance of any discussion in the family regarding the sibling's death, and feelings of resentment concerning special treatment for the sibling who had cancer. The relatively small percentage reporting a negative impact from the loss of a sibling may be attributed to reluctance of those with strong negative feelings to be interviewed. A limitation of this study was that the participants were interviewed in their homes, sometimes in the presence of parents or jointly with other siblings. Responses may have been different if interviews had been conducted in private. The use of a semi-structured interview also may have influenced the findings, as participants were obligated to answer predetermined questions posed by the researcher. None of the studies used phenomenology as a philosophical and methodological base, and none were located in which adults who grew up with a chronically ill diabetic sibling were invited to tell their stories.

THE PRESENT PROGRAM OF RESEARCH

The purpose of this study was to describe, from the adult's perspective, the experience of having grown up with a chronically ill sibling. As different chronic illnesses could predispose siblings to different psychosocial outcomes (Ferrari, 1984), the specific illness examined in this study was Type I, or insulin-dependent diabetes mellitus (IDDM). IDDM is the most common metabolic disorder of childhood, affecting one child in every 600 (Grey, 1992). To be eligible for inclusion in this study, participants had to meet the following criteria: (1) grew up with a sibling having insulin-dependent diabetes mellitus; (2) did not have a chronic illness of their own when growing up; (3) did not have a personal or family history of a major mental illness; (4) had not lived with their chronically ill sibling or family of origin for at least one year prior to the study; (5) verified that their sibling with IDDM was still living; (6) were willing and able to discuss the experience; and (7) were older than 21 years of age. With regard to criterion four, it was believed that individuals who no longer lived with the family of origin would be more likely to discuss the experience of growing up with a chronically ill sibling, having had time to reflect on the experience and, by reflecting, to know what it is they have lived through (Oiler, 1982). Participants were recruited by placing an ad in the newspaper, by contacting the American Diabetic Society, and by word of mouth. A single basic question, "Tell me what it was like to have a chronically ill sibling" was posed to all 14 participants.

All participants were volunteers and unknown to the researcher at the time of the interview. Of the total group, 10 participants were female and 4 were male; their ages ranged from 22 to 45. Socioeconomic status, marital status, and type of employment varied. Participants' ages at the time of diagnosis of their sibling's IDDM diagnosis ranged from 1 to 19 years; the length of time lived with the diabetic sibling ranged from 1.5 years to 18 years. In accordance with the steps recommended by Pollio et al. (1997), the researcher (Smith) was herself interviewed prior to interviewing any participants. The following insights were gleaned from the bracketing interview:

Bracketing Interview

My interest in knowing what impact a child's chronic illness has on the well siblings began as a result of the personal experience of having a chronically ill child. When my second child, at age 10, became ill, I was totally consumed with thoughts of her having permanent disabilities or maybe even dying. I could think of little else except what I could do to help my child. Concerns and thoughts for my other four children were put on the back burner. I knew I was ignoring the other children but felt I had no choice. I was not aware that my child's illness was also having an impact on her well siblings. This recognition only occurred when one of the well siblings asked if their sister was going to die. It was this question that made me reflect upon what, if any, long-term consequences this experience could have on the healthy siblings.

This experience with my own child made me acutely interested in other people's experience with chronic illness. As a psychiatric nurse, my interest peaked when adult patients would vividly and emotionally recall childhood experiences of having a chronically ill sibling. For example, in a group therapy session for hospitalized psychiatric patients, a middle-aged woman expressed resentment of her mother for showing her chronically ill sibling more attention than she felt she received. I have also spoken with adults who were not psychiatric patients who shared both negative and positive aspects of their experiences while growing up with an ill sibling.

Through my bracketing interview, I learned that I believed that parents of chronically ill children would have a tendency to treat these children in a special manner. The multiple perspectives of the phenomenology group members assisted me in bracketing my biases throughout the investigative process, both during the interview phase and the interpretive phase.

FINDINGS

Phenomenologically, the experience of living with a chronically ill sibling presents itself clearly in two periods of a participant's life: the past and the present. These two periods were not described as distinct and separate, but were seen to be interrelated and interdependent across the two periods. Past themes provided the background for themes of the present. Participants usually spoke of the past for only a brief segment of the interview and seemed more interested in relating their experiences of the present. For some, the present was perceived as more stressful than the past. Changes in family patterns and relationships with the sibling and parents were thematic in both periods of participants' lives.

THEMES IN PERIOD ONE: THE PAST

Changes in Family Patterns

The diagnosis of the diabetic sibling precipitated many changes and disruptions in participants' lives. For example, the daily patterns of the family were altered:

> "When M became a diabetic, we all became diabetics. . . . We all ended up having to wear shoes outside. . . . We couldn't do a lot of things because of having a diabetic in the family. Cost was a big factor in it, with having so many children in the home, plus having a diabetic. Family vacations were no more."

> "It changed all of our lives. You just can't get up and go like you would like to or even out to eat when you want to. It is all on a set time schedule. . . . You always have to think of snacks, meals, on down the road. You always have to pack, looks like you are taking everything but the kitchen sink with you."

> "Mom fed us all like we were all diabetics. There were never any sugary things in the house. We never had cokes. My mom never fried anything. She baked everything."

Other family patterns that emerged in response to the diagnosis of IDDM included: (1) vigilance of the diabetic sibling, (2) minimizing the diagnosis, (3) working together and sharing responsibility, (4) routinizing and keeping the illness in balance, (5) maintaining the family secret, and (6) over-vigilance toward the well siblings in the form of frequent urine testing to see if they, too, had diabetes. Participants used the metaphor of a *protective shield* to describe the family's perpetual vigilance regarding the diabetic sibling, as expressed in the following verbatim quote from the data: "They never broke off that protective shield that she [the mother] had woven around him wherever he went. On the church trips if he went, she had to go. . . . I am sure it would be difficult to let your child go, knowing that they could face a problem with the diabetes."

Changes in Sibling Relationships

The level of impact the illness initially had on sibling relationships varied a great deal among participants. Some felt that the diagnosis brought them closer; others felt more protective of their diabetic sibling. The following remarks are illustrative:

"We didn't always get along, but that sort of brought us closer together with that happening to him . . . we were able to talk to each other more."

"We quit picking on her about that time. You know how the oldest kid tries to pick on the youngest one, bumping them, hitting them, pinching them, stuff like that. . . . I pretty much cut that out with her because I didn't figure she could take it. I looked out after her a little more. Probably got more protective of her at that time."

"I was protective of him at school . . . and we were always checking in his bag to make sure that he had his little sugar cubes that mother packed in aluminum foil or a mint or something in case he felt . . . weak spells coming on."

Wondering How the Sibling Became Ill

A second theme participants described during this period was wondering how the sibling became ill. They needed to discover who in the family ancestry had diabetes, who was "to blame": "It was a major shock to the whole family because she is the first one on either side of the family, as far back as even great, great grandparents . . . there are no diabetics. . . . We just couldn't understand how it just triggered all of a sudden."

Preferential Treatment of the Ill Sibling

Words such as "spoiled," "pampered," "babied," "singled out," and "catered to" were used to describe the preferential treatment participants perceived their diabetic sibling to be enjoying as a result of the illness. One participant remembered that, when lined up for spankings, her sibling only got "one or two whacks to my five." Another recalled her brother getting out of chores such as mowing the lawn. This woman even viewed her brother's food as more appealing: "I do remember some times that I thought his food looked better than mine. . . . He would get something grilled in the oven and we would be having beans."

Jealousy/Feeling Sorry

Conflicting feelings of jealousy and sorrow were depicted in participants' narratives. Jealousy and resentment about preferential treatment tended to abate as participants observed what the ill sibling and/or parents had to endure. Meg acknowledged being jealous "because she was always getting toys and so forth when she was in the hospital. I didn't get the attention that she got. . . . Even though I loved her so much, I still felt the jealousy." Karen related a story about her diabetic sibling's hypoglycemic reaction during a rafting trip:

> J got low blood sugar, of course, in the middle of the river. Somebody in another boat had some candy and they threw it over to us. . . . At that point I felt a little jealous that J got to eat this candy and I didn't.

Exemplars of abating jealousy included the following:

> I think I was grateful I didn't have to have the shots and that I could eat what I wanted to. I think that is what balanced the scales. . . . I felt fortunate that I didn't have to put up with what he had to put up with." "I just remember thinking that was so sad and seeing how sad my parents felt. . . . I felt sorry for my mom and dad, and I wish[ed] there was a cure for it. I always felt sorry for mom and dad because I knew they were sad that he was having to live with this.

Feeling Scared/Alone

The fifth theme concerned feelings of being scared and alone. Participants vividly remembered when their sibling was first diagnosed or taken to the hospital. Many feared that their sibling was going to die: "They took her in immediately. She was apparently pretty bad off. That was really scary. I got home from school and nobody was home. That was really odd." Another comment emphasized the aloneness while awaiting word: "They were gone really the whole day. . . . I was left by myself wondering if my sister is going to live."

One woman described repeated hospitalizations of her sister and having no one to talk to about her own fears:

> My sister was constantly in the hospital. And my parents were working or at the hospital with her. . . . I would have to get on the bus by myself. . . . It is like you have no one to turn to then. Everybody is gone . . . It was real distressful for me. And I grew up more or less constantly worrying. You know a child really knows more than what you think they do. . . . I knew that she was real bad off. . . . I knew that something was going on around me because I could feel the stress coming from my mother and father. I was really upset yet I had no one to talk to.

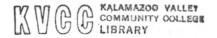

Most participants felt poorly prepared for their diabetic sibling's first hypoglycemic reaction and remember being very frightened when they observed it: "It was like someone being drunk or something. She just couldn't do anything. Her eyes would roll back into her head. She didn't know where she was. . . . It is a tense situation until she . . . comes out of it. . . . It is scary. . . . It makes you think that you might lose them there for a second."

"I honestly thought she was possessed. When I saw her having a seizure I really thought she was possessed. . . . I just remember how white she was and all the blood. She bit her tongue. There was a lot of mucus. . . . Actually I ran and hid from her. I locked myself in my room. . . ."

The fear concerning a sibling's hypoglycemic reaction was not only based on what could happen to the ill sibling but also fear for oneself because of the diabetic's irrational behavior: "He would throw things at you . . . one time he threw a phone at me and it hit me in the ankle. . . . He would break a lot of things in the house at times." One participant admitted that he was so scared by his sister's behavior when she would "go low" [hypoglycemia] that he began to avoid her: "I didn't take her as many places as I used to. . . . I would shun her. . . . I didn't know how to really handle it."

THEMES IN PERIOD TWO: THE PRESENT

The changes and disruptions in family relationships described by the study participants are both abrupt and unending: past themes set the stage for the present ones. The vigilance and protectiveness of the ill sibling that began in childhood continued and intensified as the ill sibling entered adulthood. As adults, participants report being more acutely aware of the severity and complications of insulin-dependent diabetes mellitus. Some participants also feel a shift of responsibility for the ill sibling from parents to themselves. We turn now to discussion of the themes that emerged in reference to the present time.

Changes in Relationships

Directly or indirectly, relationships of participants with their chronically ill siblings were transformed. Three issues were prominent in the data: role reversal, endearment vs. rift, and failure of the diabetic sibling to reach potential. *Role reversal* was evident in a number of cases wherein the participant, although younger, had become the caretaker of the older sibling. Carol provides a clear explanation of role reversal:

She is still in childhood. I think being a diabetic she missed some of her childhood. . . . I am more the older sister. I am younger than her, but I am still the older sister. I still . . . make sure she gets her shots. . . . I would just think, 'It is time to eat. You're acting a little funny, M, what do you need?' I watch after her. It really drives me crazy.

As in childhood, their sibling's illness seemed to bring some adult siblings closer while creating distance between others. *Endearment vs. rift* was exemplified in these descriptions of the relationship quality in adulthood:

"I think I pay more attention to that relationship. Maybe because I want her to know how I feel about her. . . . I quit thinking about myself so much and thought more about her."

"It has amplified those differences enormously. We have always had those differences. He was always Type B and I was always Type A. As the first sibling I acted the role perfectly. But it has made the differences even more huge. . . . I am not going to deal with him. He is not going to be my friend. We are never going to be compatible. I don't like him."

Because of the chronicity of their sibling's illness some participants perceived that the illness had prevented the sibling from reaching his or her potential. The siblings were viewed as arrested in their development and/or too dependent on parents, indirectly affecting the sibling relationship. *Failure of the diabetic sibling to reach potential* is illustrated in the following quotes from the interviews:

"J (age 22) has never been able to leave home and succeed or be independent, manage an apartment and a job, money, food, and clothing. . . . Anytime he has lived away from home he has ended up back. . . . I definitely think he is stuck."

"It just seems like my brother can't make a decision about anything without calling my mother first, checking it out with her. . . . Even to this day I have felt she is more protective of him. She has a closer relationship in a lot of ways with him than she does with my older brother and me."

"All these years way up to age 38 . . . the relationship [with the mother] hasn't changed that much from when he was a little boy, the way I see it. And I feel sorry for both of them."

Worried/Responsibility Without Power

Participants worried about, and felt responsibility for, their diabetic sibling but often perceived themselves as having little power over the situation. As adults, the healthy siblings understood more about the seriousness of diabetes. One woman, only seven years old when her 13-year-old sister was diagnosed, never realized the gravity of the illness until years later when a hospital radiologist told her, "Your sister may or may not make it through this [pregnancy]." In some cases, worry intensified when the diabetic sibling moved out of the parents' home. Participants voiced concern about the potential for binge eating, overdoses of insulin, cuts on the foot, elevated blood pressure or cholesterol, kidney failure, problems with circulation, and the abbreviated life span of the sibling. Participants were painfully aware that they would outlive their ill sibling. Heavy responsibility was placed on some of them by the ill sibling: "She told me many years ago, I guess we were in our 30s, 'If I ever go into a coma . . . then you are to make sure that I don't just lay there. You are to unplug the machines.'" They felt powerless to decline these responsibilities. Participants also spoke of their inability to control their siblings' behavior when noncompliant with the prescribed diabetes treatment regimen: "She drinks regular cokes, one after another, one after another. She just does not take care of herself."

Participants perceived that they and/or their parents managed their fears by becoming over-vigilant toward the adult ill sibling. Some explicitly stated that the protective shield continues into adulthood: "Mother never broke off that protective shield that she always had woven around him wherever he went." Participants described frequent phone calls and visits to their siblings to monitor their condition: "If she doesn't call me, I call her." "I make her check her blood three or four times if I think she is low. . . . She'll sit there and argue with me, 'I'M FINE,' but I'll still make her check it." Protective behaviors became a part of participants' daily routine: "Maybe before this interview I thought [this] was normal. I guess maybe I never realized how much I looked out for her, how much I worried about her. . . . Even through the week, if I go over there in the mornings, I still fix her shot for her if she is in a hurry or something, fix her toast for her, or get her some orange juice or whatever. It is just habit." The caregiving ability of individuals who were not members of the family of origin was questioned: "Is his wife preparing his meals the way they should be prepared?" "Somebody in that state of mind could not be handled by somebody her size." "They all knew that A was a diabetic but . . . I know that they were drinking that night."

Empathy/Sadness/Guilt

Mixed emotions of empathy/sadness/guilt comprised a third major theme in participants' descriptions of their experience in adulthood with their ill sibling. Empathy toward both the sibling and the parents was evident: "I am real sorry it had to happen to her. I wouldn't want anyone to have the problem of that disease, especially with the attitude toward shots that I have. I hate to take shots even though I am 43 years old, weigh 250 pounds." "I wouldn't want to have to go through something like that every day. It does not look like something that would be enjoyable." "It bothers me that my mother worries about it too. And I worry about my mother worrying about it." Participants felt guilty about their own good health and freedom in comparison to that of their brother or sister with diabetes: "I'm fine, I get up, go hop in the shower, go to work or whatever. She has to stop and take time and take her shots and . . . make sure she has the right foods to eat . . . good shoes . . . good glasses." "I am physically stronger. I don't have the threat of blindness or amputation." "She has already had more sickness and pain than most people have all their life. I never had to deal with that kind of pain."

Burdened

The fourth theme pertained to participants' perceptions of burdens resulting from their sibling's illness. They described sacrificing their own time, health, families, and careers to care for their adult diabetic sibling. When Joyce's sister is in the hospital, she stays with her for more than 12 hours per day, despite having children of her own who need her attention. Tyler becomes depressed when his diabetic sibling talks of suicide: "It pulls you down. . . . It wears on you. . . . You can't go to sleep. . . . Be thinking about her at work. . . . You are trying to do your job, and you are thinking about something like that." Meg states she has put her career on hold for her sister: "She works every day and I've pretty much put my career on hold so I can help her and stay home and watch her little boy. She has a lot of stress if she doesn't have anybody to watch him. . . . It is stressful on a person. I am 26. I am on blood pressure medicine, nerve medicine, and that is quite a bit for a 26-year-old." One insightful participant recognized that caretaking of her ill sibling, although burdensome, served to ease her guilt.

Can't Talk About Feelings

Participants believe that they cannot truly express what they are feeling to their ill sibling or other family members. They articulated various reasons for suppressing their feelings, including fear of damaging family relationships or precipitating the sibling's suicide. The sibling is perceived as fragile ("he could suffer a severe illness at any time"), and the consequences of expressing feelings of a strong emotion like anger are seen as potentially destructive: "With me and C it is not that I can't express my anger, but I don't want to. . . . The least little thing will set her off. I don't want to do anything that upsets her or anything because of the way she talks now. . . . If something like that erupts, she won't eat."

The above themes are not isolated, distinct themes but connected to each other; each theme influences the other. For example, changes in participants' relationships with their ill sibling create feelings of empathy, sadness, and/or guilt. Worry, concern, and responsibility contribute to participants' experiences of burden. Contributing to their burden is their perception of powerlessness. Finally, their inability to talk about their feelings reinforces both burden and the sense of powerlessness.

The present themes are also related to themes from childhood. Although described differently, present themes are often the past themes brought forward. For example, participants described changed relationships beginning at the time of diagnosis and continuing into the present. The wondering of a child is described in adult terms as worry and responsibility. The child's feelings of being jealous and sorry are evident in the sadness and guilt of the adult. The scared feelings of the child evolve into the adult burdens and "what ifs" concerning deterioration of the sibling's health and vulnerability to an earlier death. Finally, "feeling alone" is brought forward into the present by participants' continuing inability to express their feelings to their siblings and/or to other family members.

DISCUSSION AND CONCLUSIONS

The phenomenon of having a chronically ill sibling was described in terms of two interrelated periods (past and present) in which relationships with the sibling and other family members were transformed. Participants became more acutely aware of changes in family relationships with the passage of time and accumulation of worrisome experiences with the chronicity of insulin-dependent diabetes mellitus. According to Minuchin (1974), a family is a "system that operates through transactional patterns. Repeated transactions establish patterns of how, when, and to whom to relate, and these patterns underpin the system" (p. 51). The diagnosis of a child with a chronic illness has a major impact on the family system, causing patterns to be disrupted. Participants in this study spoke of how they and their families worked toward protecting the ill family member. This protection, or "protective shield," was not removed even when the ill member entered adulthood. In fact, it was even brought to bear over the protests of the diabetic person in some cases. When one man expressed concern to his sister about not returning their mother's telephone calls, she "got mad about it. She said, 'You don't even let me breathe.'"

Some of the families in this study appear to exhibit characteristics of families that encourage somatization: enmeshment, overprotectiveness, rigidity, and lack of conflict resolution (Minuchin, Rosman, & Baker, 1979). Lacking longitudinal studies, it is not known whether a chronic illness such as diabetes creates these characteristics in a family or crystallizes them.

This study's major theme, that changes in relationships occur within families having an identified ill sibling, is congruent with findings of nursing studies done by Gerace et al. (1993) and Lively et al. (1995). It is extremely interesting how these two studies involving a family member with mental illness yielded similar themes to those of the present study of adults whose siblings have a physical illness. The long-term impact of a child's illness on well siblings is consistent across all three studies.

Preferential treatment of the ill sibling by parents was a second important theme in this study. Researchers agree that perceived preferential treatment of siblings affects the quality of sibling relationships and parental interactions (Dunn & McGuire, 1992; Powell & Gallagher, 1993). Given the likelihood that well siblings, in most cases, will outlive their parents and, to some degree, may feel or be responsible for the care of their ill sibling, future research should explore the nature of interaction between the siblings, quality of caregiving by the well sibling, and the effect on the mental health of both the ill and well sibling.

Lazarus and Folkman (1984) contend that "the persistence of a chronic stressor can give the person the opportunity to learn to deal with its demands, or to deal with it by avoidance or distancing" (p. 100). Although most participants in this study chose to deal with the stressors associated with their sibling's illness by trying to meet the demands of that illness, a few chose to avoid and distance themselves from their ill brother or sister. In the sample studied by Gerace et al. (1993) distancing from the mentally ill sibling also was evident. Siblings admitted feeling guilty about wanting to get away yet compelled to do so for their own well-being.

Similarity to one's ill sibling has been hypothesized to be an important variable in the ultimate adaptation of the well child. Writes Bush, "Well siblings' perceptions of similarity or identification with their ill sibling relate to their psychological adjustment. Adjustment is expected to be poorer among siblings who perceive themselves as either extremely similar or extremely dissimilar to their ill sibling than among siblings who demonstrate more balanced perceptions of both similarities and differences. The rationale for this hypothesis is that siblings who perceive themselves as very similar to their ill brother or sister are more likely to be over identified with them. On the other hand, siblings who perceive themselves as very much unlike their ill sibling may be defending against underlying fears of identification which may reflect a maladaptive level of anxiety" (Bush, cited in Drotar & Crawford, 1985, p. 359). The present study provides some support for the above hypothesis. In general, those participants appearing to have the most difficulty coping with their siblings' illness were those who described themselves either as very similar to or as very different from their sibling. One participant, who had described herself as very much alike and very close to her diabetic sibling, became so distraught during the interview that she could not finish. Another participant who described herself as being very different from her sibling was consumed with anger towards her brother and his inability to take control of his illness.

The findings of this study provide a greater understanding of the long-term impact chronic illness has on the entire family, in particular on the well sibling. The adult well sibling's viewpoint has long been a missing link in our understanding of the stressors involve in a chronic illness. The method used in this study allowed participants to clearly articulate the stressors and burdens they perceive as generated by their sibling's insulin-dependent diabetes mellitus. The study findings may surprise many nurses, for seldom are adult well siblings viewed as vulnerable to the stressors of their sibling's illness.

IMPLICATIONS OF THE STUDY FINDINGS FOR NURSING PRACTICE

At first, most of the participants in this study were confused about why a nurse researcher would be interested in talking to them. They wondered why the research was not being done on the ill sibling, "the designated patient." Through the years, health care professionals had focused almost exclusively on their sibling, failing to include them in educational sessions. Only one participant remembers having a family meeting with a physician who explained diabetes. Participants learned what they could by reading books and hearing their parents talk about the disease. Frightening episodes when their sibling's diabetes was out of control gave clues regarding what they should be looking for and doing:

> When she started screaming and acting really wild, I got really scared. And later I thought . . . no one prepared me that this might happen. I just happened to put two and two together and know that I should do that. So what if I hadn't thought that this was what it was? And I realized how close to death she could become. . . . Looking back, if I would say anything should have been done, I should have been included in [instruction about] all the different dangers that were there. Which I don't remember anyone telling me.

This woman's words are a clear mandate to all nurses who work with families of chronically ill individuals. The exclusion of families from instruction not only offends them but also creates the likelihood that the ill individual may not receive the proper assistance in a frightening crisis situation. The importance of communicating directly to all family members was demonstrated in the study of families of schizophrenic patients conducted by Main et al. (1993). Lack of communication and education by health care providers were two of the major obstacles that prevented families from obtaining the information necessary to assist them in caring for the schizophrenic family member. Other studies have shown that when siblings are not kept informed, they often fill in gaps with misconceptions (Kramer, 1984; Sourkes, 1987).

Nurses cannot assume that adults who have grown up with a diabetic sibling possess correct information concerning the illness. It is imperative that nurses continuously assess the knowledge level of well siblings and supply them with accurate information, anticipatory guidance, and counseling, as appropriate. Beyond helping siblings understand the illness and empathize with what the ill person is enduring, nurses should recognize the struggles and hardships entailed by their caregiving responsibilities. Attentively listening to family members is a first step in establishing a trusting relationship in which the family will be able to reveal true concerns and feelings. As shown in this study, well siblings may have long-suppressed guilt and anger that needs to be expressed.

It is difficult to convince some family members to relinquish control of caregiving because they feel that only they can provide proper care (Smith, Smith, & Toseland, 1991). This is an area that nurses must evaluate in regard to adult well siblings. Helping family members to give up some of their burdensome responsibility and thereby give control to others is a challenge to all health care providers.

POST-STUDY REFLECTIONS FROM MARILYN SMITH

Because of my own life experiences I have always been interested in family responses to life's stressors and traumas. Having a sibling with a chronic illness is a serious family stressor. Through the process of dialogue, participants taught me a great deal, not only about the experience of having grown up with a chronically ill sibling but also about their current experiences with a diabetic brother or sister. Although nurses have espoused holistic nursing for many years, this study reminds us that we still have a long way to go. As nurse educators we have urged our students to include the entire family in their nursing care plans. We have taught students for a long time that an illness of any family member may affect all members of the family system. But many of the siblings studied in this research project had been virtually ignored by health care professionals to the point of wondering why a researcher would want to interview them. No one had recognized how scared and alone they felt as their parents focused on the health crises of their diabetic siblings. Rarely were they given information concerning their ill sibling. It is my hope that nurses in a variety of settings will benefit from what these individuals shared and use this knowledge to promote optimal family adaptation to chronic illness.

8

"Walking in the Dark": The Experience of Living With a Daughter Who Has an Eating Disorder

"Every mother contains her daughter in herself and every daughter her mother, and every woman extends backwards into her mother and forwards into her daughter."

—Carl Jung, 1959

Recent years have seen a tremendous increase in the incidence and awareness of eating disorders. These disorders are frightening and poorly understood. In addition, their devastating consequences to physical health, including endocrine, cardiovascular, renal, and hematologic complications and the possibility of death, make the exploration of eating disorders an important concern for all health professionals. Nurses know from clinical practice that dealing with eating disorders exacts a tremendous emotional and financial toll on patients' families, although researchers have directed little attention to the experiences of the family members. When families are discussed in the literature, the language—particularly toward the mother—is often accusatory as to the etiology of the disease.

* This chapter is based on a study conducted by Mitzi Davis, in collaboration with Becky Fields, Johnie Mozingo, and Sharon Sarvey, at the University of Tennessee, Knoxville.

RELATED LITERATURE

Eating disorders are characterized by unusual self-imposed dietary behavior, odd ways of handling food, preoccupation with body shape and size, and a marked fear of gaining weight or becoming fat. (See Chapter 3 for examples of the distorted perceptions of body image by patients with these disorders.) Incidence is more common in women, being especially high in white, middle and upper socioeconomic, high-achieving women with onset in early adolescence for anorexia nervosa (AN) and mid- to late adolescence for bulimia. Epidemiological studies reveal the prevalence in American females as 1:100 or 1% for AN and 2% to 8% for bulimia, with a mortality rate ranging from 5% to 20% depending upon treatment (ANRED, 2000; Kaplan & Sadock, 1991; Love & Seaton, 1991). Treatment is aimed at restoring healthy body weight and eating habits and resolving psychological issues. It is multifaceted, reflecting the mixed aspects of these disorders, including individual and family psychotherapy and psychopharmacologic interventions. Long-term treatment may be necessary (Becker, Grinspoon, Klibanski, & Herzog, 1999; Muscari, 1998). With treatment, 51% of these individuals fully recover, 21% partially recover, and of the remaining 28%, 15% die (Zipfel, Lowe, Reas, Deter, & Herzog, 2000).

The etiology of eating disorders is usually conceptualized as multifactorial, resulting from biologic vulnerability, societal pressures, and family issues. Research has shown a high incidence in monozygotic twins and female first-degree relatives (mothers, sisters, daughters) (Kendler, 1991; Wade, Bulik, Neale, & Kendler, 2000). Dysfunctions involving the neurotransmitter serotonin and the hormone leptin are thought to predispose individuals to AN (Walsh & Devlin, 1998). Other metabolic and neuroendocrine dysfunctions are associated with AN but none provide a demonstrated causal link. There is also a substantial body of literature indicting Western society's preoccupation with thinness as an essential component of beauty in the idealized feminine body (see White, 2000 for a review). Eating disorders are most likely to occur in groups that place high value on thinness, such as gymnasts, models, and entertainers (Smolak, Murnen, & Ruble, 2000). Rodin (1993), for example, found that dancers have a notoriously high rate of anorexia.

Family dynamics are often posited to influence the development, maintenance, treatment, and outcome of eating disorders. In one early explanation by a physician, Charles Lasegue, anorexia was termed a "form of rebellion . . . in wealthy children . . . stressed by all the dinner table rules and regulations [and] suffocating and manipulative parental love" (cited in Decker & Freeman, 1996). Bruch, who began therapeutic work with anorexics in the 1940s, believed that parents seek to impose an identity on the daughter. She viewed the parents, especially the mother, as rigid and intolerant of the daughter's independent behaviors. As a result, the daughter fails to develop a sense of self, making it impossible for her to mature. In the daughter's struggle to achieve her own identity, she adopts "rigid discipline over [her] eating . . . [and] the visible weight loss gives these adolescents the experience of being effective in control, at least in one area—the more weight lost, the more superior they feel" (Bruch, 1985, p. 10).

Bruch's conceptualization was echoed by a leading family systems theorist, Minuchin, who studied several anorexic clients and their families. He viewed anorexia nervosa as the result of family patterns in which families are intrusive, overprotective, rigid, and unable to effectively deal with conflict. He believed that young women with AN grew up in families that valued loyalty to the family moreso than autonomy and self-realization. As a consequence, the women learned to subordinate their own needs and assert the only power they have—refusal to eat—thus regaining control over one aspect of their lives (Minuchin, Rosman, & Baker, 1979).

Pathology in the mother-daughter relationship has been emphasized since the first identification of anorexia nervosa. In 1895, *The Lancet's* report of the first death from the disorder stated that "the attending physician attempted to keep her family, particularly her mother, away from the girl" (cited in Brumberg, 1988). Since that time, various aspects of poor mothering have been cited as critical in the etiology of eating disorders (Johnson & Connors, 1987; Palazolli, 1978; Rampling, 1980). In the literature concerning the dynamics of the mother-daughter relationship, recurring elements are enmeshment and poorly defined boundaries, yet little intimacy. Chernin (1985) attributes the daughter's refusal to eat to her fear of becoming like the mother. For the daughter "whose mother's life has made a negative impression on her, the act of eating will be fraught with peril. With every bite she has to fear that she may become what her mother has been" (p. 42).

Given the pejorative nature of the literature about the mother's influence on her daughter's eating disorder, many professionals hold scant sympathy for the mother. While recent reports have managed a somewhat less condemning tone, the mother continues to be seen as crucial to the genesis of the disorder, either as an overly intrusive parent or a transmitter of the cultural obsession with thinness (Hill & Franklin, 1998; Pike & Rodin, 1991; Rorty, Yager, Rossotto, & Buckwalter, 2000; Shoebridge & Gowers, 2000). To date, no studies have explored the mother's experience of parenting a child with this tenacious and life-threatening disorder. The mother is faced with a child who will not eat (or who surreptitiously purges what she has consumed). Historically and culturally, a child's eating is regarded as a reflection of maternal nurturance. Consider the approval that is generally dispensed to "good" mothers whose babies are plump. Hence, observers of an emaciated child wonder: what kind of mother cannot keep her child adequately fed? A better understanding of the mother's experience could assist nurses in providing sensitive and appropriate interventions.

THE PRESENT PROGRAM OF RESEARCH

The purpose of this study was to describe the experience of women whose daughters have been diagnosed with anorexia nervosa or bulimia. As a maternal-child clinical nurse specialist and a PhD-prepared nutritionist, I (Davis) had a long-term but super-ficial, cognitive acquaintance with eating disorders and regarded them, and the girls who had them, as strange or weird. I could not understand how the girls could not know how they "really looked" and how "crazy" their behavior was. While growing up, I did not know anybody with an eating disorder and could not imagine myself with one. I did have some sense of vulnerability because I was careful in modeling eating behavior with my daughters and refrained from comments that I assumed might pertain to the development of eating disorders. I gave little thought to the mothers. I had read that eating disorders were the result of overcontrolling mothers and adopted that belief, having no reason to question its validity. Eating disorders remained an interesting oddity, encountered mostly on TV or in magazines, until I went to my niece's college graduation.

I turned the corner to see that beautiful, successful, bubbly girl I had loved since birth and literally gasped at the emaciated, sickly, scary person before me. She was skin and bones in a short, sleeveless dress. I was shocked at her and at the fact that my brother had not shared this with me. Although not geographically close, I subsequently watched as he and my sister-in-law dealt with their daughter, her illness, her prolonged treatment, and her uneven recovery. I saw their pain. I wanted to help them and went to the library to see what was known about parents of girls with eating disorders. I found descriptions of pathology that didn't seem to fit this family. I found nothing that described their first-person experience. Thus, this study was born.

Bracketing Interview

My bracketing interview indicated that I (Davis) was puzzled by eating disorders and frustrated by the lack of answers. I needed to know what caused these disorders and how to cure them. I was not particularly open to the idea that family dysfunction was involved in the etiology. I was most surprised, however, when a colleague in the phe-nomenology research group gently asked if I didn't see similarities with the way I viewed my experience as the mother of a handicapped child. There were, indeed, sim-ilarities. I anticipated that the experience would be painful for the mother because she would grieve over what her child lost and her inability to do anything about it. I thought she would be aware of others looking at her child's altered physical appearance and then treating the child differently, even shying away or rejecting her. I thought she would be concerned over the daughter's inability to safely care for herself and the resul-tant need for increased parental supervision and vigilance. I thought she would be scared for her daughter's future. Clearly, I had a lot to bracket.

Sample

Nine mothers, recruited by word of mouth and snowball sampling, volunteered to par-ticipate in the study. The mothers ranged in age from 36 to 60 years and their daughters from 15 to 31 years. Because of the initial secrecy maintained by their daughters, exact duration of the eating disorder was hard for mothers to accurately describe. Estimates of duration ranged from less than 6 months to over 15 years. All mothers but one were currently married to the father of the daughter with the eating disorder. The participant not currently married to the father was in the process of getting a divorce. All mothers were Caucasian and middle class.

Participants were interviewed at the site of their choice by the principal investigator or a graduate student trained in phenomenological interviewing. After informed consent was obtained, participants were asked to "think of a time when they were aware of their daughter's eating disorder," although the exact wording of the question seemed almost irrelevant. The mothers had given thought to the story they wanted to tell. They started the story at the beginning of symptoms, or even in some cases at the daughter's birth, and they talked with essentially no prompting until they had provided an exhaustive account of the current situation. Interviews tended to be lengthy, in some cases yielding as many as 30 or 40 pages of typed transcript.

FINDINGS

"Walking in the Dark"

Although each mother's story was unique, there were remarkably consistent patterns. The participants described the experience as a long journey, one which they traversed feeling bewildered and alone ("walking in the dark"), starting with their initial suspicion of an eating disorder. The process is presented here in a sequential manner but was described as more dynamic with events and emotions occurring simultaneously and often in non-linear fashion. Following their initial suspicion that the daughter might have an eating disorder, participants described seeking acknowledgment from others, assuming responsibility for fixing the problem, being consumed by the disease, struggling and coping, and finally relinquishing responsibility. Long-term effects were described as well. After discussing these aspects of the "journey," we will turn to a delineation of figural themes contained in narratives provided by this group of mothers.

Suspicion/Normalization

The mothers reported initial, reluctant suspicions of the daughter's eating disorder. A number of clues were observed such as increased rigidity in vegetarianism or baggy clothing. The following quotes are illustrative of behaviors creating a mother's first suspicions: "She would stop eating with us—would make a point to eat either before we ate or after we ate . . . just sort of, kinda separated;" "She began to avoid certain foods that I know she used to like;" "I noticed she was doing a lot of exercising even though she had this back problem and so much pain."

The mothers reported that they didn't want to believe the possibility of an eating disorder but the evidence before them, along with their intuition, led them to consider it. Concomitantly, they considered the possibility that the behavior was normal. Exemplars from the data depict the tension between suspicion and normalization:

"I was all by myself, but I knew. I knew. I don't know how I knew, but I knew what was happening wasn't healthy."

"How could she be caught up in it? So my retort to myself was: You're over-reacting. Don't say anything, just keep an eye on it."

"I remember the time when I first noticed she was taking her experiences with food a little differently. She was a little more worried about ingesting red meat. This isn't unusual for college kids, though, especially if their food at school is not good—and she said it was pure grease."

"I began to notice that she began to act moody and depressed and upset easily. And we thought—she was our oldest child—this is normal teenage stuff."

"We knew something was wrong. I couldn't quite put my finger on it. And she was deteriorating. She looked awful. Her hair was falling out. . . . I thought of all the things that might be wrong, but I didn't know what."

Seeking Acknowledgment from Others

The mothers reported that they sought acknowledgment from others that something was wrong with their daughters, but it was often a disappointing experience. They described difficulty in getting others to listen to their concerns. Unhelpful advice or reassurance was received from friends and physicians, as depicted in the following comments:

"Just to not have anybody really listen to what I was trying to say was very hard."

"And I had a few friends in town that I would talk to. And it would be like, 'Oh, she'll be okay. She's coming home and you now, you'll fatten her up.' And they would make light of it. . . . Finally, I, out of frustration, sometimes would burst out, 'Will you stop? It's not okay, she could die. This is a life-threatening thing.' I'm having to pound people's heads and then I would think, 'back off.'"

"And he [doctor] said, 'What are you suggesting?' And I said 'I'm suspicious. . . . I think she's caught up in the depths of anorexia.' And he looked at her again and he says [to her], 'Now you know, young lady, that's not a healthy way to live.' . . . . So she got a little lecture about how she had to eat right. I was livid at his behavior."

Assuming Responsibility

Once the mother's suspicions were confirmed either by others or by her own experience, she immediately assumed, or was given, responsibility by other family members for remedying the daughter's condition:

"He [husband] was telling me to make it happen, make it better."

"Much as I love my husband, he did not want to deal with this."

"Her dad, her step-dad, they're just out there. . . . They were so useless, so counterproductive. It was just like, 'Get over it. Look in the mirror!' 'She can see she's not fat. If she thinks she's fat, she's crazy.' Well, duh, that's part of it. She is crazy. That's a given, okay? Now let's move on."

"Our older daughter said, 'You've got to fix her.' Mothers fix everything, but I couldn't fix this. I had a sister-in-law call from another state and say, 'Are you aware of how bad she is? I heard her throwing up. Well, there is a girl in our church who died from anorexia. You've got to do something.'"

Some of the mothers were able to enlist their husbands as allies in the struggle against their daughter's eating disorder, but none reporting finding cooperation from the daughter. Indeed, as part of the disease, mothers reported that the daughter resisted their efforts to help, sometimes quietly but sometimes defiantly, by overt behaviors such as vomiting in the mother's presence:

"Then one night she's crying again and she's saying, 'You can't make me stop throwing up. I like to, I want to, and I'm not going to stop.'"

"I took it as a personal . . . that she didn't love me, so this was her way of showing me that she could hurt me. The vomiting was a way, I thought, of showing me, 'I'll show you.'"

Being Consumed by the Disease

The daughter with the eating disorder and the related efforts to combat it become the almost exclusive focus of the mother, and to a great degree, of the entire family. The word "consumed," taken directly from a mother's transcript, is an interesting choice of words, given that the disease involves *refusal to consume*. The following interview excerpts depict being consumed by the disease:

"I mean I was so focused on her and the problem that she was going to have to face, and what am I going to do? Am I going to lose her? I know people could die from this. I'm self-employed so I quit accepting jobs. I gave up my own life because I was willing to give that up at that time to make her life happen."

"She was the center and everybody revolved around her."

"My husband was devastated. My younger daughter cried every night because she thought her older sister was going to die. The whole family was in crisis."

"For a while our entire family was obsessed with helping her get better and it disrupted the whole pattern of everything. She was in all our thoughts constantly. I feel I've neglected our other two daughters because this one required so much emotional support."

Struggling and Coping

During this time, the mother is actively and fully engaged in the struggle against the eating disorder, a struggle in which she feels alone much of the time. As one woman put it, "It was like walking in the dark . . . alone, very lonely, very lonely, just feeling isolated." All of our participants reported desperate attempts to understand the baffling disease. Where did it come from? They frequently saw the genesis in themselves:

"I had done something wrong as a parent."

"I failed. I didn't do it the right way, the perfect way."

"She's trying to do everything she can do to not be like me because I typically had an overweight problem."

Study participants also sought expanded explanations through reading or scanning the Internet. Psychological, spiritual, and physiological etiologies were proposed:

"When stress factors came back, that was her way to cope with stress."

"What it was in her case, she was addicted to serotonin."

"We now know that there might be synapses in the brain that actually cause this. It might be like diabetes or something like that."

"Satan, I really believe, uses this illness to blind their minds and to destroy their bodies."

Some mothers disclosed their daughter's condition only to immediate family or impersonal agencies. For example, a mother who had been dealing with her daughter's eating disorder for over 15 years spoke of the "family's secret": "So I have pulled into myself. I don't talk to people. This is the first time I've written my feelings down or talked about them. It's our family's secret." In most cases, however, the mothers reported attempts to seek help from friends, support groups, and therapists:

"I attempted to call friends and tell them 'I know you don't know what she is going through, but please try to be patient.' I was too interfering, but I wanted so much to help."

"I had to ask teachers to have some compassion for my child: 'Call us if she runs out of class. She is ill.' I went to bat for her and did everything I could think of doing."

"I talked to the insurance people for months on end. I finally got some top person and literally begged them for the life of my daughter: ' Please pay for this counseling.' We're going to all of this [counseling] and fighting insurance companies and we have a kid dying and they say, 'We don't cover that.'"

The mothers described trying various coping strategies, such as exercise and prayer, but attention to their daughter's disorder came at a price to their marriages and careers. Participants felt they were neglecting their partners and other family members. Most striking were the physical changes described by some of them. Weight loss was an interesting parallel to the daughter's pathology:

"I couldn't sleep at night. I didn't eat. I lost 50 pounds. . . . I didn't want to talk to anybody. I wanted to be left alone. I turned her picture upside down. One of them I cut up. I was vengeful. It consumed my every waking thought."

"Physically I'm losing weight, mentally I'm a drain. I'm trying to stay strong for her and having to deal with all these other things and be referee. I even used that word with my husband: 'I can't do this. I can't be the referee between you two or between you and your brothers.'"

Although the mothers described confusion about their limitations and concerns about making the disease or the relationship worse, at some point they confronted their daughters:

"Now I became the mother and I'm telling a little girl, 'Don't lose any more.' I hugged her and looked at her and said one last time, 'One more pound and we start to see doctors.'"

"One day I finally called her and I said, 'We have two options. You've either got to find a psychiatrist that will help you. . . . We can pay either the psychiatrist bill or the mortician's bill, because they are going to come about the same.'"

Relinquishing Responsibility

The mothers in our study described a willingness to assume responsibility for their daughters' recovery but were ultimately faced with their inability to bring about the changes they wanted in the lives of adolescent or adult daughters. They eventually realized they had "no control whatsoever" and relinquished responsibility. One mother's detailed description of her failed attempt to intervene is particularly poignant:

I remember one day I fixed her some peas, that she used to love, and I had put a little butter on them. And she knew it. I would try to sneak fat into her meals and she would know it. I added whole milk to skim, but she would sense it right off the bat. She started to eat this and she began to gag. There was a physical reflex. She put another bite in her mouth and she looked at me and tears were just rolling down her cheeks. And she opened her mouth and they fell out. And she said, 'I can't swallow this.' We held each other and cried.

Forced to recognize their limitations, the mothers had to "let go" and shift responsibility for recovery to their daughters, but it was very difficult: "That's real hard as a mother, when your whole role in life is you take care of them. Do you have enough to eat? Are they taking their medicine or getting sleep? That's a mother's job. For 14 years my whole relationship with my child is to come and do these things. I would just have to sit there and bite my tongue and walk the streets and cry. It was all up to her."

Experiencing Long Term Effects

All of the daughters were in at least partial recovery at the time their mothers were interviewed for our study. But each mother described continuing effects of the disease on themselves, their families, and the daughters. One participant described herself as "never quite relaxed" and speculated that "maybe 10 years from now I will be." The mothers remained vigilant, unsure of the recovery, and expressed concerns regarding "permanent damage" to the daughter's body:

"It's something that kind of hovers over us and always will. We know it's there. It's like any addiction. You don't want to ignore it and you don't want to talk about it every day, but you've got to face it and deal with it."

"I'm still afraid, because at one time I was naive and thought this was all behind us . . . and I suspect it might be a lifelong thing, that every time the pressure gets on, this will reemerge."

THEMATIC ASPECTS OF THE PARTICIPANTS' DESCRIPTIONS

Heartbreak

Heartbreak and devastation characterized mothers' descriptions of the experience of parenting daughters who had an eating disorder. Over and over, mothers spoke in terms of their hearts being broken, expressing great emotion during the interviews as they told their stories:

"It broke my heart. It broke my husband's heart."

"This person was at the bottom of the hill, and I thought, 'Who is that?' And it was my daughter. I didn't even recognize her. She was so thin and so tiny. And I just . . . it just broke my heart."

"It really broke my heart when she said she would be in bed crying because she would be so hungry. But she couldn't bring herself to eat because of the secondary gain she got [from not eating]. Having the control not to eat was more important than the physical hunger. That's really hard to bear."

Interrelated themes of anger, guilt, fear, and confusion/ineptness/helplessness also characterized the participants' experience as they moved through the above-described "walk through the dark." Each of these themes is described below along with verbatim quotations from the mothers' transcripts.

Anger

Anger was a universal emotion described by all participants. They were angry at health care providers—doctors and therapists. (Absent in their accounts was any mention of nurses.) Mothers were angry at doctors when they could not engage them as allies in the battle against the disease the mother recognized or feared: "I wanted to call some of these doctors she has been to and just say, 'You're worthless. You're a jerk.'" Psychotherapists evoked mothers' frustration and anger when they did not provide useful feedback. Some mothers saw therapists as excluding them.

Mothers also were angry at others in the family, most often the father, who was not always seen to be in the same place emotionally in dealing with the daughter's eating disorder or not behaving in a way the mother thought helpful: "I was really mad at him for his lack of educating himself when this ability to do this was in front of him and causing more problems by not. In fact, at that time quite honestly I thought of taking her and leaving him, just . . . or asking him to leave until we got through this, because he was creating more stress for her and that was not helping. And of course I was accused of coddling her."

Mothers also related feeling anger toward the daughters, but always with reservation: "I have been angry at her because she has caused it. Because I think she's betrayed a trust, but the more I understand about this . . . it was not an intentionally inflicted thing." Even in the face of what might be seen as an overtly hostile act (daughter throwing up out a second floor window in view of the mother), the mother found it distressful to express anger at her daughter: "It broke my heart that I said that, but I was so angry that she would have the audacity to throw up out of the window that was over my head. I was so angry." One mother purposefully redirected anger away from her daughter:

I made a pact with myself. I was not ever going to get mad at her. And I didn't. . . . I got mad at the monster [the disease]. . . . I was not going to let her die. . . . I was going to fight this thing. And because she wasn't, I was going to fight it for her. . . . I became mad that this thing had interrupted our lives. How dare this monster come into our lives. I let it out. I'd cry, slam my fist into the wall. Sometimes I would go outside and hike. I would just pound the earth. I would never take it out on my daughter.

Guilt

The commonly held notion that individuals with eating disorders come from unhappy, dysfunctional families is unsettling to mothers and causes them to struggle to understand what they may have done to contribute to their daughters' illness. In effect, it calls into question the mother's entire experience of parenting. All narratives, except one, included descriptions of guilt among the mothers. One mother attributed her sense of guilt to a therapist who "made me feel it was my fault. . . . I felt she was saying, 'If you were a better parent, this child would not have had such a low self-esteem.'" Most, however, regretfully reflected on their own parenting abilities or styles, or on aspects of themselves such as being overweight or having a "negative gene" that could have influenced the etiology or course of their daughters' disease:

> "I think she might have been reaching out trying to provoke boundaries. I think probably I didn't do her justice by not being a stricter mother, the more rigid kind of mom. I don't know."

> "I was very concerned because I have been treated for clinical depression. So I had a lot of guilt feeling from my experience. I thought that this was some sort of negative gene I had passed on to my daughter."

One mother did not report any guilt. She was the only participant who did not talk about reviewing the past for anything she may have done to contribute to the disorder. In her narrative she emphatically excluded others, such as her daughters' coaches, from culpability as well. She is the mother, quoted in the previous section, who depicted the eating disorder metaphorically as a monster that had taken over her daughter's life.

Fear

Throughout the narratives the mothers related a sense of fear, sometimes close to the surface and sometimes much deeper, but still ever-present. The major fear expressed by all of the mothers was fear for death of the daughter: "I am by this time so upset I can hardly work at work. I am thinking, 'What can we do? We are getting all the professional help we can for our daughter and this child may die if it doesn't stop soon;'" "I became hysterical at this point, this had been very traumatic going through all of this and thinking your child is so emotionally upset that they're trying to kill themselves;'" "You see your child dying in front of you, little by little." In the following statement, a mother provides a graphic description of the visible cues of her daughter's impending demise:

When you see your daughter and see her body is disappearing before your eyes and her eyes are hollow and I saw fuzz on her face. And when I hugged her all I could feel was bone. Yeah, that's an awful feeling. . . . That's when I began to really call it the monster. That is, was, not my daughter anymore. It had inhabited her body and now taken over her mind and it was like I had a war on my hands. A tug of war and my daughter was in the middle and both of us were pulling and yet this was a powerful thing. And I was scared, 'cause I didn't know what to do.

Intermingled with this fear of the daughter's death was fear of the loss of the mother-daughter relationship: "By now I'm feeling that she's putting up a wall and I'm so fearful of losing the relationship that we have." Mothers expressed fear of doing the wrong thing, thereby making the situation worse: "We're trying to find the fine line of balancing—when not to be too harsh with her. We felt like if we were too harsh, she was going to sink back into bingeing and purging." Relationships with daughters were fragile, and mothers became very tentative in their actions: "To push or not to push, you know, it was just like walking on eggshells. It was just thin ice all the time."

Confusion/Ineptness/Helplessness

Mothers could no longer follow their instincts as parents. They cared very much about what was happening and wanted to take definitive actions, but they found themselves feeling helpless and powerless. They doubted themselves, even labeling themselves as failures, and were confused about what to do. Quotations supporting this theme follow:

"It was a very confusing time for me to know what to do with her."

"I didn't know if I was making the right decisions. . . . In my own mind, I didn't know how to deal with it and I didn't know where to go for help."

"As a mother I was thinking, now where I am overstepping a boundary here? She's not really an adult, but she is an adult. She was 18 at the time. Eighteen, where do I have the rights?"

"My ineptness—like I would say [to the daughter], 'Tell me what to do. Tell me how I'm supposed to deal with this. You are asking me to accept that you are doing 350 crunches after you're spending an hour and a half [running]. . . . Tell me how I can deal with this.'"

"Last summer was the hardest summer I've ever lived in my life. It was very difficult to see your child going through this and you could do nothing to help. . . . I came to find out how totally helpless we were; we had no control whatsoever."

"At one point she told me she hated me, and never in her life has she ever said that and uh, I think that was the worst, the worst, definitely the low point in my life."

DISCUSSION AND CONCLUSIONS

Participants in this study were women reflecting on what is widely described as the most basic, formative, and important relationship in an individual's life—that of mother and child. In previous literature, the relationship of a mother and her anorexic or bulimic child has often been described from the point of view of mental health professionals—or from the perspective of the child who reflects on the actions of the mother and their impact. The present description, however, was obtained from the vantage point of the mother. The study, thus, sheds light on the less-studied experience of the mother, an experience of bafflement and heartbreak.

What it means to experience the heartbreak of being the mother of a daughter with an eating disorder is inextricably intertwined with what it means to be the mother of an adolescent or young adult daughter. The mother-daughter relationship at this point is widely regarded as complex, unique, and emotionally charged (LaSorsa & Fodor, 1990), occurring at a time when both are confronting different developmental issues. Although contemporary scholars think the notion of separation inadequately describes the dynamic occurring between mother and maturing daughter, there is supposed to be synchronous movement away from the extreme closeness previously experienced by both members of the dyad. In contrast to this depiction of the normal transition to a mature mother-daughter relationship, the movement by mothers and daughters described by participants in our study was not synchronous. It was not predictable and did not fit the mother's imagined scenario of how it should and would be.

All mother/daughter dyads engage in negotiation processes to maintain their own transitions in status (Kenemore & Spira, 1996), but the presence of an eating disorder made normal negotiations impossible for the mothers interviewed for this study. The mothers tried to set limits, create rules, and establish consequences for their daughters' excessive dieting, purging, and exercising, but the mothers were left floundering with patterns of interaction that no longer worked. They could not proceed with developmental tasks—moving to the next level of the mother-child relationship—but neither could they maintain the old relationship with the power differential that had once favored the mother. The current state of the relationship filled them with anger, guilt, feelings of confusion/ineptness/helplessness, and a deep abiding fear for the loss of the life of a much-loved daughter.

In their description of the human experience of other people, Pollio, Henley, and Thompson (1997) found three major themes: Relationship, Comparison, and Benefit (see Chapter 6). In addition to the disturbed and asynchronous mother-daughter relationship so prominent in the narratives of mothers in the present study, echoes of the Comparison theme also appeared in our data. Comparison refers to the tendency to categorize other people as similar to and different from ourselves and/or social norms. Mothers in this study compared themselves to other mothers and their eating-disordered daughters to healthy siblings. They also compared their families to other families. The contrast was rarely favorable to the mother, often adding to her sense of loss and failure. When participants did listen to the experiences of other people with similar situations, however, as in support group sessions, they realized shared commonalities. One woman, for example, described a great sense of relief from the comments of colleagues at work that other families had problems as great or greater than hers—that no one had the perfect family she had envisioned and expected to enjoy.

The third theme evident in the Pollio et al. (1997) study, Benefit, pertains to experiencing others in terms of their ability to meet our needs. The stories of mothers in this study teem with accounts of people—physicians, therapists, coaches, husbands, and other children—who failed at times to meet the mothers' needs for support—informational support to arm them with knowledge to fight the daughter's disease, affirmational support to normalize and validate their feelings and actions, and emotional support to empathize, understand, and convey positive regard. Most striking was the daughter's perceived inability to meet the needs of her mother. Participants felt deprived of the self-enhancing experience of being a loving, caring mother, as described by McMahon (1995). Whether the mother's needs are conceptualized as simply as Maslow's hierarchy or examined in light of feminist developmental theory, the mothers' needs were not being met.

Stern (1995) describes a psychic organization which he calls the "motherhood constellation" that includes a unique set of behaviors, wishes, aspirations, and fears. Although mothers in this study were quick to absolve their daughters of responsibility ("It's not her"), this psychic organization was thrown into disarray by the daughter's eating disorder. It was a time of turbulence, unmet wishes, failed aspirations, ineffective behaviors, and pronounced fear. To experience their daughter as literally starving, "a skeleton walking up the hill," suggests failure to perform the most basic mothering function—that of feeding—and calls into question the fundamental ability to perform the role most valued, that of nurturing mother. The result was described as devastating.

IMPLICATIONS OF THE STUDY FINDINGS FOR NURSING PRACTICE

The purpose of this study was to describe the experience of mothers whose daughters have an eating disorder, and mothers provided an intimate, sometimes brutally honest description of a most difficult experience. Their voices gave life to the often flat conceptual descriptions of emotions such as anger, guilt, and fear, and force a sympathetic response from those who will listen. These were not the voices of stereotypic, self-centered, emotionally cold women seen in myth, popular culture, and much professional literature as the cause and perpetuator of the disorder. They were women in great pain. As such, they deserve better, more sensitive care from nurses and other caregivers.

Increased educational preparation of nurses may be needed. A recent study of registered nurses caring for adolescent females with eating disorders within pediatric wards indicated a need for extensive preparation, ongoing support, and continuing education programs to prepare nurses to care for these patients with greater confidence and understanding (King & deSales, 2000). There is no comparable research on nurses' perceptions of their ability to interact therapeutically with mothers of these patients. Many nurses, especially those educated in the 1960s and 1970s, were taught only those psychoanalytic and family systems theories that placed the onus on mothers for their daughters' eating disorders (Conn, 1999). New information on neurobiology, psychopharmacology, and cultural influences could lessen the tendency of nurses and other professionals to distrust and blame mothers.

Nurses were absent from narratives of the mothers who participated in this study. Some of the therapists mentioned by mothers could have had nursing backgrounds but, if so, this was neither recognized nor seen as important. Clearly, nurses must become more visible and involved in the delivery of interventions to families affected by this devastating illness. School nurses, nurses in inpatient treatment facilities, and nurses in the offices of the mothers' and/or daughters' doctors could surely have a positive impact, playing a substantive role in assisting these mothers.

POST-STUDY REFLECTIONS FROM MITZI DAVIS

I feel a personal connection with the participants in this study and am committed to using their stories to expand and improve care for other mothers in this difficult situation. I find myself looking at quantitative research findings about eating disorders from a different perspective. What appear to be objective findings imputing blame to mothers and families may be viewed in a less pejorative light when one recalls the mothers' descriptions of their heartbreak and devastation. By conducting this research, my understanding of eating disorders and mothers of daughters with eating disorders was enhanced, but the impact is perhaps greatest on my personal perspectives, my clinical practice, and my teaching. As a relative newcomer to existential phenomenology, I continue to be changed by the practice of focusing on the experience of the other person. I am convinced that interactions based on preconceived ideas and assumptions will not enable me to practice nursing at its best. I cannot practice what Swanson (1993) calls "informed caring for the well-being of others" without openness to the unique perspective of the person whose life is at issue. This approach has made me a better researcher, a better teacher, a better mother, and a better nurse.

9

"She Became an Alien": The Father's Experience of Living With Postpartum Depression

"I've lost my wife now, and I don't mean physically but mentally. . . . I didn't know if she was going to make it back from that faraway planet that she was on."

—words of a husband interviewed for the present study

A mother with postpartum depression (PPD) is overwhelmed, tearful, angry, and panicked. The downward spiral of her depression can even include suicidal ideas or attempts (Beck, 1992; Wood, Meighan, Thomas, & Droppleman, 1997). PPD is more seriously incapacitating than the transient "baby blues," and its debilitating symptoms can last for months after the baby's birth (Martell, 1990). Although this disorder has a major impact on fathers, who have to assume greater responsibility for infant caretaking while the mothers are immobilized by depression, few studies have focused on fathers' reactions to the problem. The purpose of this study was to gain a better understanding of living with PPD from the father's perspective.

* This chapter is based on a study conducted by Molly Meighan in collaboration with Mitzi W. Davis, Sandra P. Thomas, and Patricia G.Droppleman at the University of Tennessee, Knoxville. The authors acknowledge the contributions of Cheryl Sherrill, Amy Wolz, Carol Snyder, and Ed Conway to this project. An earlier version of this paper appeared in *MCN* (Volume 24, No. 4, 1999, pp. 202–208). Reprinted by permission of Lippincott Williams & Wilkins.

RELATED LITERATURE

There is scant research about the impact of PPD on the father. In a clinical paper, George (1996) proposed that male partners influence the woman's recovery from PPD but contended that few husbands understand the condition or know how to support their depressed spouses. George also proposed that a depressed spouse could have a significant impact on the non-depressed partner. Not only are interactions more negative, but living with a depressed person also tends to decrease cognitive and problem-solving abilities of the non-depressed spouse. It is not known how often separation or divorce occurs as a result of PPD.

Several researchers (Boyce, 1994; Holden, 1994; O'Hara, 1995) have noted a relationship between depression and marital dysfunction. These studies, however, did not establish whether depression was the cause or the result of marital difficulties. Of particular interest are studies revealing that a significant number of the spouses of women with PPD were also found to be depressed (Ballard, Davis, Cullen, Mohan, & Dean, 1994; Harvey & McGrath, 1989; Lovestone & Kumar, 1993). Lovestone and Kumar (1993) compared three groups of men, which included husbands of wives admitted for postpartum psychiatric morbidity, husbands of women admitted with lifetime psychiatric problems, and husbands of wives who were tested and found not to be depressed. The men whose wives were suffering from postpartum psychiatric problems had significantly more symptoms indicative of psychiatric disorders than the other two groups.

The husbands of 40 British women admitted for a postnatal psychiatric disorder were interviewed and assessed for psychiatric morbidity by Harvey and McGrath (1989). Forty-two percent were found to have anxiety disorders, major depression, or evidence of poor social adjustment compared to only 4% of men in a control group. In another British study of 200 postnatal couples, 27.5% of mothers and 9% of fathers screened positively for depression at six weeks postpartum, and 25.7% of mothers and 5.4% of fathers were depressed at six months postpartum. Postpartum fathers were more likely to have psychiatric morbidity at both six weeks and six months if their partners also screened positively (Ballard et al., 1994).

While the literature documents that fathers can experience dysphoria after childbirth—especially if their wives are depressed—in-depth interviews about their lived experience have not been conducted. Extant studies have relied on structured questionnaires or clinical interviews designed to detect psychiatric morbidity in the men. These approaches to data collection do not permit a full description or elaboration of a man's pre-reflective perceptions or immediate thoughts and feelings about his world.

THE PRESENT PROGRAM OF RESEARCH

In this study, interviews with eight men whose wives suffered from PPD were audio-taped and transcribed for analysis. Some of the participants were contacted initially through their spouses who had been in a previous study about PPD (Wood et al., 1997). Others were contacted through health care professionals and by word of mouth. Interviews were conducted in participants' homes. Interviews began with a broad, open-ended question about the husband's experience with his wife's PPD: "Tell me what it was like when your wife experienced postpartum depression." Themes were condensed and common factors identified in order to distill the essence of the experience. All themes were supported by participants' own words from the text of their interview transcripts. Prior to initiating the study, the principal investigator (Meighan) reflected on her bracketing interview.

Bracketing Interview

I had not thought about my own experiences following childbirth for several years, but the bracketing interview brought back a flood of memories for me. Although I did not have postpartum depression and viewed the birth of my first child as a joyful event, I did have "the blues," a common event for many new mothers. I was hurt and angry with my husband because he didn't understand my tearfulness. I felt misunderstood and truly alone. Reconnecting myself with those feelings through the bracketing interview brought back the anger and hurt that had been pushed into the far corners of my mind. This reawakening made me realize how easy it would be for me to stereotype other men as non-caring based on my own previous experiences.

Bracketing those personal thoughts and feelings, along with other experiences from my clinical practice, made it possible for me to start with a clean slate as I interviewed men whose wives had postpartum depression. I know it would not have been possible without going through the bracketing process. I never realized how important that step would be for me or how impossible it would have been to truly listen to the stories of those men.

In addition, bracketing provided an opportunity for me to experience the interview process from the participant's perspective. As I engaged in the dialogue with the interviewer, I felt a range of emotions from joy to anger to sadness. The bracketing interview was followed by a sense of relief from sharing my story with someone who listened intently and wanted to understand. Later, I remembered how I had felt during my bracketing interview as I tried to actively listen to fathers talk about living with postpartum depression.

FINDINGS

Experiences related by the participants in this study were similar in several respects and a common thematic structure emerged, contextualized by the former marital relationship and its known patterns of partner interaction. The birth of the infant brought about a bewildering loss of the partner the husband had known and loss of the relationship he once shared with his spouse. The men also described other losses, including loss of control, loss of intimacy, and loss of how things "used to be." Attempts to find someone in the health care system who could help were unsuccessful in most cases. Most of the men and women had sought professional help in the first few weeks after the onset of the depression.

The first of seven interrelated themes in narratives of the fathers was **"She becomes an alien."** Prior to the birth of their infants, respondents had established familiar patterns of interaction and behavior with their partners. None of the participants had noted symptoms of depression in their wives before delivery of the infant. The men had expectations about the future based on previous interaction patterns and mutual dreams and plans. Following delivery of the baby and the onset of their wives' depression, husbands reported that their wives were significantly changed, to the point of no longer being themselves. One young father described his initial impression that his wife had seemed so maternal, wanting children before their marriage, and the hurt he now felt to see her so differently after the birth of their child. A father of two children sadly remarked, "She . . . within one afternoon became a completely different person." Another said, "It amazed me to see my wife change overnight." Another man stated, "I thought she had become an alien."

Obviously, one cannot interact in the same way with an "alien being" who seems to be on a "faraway planet," and the husbands' early experience with their wives' depression was one of confusion, fear, and concern. Men used words such as "nightmarish" to describe incidents such as a wife kicking a hole in the wall or sobbing hysterically. One man said, "At first I was just scared. . . . I didn't know what it was and she didn't know what it was." Participants did not know what to do to keep their wives and babies safe. They wondered whether their wives would ever be themselves again.

He Attempts to Fix the Problem

Respondents reported attempts to help their spouses recover, to find a cause, and to "fix the problem," often speaking in very detached mechanistic terms. As one father stated, "I knew it was an imbalance of some kind . . . either hormonal or chemical or emotional, and all we needed to do was pull it back in line." Another man said, "I was trying to find something wrong, you know, I wanted a wrong we could fix." Some participants lavished their wives with material goods (new house, new car) in a fruitless attempt to brighten their spirits. Realizing that his efforts were not working, one respondent said, "The hardest thing was that I couldn't fix it. Nothing that I could do or was doing at the time was helping her." Aptly summarizing the frustration expressed by all of the participants, one man lamented, "I couldn't hit it and make it go away . . . I couldn't scare anything off . . . or I couldn't beg it or give it money to go away."

Eventually, the men concluded that they were unable to "fix the problem" and found themselves subjugating their own needs to help the family survive the crisis. Gone was the former reciprocal relationship with the partner and helpmate and gone were the fantasies about new fatherhood. The following comment is illustrative: "It's like . . . 'You take the baby,' and I'd take the baby, and she'd start screaming, and my wife is crying, and I'm going, 'What do I do?'"

He Making Sacrifices

The men in the study described a strong sense of responsibility and willingness to sacrifice for the good of the family. According to one man, "I had to do whatever it took to get through this."

Grim stoicism was evident in language such as "had to stick it out" and "just suck it up and go on." One respondent described his role in military terms: "It calls for a certain bunker mentality. . . . I felt like I was hunkered down for the duration." The strong sense of responsibility was described by another father: "It was up to me to hold things together. . . . I had to take care of them . . . my needs were last." "Taking care" included care of wife, child, and household. The men also had to continue working.

Many of the respondents described exhaustion and lack of sleep: "I would get tired and I remember feeling like I went into overdrive. . . . It was almost . . . it wasn't me . . . it was superhuman." When the fathers were at work, their concentration was frequently disrupted by anxiety about what was happening at home. A desperate call could summon them to return home: "She would call sobbing and say, 'You've just got to come home . . . I can't take it another minute." This statement from the data typifies the men's personal sacrifices in this difficult situation:

> I guess I just felt like—do whatever is necessary to get through this . . . I also tried to make it peaceful . . . peace at all costs, even if I had to sacrifice my own feelings. . . . I didn't want the children to suffer. . . . I tried to protect them. . . . It was part of the weight I was carrying.

World Collapsing

Fathers described their world collapsing around them as their sacrifices for the family took an emotional toll. Participants described feelings of anger and resentment. As one man stated, "I felt pushed to the edge—didn't know how to express it. I didn't like it . . . I was angry at the situation, angry at depression, angry at her for being depressed." There was no outlet for emotional release or escape from the family demands: "I was there

24 hours a day, 7 days a week, really no time for myself . . . I needed sunshine, breathing room." One man admitted, "Most of the time I just wanted to say 'I'm leaving'. . . . I wanted to leave . . . escape, but I couldn't leave the child . . . not with her." Another respondent who had struggled with his mate's threat to kill herself stated, "I thought her suicide would be an answer, then I felt guilty for [having] those feelings." Unacceptable feelings such as these had to be suppressed: "I had to swallow it, bury it."

Despite its heroic dimensions, the father's effort was often ignored or unacknowledged by either the partner or the extended family. At a time when the husband was overburdened with responsibility, unappreciated, and scared, he also lost the one to whom he had historically turned for help, comfort, solace, and intimacy. The Other was not noticing his pain or his superhuman efforts. One participant remarked, "There was nothing in particular that I ever did that L [his wife] just brightened up and said 'that's great.'"

Loss of Control

The world became unpredictable and out of control for these participants: "I dreaded going home because I never knew what to expect. . . . Some days were good and some very bad." The unpredictability and loss of control led to feelings of being trapped. All of the fathers in this study described being afraid to leave their wife alone for fear that she might harm herself, harm the infant, or be unable to care for the infant. One man said he told his boss, "I can't go on the road now. . . . I'm afraid to go on the road. . . . My wife is unstable right now." Four of the eight men explicitly described their fear surrounding potential suicide:

". . . I might find her dead."

"I had to condition myself every day when I got home . . . if you go in and she's on the floor, call 911, check for vital signs, try to remember those things in first aid."

"I was afraid to leave because she said she wanted to die—to just get in the car and drive off into a tree."

Loss of Intimacy

Participants described a loss of intimacy in the marital relationship as well as a loss of the way things had once been. The relationship became guarded and nonreciprocal. During the height of his wife's depression, one man stated, "There was no relationship between us. . . . We were just living day by day." "I've lost my wife now, " another man said. "And I don't mean physically but mentally. . . . I didn't know if she was going to make it back from that faraway planet that she was on." Loss of sexual intimacy was particular painful, as shown in this excerpt from a transcript:

I would approach by simply just laying a hand on her shoulder or rub [bing] her back and wait [ing] to see if there was any reaction . . . in those first 3 or 4 years, 99% of the time there was no response . . . [I would] swallow that hurt, that rejection. . . . I remember times of sobbing and trying not to let her hear it. The head says: I understand that there is a medical reason or a hormonal reason, it's not because she doesn't love you, but for the heart and those natural desires that a man should have for his wife—to be rejected continually, that's a tough one.

Bluntly, one participant summarized, "Our relationship went to hell." It is not surprising that the husbands often became depressed. One father recounted how he reached a state of not caring about himself or his surroundings. Another man admitted that he was still dealing with it and trying to learn to be stronger. He explained, "I got into a pattern . . . a pattern of me not standing up [to her] . . . always being the one to give in . . . ever since then, I'll find myself still being the one who gives in more." This man's words provide an appropriate segue to the next theme.

Altered Marital Relationship

As indicated in the above quote, an altered pattern of interacting with wives evolved. The wives' depression lasted for varying lengths of time, ranging from months to years, but ultimately abated in all cases. Resolution of the depression, however, did not mean that the marriage returned to its former state, and many of the men indicated that they have never fully recovered their losses. One participant, speaking of the emotional separation during his wife's PPD, sadly said that he is still suffering from its "long-lasting effects."

The men continue to see their wives as vulnerable or fragile. One asked, "Is she always going to have a weak spot with depression . . . or some kind of emotional weak spot now because of this?" Another man voiced similar concern, fearing the onset of menopause with its hormonal fluctuations. The men are sometimes frightened by the prospect of doing something that will precipitate another depressive episode and continue to expect, and accept, less than the full partnership or happiness once experienced in the relationship. Plans for other children were sometimes abandoned because of fear of a recurrence of PPD.

Postpartum Depression: A Real Thing—A Crisis

Participants in the study described other people's lack of understanding of PPD. Often, the woman had confided to her physician, midwife, or nurse that something was wrong at the onset of her symptoms. If that did not yield a helpful response, the man tended to look for help elsewhere in his attempt to "fix the problem." More than 50% of the men reported that health care professionals and others tended to minimize the problem. In some cases, the failure of health care professionals to respond resulted in the couple trying to conceal the problem from anyone else, fearing that no one would understand. "I felt like I was out there all on my own, without anybody to guide me, or anybody to talk to," said one of the men in the study. "There was no one that I could go to," he lamented. A second man stated, "People don't take it seriously. It's like having a terminal disease and . . . people [either do not understand] or they don't know enough about it . . . and I'm talking nationwide." "Depression is a real thing," a third man said. "It's not as her doctor said, 'It will pass . . . you'll go through and you'll get over it and you'll be fine.'" Participants were adamant that postpartum depression is a crisis, "an absolute illness," and one man served as spokesman for the group in expressing "hope that this project can make some changes or turn some people on to [PPD] and make it better known."

DISCUSSION AND CONCLUSIONS

Against the contextual background of their former loving marital relationship and the hopes and dreams regarding the impending birth of their child, fathers in this study described not only shattered dreams but irrevocably altered relationships with their mates. Thoughts of the future were clouded by uncertainty and fear of recurrent depression. As discussed in Chapter 6, one of the three dominant themes in the human experience of other people is relationship synchrony/asynchrony. Participants in this study described a profound asynchrony and inability to relate to wives who had suddenly become distant strangers. Depressed wives were cold and rejecting toward their husbands and unable to nurture their babies. Husbands described many losses: loss of intimacy, loss of the relationship once shared, and finally loss of control. Committed to their wives and determined to hold the family together, they made incredible sacrifices. However, when they were unable to "fix" the problem despite heroic efforts, their world collapsed. The behavior of wives prone to unpredictable hysteria and suicidal impulses had brought about a crisis situation.

IMPLICATIONS OF THE STUDY FINDINGS
FOR NURSING PRACTICE

Childbirth is itself a crisis or a turning point for couples. Even in the absence of postpartum depression, alteration in marital relationships is common after the birth of a child (Boyce, 1994; O'Hara, 1995). Under usual circumstances couples are able to rely on each other for assistance and support following childbirth. In PPD, this is not the case. Fathers in this study described being alone and in a nonreciprocal relationship with their mate. Often, the father felt he had no one to whom he could turn. The lack of support from his wife—the person upon whom he customarily relied—greatly impacted his adaptation to parenthood and reestablishment of the marital relationship following the crisis of childbirth.

Clearly, the presence of PPD adds tremendous strain to the already-stressful postpartum period. Fathers in this situation need additional support in order to cope. Because PPD has not consistently been viewed as a serious complication by health professionals, few early interventions are in place. Expectant couples should receive information about PPD in prenatal classes or prior to hospital discharge and should be given advice about what steps to take if they encounter it. Some participants in this study had never heard of PPD and had no idea what has happening to their mates. When screening, nurses should be aware of factors that may predispose the couple to PPD such as being very young, lacking family support, or previous depressions following delivery. Prenatal teaching should be reinforced by providing both verbal and written information about PPD at the time of discharge. Follow-up telephone calls from nurses, home visits, or hotlines could be especially helpful to young couples who have little or no family support and could serve to screen for early symptoms of PPD and minimize its impact.

Most of the men in this study indicated that they suffered in silence for fear of what others might think. Because some stigma is attached to PPD, both obstetric and pediatric health care professionals must be sensitive to the signs and symptoms. PPD may be greatly underdiagnosed. This study of husbands revealed that pervasive changes in a couple's relationship occur and can be extremely troubling to the husband. Timely referral and treatment can prevent parenting problems and potentially save a marriage. Fathers must be included in screening, education, counseling, and treatment of PPD. Husbands in this study suffered along with their depressed wives. A support group for men whose spouses have PPD could help new fathers in the midst of this crisis. Many participants in this study expressed a willingness to share their experiences and offer support to others.

POST-STUDY REFLECTIONS FROM MOLLY MEIGHAN

As an experienced maternal-child nurse, I was aware of the signs and symptoms of postpartum depression, and I had a great deal of sympathy for women experiencing the phenomenon. I was unaware, however, of its dramatic impact on their husbands. Fathers in this study expressed helplessness, frustration, and personal loss. I learned how painful PPD can be for a new father, and I became much more aware of the emotional impact of childbirth on fathers, even when the birth process and postpartum transition is considered normal. Conducting this study made me realize the importance of including fathers in the care provided for mothers and infants, and it led me to do my doctoral dissertation research on fathers (Meighan, 1998). Now, I make more effort to consider the father as well as the mother in all my practice settings.

Doing a phenomenological study changed my approach to clients and their families as well as to students. The study sensitized me to the importance of listening to people's stories about the life events they face. It made me realize that the act of listening is therapeutic in itself. It is an essential part of the dialogue between client and nurse. Participating in phenomenological research has heightened my awareness of the meaning of an event for clients and their families. Now, I encourage people to tell me how they feel, and I am able to act more on their feelings rather than applying my own inferences. With my students, I find that listening first not only facilitates communication but also provides a starting point for learning.

IV

Nursing and the Human Experience of Time

The Time Being

A man coming forward
leaves a hole in time
He cannot see any more
than the hole in space
where he just was.
He can pivot, flex,
bend, reach, spin,
chase himself in circles,
and never see it.
He leaves it all behind,
the print of the face,
the work of the hands,
the mark of the nerves,
like a trail of coins
dropped for someone else
to collect or spend.
He peels the past forward,
rips the future back.

He is a wedge in space,
his life a wedge in time.
He moves at angles
to everything
splits time
into the geometry of dance.
His sweat
has the smell of forever.
Too much energy
to stay quiet
on any surface,
he reaches up, and out,
to eat the stars.
For him
the sun is gold,
the moon is silver,
the earth is round
and worth saving.

—John Calvin Rezmerski
Reprinted from *An American Gallery*, Three Rivers Press, 1977.
Used by permission of the author.

10

The Human Experience of Time

A nursing student has two classes on Monday morning. The first class runs from 9:00 A.M. to 9:50 A.M. and the second from 10:00 to 10:50 A.M. The student enjoys the first class but dislikes the second one. Although it may seem odd, since both classes are 50 minutes long, it will come as no surprise that the student perceives the second class as much longer than the first. We may smile and shake our heads in recognition of a similar experience because psychological time is often out of synchrony with clock time. We all remember waiting in line for 45 minutes to get tickets to a two-hour concert that went by much faster than the wait. Likewise, if our team is losing by only a few points, the last two minutes of the game go a lot faster than if our team is winning when the game seems never to end.

A different situation in which clock time and lived time are relatively distinct concerns the experience of some hospitalized patients. The specific patient we have in mind is sitting outside an x-ray room in 1960 waiting for the test that will indicate the progress of his tuberculosis. In the following excerpt, the patient is speaking to someone sitting next to him:

> You know, I was supposed to get this x-ray five days ago, but somebody slipped up. You have to keep after these people or else they forget all about you. When there is a delay in your x-ray once, it's passed along to the next time, and so on. It means you get out of this damn place that much later. Every day an x-ray is delayed is another day of your life (Roth, 1963, p. xv).

For this patient (who is in no sense atypical), being in a hospital is experienced as "doing time," and the patient wants to know when it will end. Because there are no precise markings in this situation, patients deal with uncertainty by structuring their time on the basis of a series of what Roth (1963) called benchmarks. Some of these are formal such as a change in the person's health category; others are informal such as getting the first pass to the exercise room. By means of both kinds of benchmarks, the course of a hospital stay is carefully monitored by the patient and indicates whether progress is, or is not, being made. Benchmarks serve not only to mark out progress toward a goal but also to segment time into manageable units. If the present is frightening or uncertain, one way to make it manageable is to develop norms that enable you to evaluate progress toward a better time.

In other contexts we use different markers. Although birthdays take place each year, some seem more important than others. We manage to make a big deal out of being 13, 16, 18, 21, 30, 40, 50, and 65. Thirteen is important because the child becomes a teenager; 16 because you can drive a car in some states; 18 because you're really an adult; 30 because you can't be trusted anymore; 40 because you get to do one more stupid thing before you enter middle age; 50 because you're a half a century old; and 65 because many employers say you have to retire. There is no simple way to organize this collection of important ages. Some have to do with numbers (10, 50), others with legal matters (18, 21), and still others with the end of one phase in a life and the beginning of another (13, 65).

In passing from one phase of a life to the next, some societies have special rites. In our society the retiring employee (age 65) has this occasion noted with a check and a gold watch. The 13-year old Jewish child gets a public celebration and a fountain pen. Not all significant changes in a life, however, are as publicly marked. For this reason, we often commemorate personally significant events with anniversaries or family observances. In the case of marriage, not only do we celebrate the yearly date of the wedding but also we single out 10, 25, and 50 years of marriage as having special significance.

Clearly defined units also mark a student's progress through various educational institutions. We divide learning into elementary school, junior high school, high school, college, and, for the particularly masochistic, graduate school. Each phase has its own subdivisions, some simply marked by a number—third grade—and others by a change in status—freshman to senior. Finishing college (and later graduate school) is also marked by a formal change in status: Jane Doe, BSN, MSN, PhD.

Professional careers are also marked in this way. Here, success is usually correlated with age and experience. Although college instructors usually do not achieve the rank of professor before 45 or 50, a number of extraordinary scholars have been promoted to full professor at age 25 or so. In the military, enlisted personnel have their time marked out from private to sergeant, while officers have their time marked out from lieutenant to general. Not every member of the professorate or the military reaches the highest rank; even so, everyone has some expectation to advance to a higher level after some time. Progression in rank is not directly related to chronological age; an outstanding achievement in research or battle may speed up a promotion, while a crowded field may slow one down.

Although benchmarks structure progress toward a goal, some situations do not allow for such orderly marking. One example in which clock time and lived time were widely discrepant was described by the French psychologist Paul Fraisse (1963) and concerned an accident in which three brothers were buried in a mine shaft under the rubble of an earthquake for 18 days. When they emerged from the shaft, the brothers spontaneously volunteered that they were glad to be out after "four or five days." Needless to say, they were extremely surprised to learn they had been buried for 18 days. In car accidents, clock and personal time are also out of synchrony. Although some individuals report time speeds up during the accident, the more usual experience is that everything, the car included, moves more slowly.

TIME AND PERSONAL CHANGE

These experiences all involve physical events that are external to us. What about cases that involve changes inside us? Here we need only think of the ways in which time is experienced in states of consciousness induced by drugs, alcohol, hypnosis, meditation, marijuana, and so on. Under the influence of some of these substances (alcohol), time is regularly experienced as speeding up; under the influence of others (meditation), time is perceived as slowing down. An early investigator of mescaline (Ludwig, 1966) found that one of its major properties was a "distorted time sense": clock time can be speeded up, slowed down, reversed, or made irrelevant. Occasionally, the same episode exhibits two, three, or all four possibilities.

A person's age also affects the perception of clock or calendar time. The usual experience is that time passes more slowly for children than for adults. Even at age 20 or 25 we sense that the six years it took to get through high school and the first two years of college went by much more quickly than the first six years of elementary school. As long ago as 1890, William James noted that the same duration of clock time invariably seemed shorter when the person was older. The speed with which time passes continues to accelerate, so that parents do not exaggerate when they tell their children "it seems like only yesterday that you were a little child."

Many explanations have been proposed to account for this phenomenon. Pierre Janet (1877) thought it was a ratio effect: 6 years of 12 is a larger proportion than 6 of 25. James (1890) explained it in terms of vividness. In youth, events are vivid and exciting; hence, everything has more detail as the person lingers over each event. Lecomte du Nouy (1936), drawing on the fact that physical wounds heal much more rapidly in infancy and childhood than in old age, suggested that we need more time when older to do the same work; hence, six years for the child amounts to more time, biologically and psychologically, than six years for the adult.

Not only our experiences of time's passage are affected by age; so too is our understanding of time. An early example of the infant's understanding of time occurs at around four months of age. At this time, most infants will look for absent objects but not for too long. At about six months of age, most infants will look at the location where mother was last seen, whereas at a year they will not search in two different places for an object previously found in one of them. Between 18 and 24 months, not only do infants search for absent objects persistently but they also begin using words referring to time. The earliest words are "now" (18 months), "sometime" (24 months), "tomorrow" (30 months), and "yesterday" (36 months) (Ames, 1946). The overall progress of these achievements suggests that the first thing an infant learns is that there is constancy to people and things; more formal meanings of time begin with the *present*, which is different from *sometime*, and then go on to include the *future* and then the *past*.

Another way of looking at the child's ability to "talk time" concerns grammatical terms. From a careful examination of children's conversations, Cromer (1968) noted a strong increase in the child's command of tense at around four years of age (from 4.0 to 4.6). It was at this point, for example, that one of his children began to use different time references in the same utterances: "I will show you what I got for Christmas" (age 4.6). Even more significant are reversals, that is, sentences in which time references are not in the same order in which they were experienced. In the Christmas sentence quoted above, the child mentioned what she is going to do (future) before mentioning what happened some time ago (past). All in all, the child's sense of time (as reflected in language) takes a good-sized jump in the fourth year. Even though tense is not always used correctly, the child can talk about imagined as well as real events. Children of this age can even combine tenses in the same statement. Taking these findings in combination with those regarding vocabulary development, we can conclude that time becomes increasingly significant to the child between four and five years of age.

When and how do children learn to tell time? Here, a set of early studies by Springer (1951, 1952) is still quite instructive. In the first of these studies, children ranging in age from four to six were asked to draw a clock (remember, this is before digital time pieces). About 41% of the four-year-olds did not know what clocks looked like and only 11% knew at age five. In a second study, children were asked "Why does a clock have two hands?" For the answer "One is for minutes, one is for hours" the values were 0%, 8%, and 10% for children aged four, five, and six, respectively. Taking into account other answers that were almost as good (for example, "one for hours, one for 2:30, 4:15" or "you need two hands to tell time"), the values rose to 9%, 31%, and 58%, respectively. Other answers produced by four-year-olds included: "One to go to one place, one to go to another place," "To pass the numbers by," and "God thought it would be a good idea."

Children do not know how to deal with the calendar early in life. Although there has been no single, large-scale analysis of this topic, there have been some fairly well-documented anecdotes. Werner (1948) reported that many children believe calendars "make" time, and that if you rip off a calendar sheet you have lost the day. Katz and Katz (cited in Werner, 1948) asserted that, for children, calendars are useful not only to give the date but also significant in their own right: "Sunday is the day when the calendar is red" or "A weekday is when the number is black." Similarly, a six and a half-year-old boy was observed to say after tearing off June 30th, "Look, no more June bugs" (Scupin & Scupin, cited in Werner, 1948).

For the child, even one of five, six, or seven, time is not the continuous system adults understand it to be. It is much more personal, much more individual, much more discontinuous. Events are organized into personal meanings ("Snow equals winter," "June bugs go away on July 1"), and sequential events such as the seasons are not seen in any ordered relationship to one another. There seems to be no overall concept of time for the young child, only the experience of a highly personal time organized in a unique way. One of the best illustrations of the difference between a "personal" and an "abstract" sense of time is given in the following observations. Sturt, in 1925, asked children ages 4 through 10 two questions: What time is it for your mother at home now? and What time is it in another nearby city? At age four, 50% of the children answered the first question correctly, while only 14% answered the second correctly. Even by age 10, when all children answered the first question correctly, 14% still did not answer the second question correctly.

For small and not-so-small children, the idea of time is not an easy one to grasp. Research suggests two critical ages at which the child comes to handle time and concepts of time: the first occurs between four and five, the second between 11 and 13. Although four- and five-year-old children begin to use time words, the idea of time as a system is still well beyond their ken. The ability to redefine time from personal to abstract occurs at around age 11. Only at this age does the child understand that seasonal change is cyclic, that years form a continuous series, and that different locales have one and the same time. Time, as a fact in the child's life, has clearly moved from a strictly personal event to one of more general significance, and everyone is now understood to live within the same system of temporal reference.

DISORIENTATION IN TIME

But we are not always able to use the clock (or calendar) to organize our lives. Sometimes, when we are confused, we have a great deal of difficulty in regard to time. A person being tested by a nurse for admission to a psychiatric unit must correctly identify the day, date, hour, and year. If the person is unable to answer one or more of these questions correctly—that is, if he or she shows disorientation in time—the nurse may recommend admission to the hospital.

Some patients exhibit much more profound disorientation in and about time. To appreciate what such temporal disorientation is like, we must examine it in clearly defined styles of abnormal behavior such as occur in mania or depression. Slowness of movement and speech are prominent aspects of the clinical picture of a severely depressed person. Patients often sit in one place with folded hands, unable to summon the energy to perform even the simplest tasks. If questioned, they speak slowly, in a low tone, and with great economy of words. Ideas do not come readily to mind, and problem-solving seems impossible. The manic, in contrast, shows an incredible excess of frenetic activity. Outstanding among these is talking, which never seems to stop. For short periods, such talk may seem coherent, although change from topic to topic takes place constantly. Patients with mania also are quite distractible. Whatever they see or hear may divert their attention completely.

How is time experienced by the depressed individual? Here are the words of one patient: "The hands of the clock move blankly, the clock ticks emptily . . . they are the lost hours of the years when I could not work. . . . The world is of a piece and cannot go forward or backward . . . this is my great anxiety, I have lost time" (Jaspers, 1968, p. 84). Time, for this patient, existed only in the past; the present never seemed to move forward toward the future. The patient behaved as if he did not want time to go on—as if, for him, the future was totally closed down. Not only the future, however, is at issue. There may be similar disorientation in regard to past and present. The clinically depressed patient experiences the past and present in a way that can be summed up best by a patient who said, "There is no beginning and no end to things" (Straus, 1947, 1964). Events that happened this morning are forgotten, and yesterday's events are as remote as those of years ago. The basic structure of time has broken down, and the patient can find no place for himself in the void of this formless structure.

But how did this come about? Why is the depressive lost in time without the familiar landmarks known to us all? According to Straus (1947), in severe depression the person no longer experiences any possibility of becoming. The depressed person is at a standstill and any projection into the now-empty future is impossible. We might therefore expect the depressed patient to be thrown back on the past; yet, here there is no refuge, for it was in the past that the person lost his way. The depressive patient is trapped: if bad things were done or good things left undone in the past, then some punishment must await in the future. The past—done or undone—is an area of failure that can be set right only by punishment. As one patient envisioned: "I will be condemned to live covered with vermin, in a cage with wild beasts, with rats in the sewer until I die. The whole world knows of my crimes and knows that punishment awaits me" (Minkowski, 1970, p. 180).

Like the depressive, the manic also has lost contact with the past and the future; all that now exists is the present (Fraisse, 1963, p. 184). Although being able to live fully in the present is a good and healthy way to be, the manic lives in a present torn out of the usual fabric of time. It is an "instantaneous present;" it has no location in "before" and no projections into "after." What the manic patient lacks is an "unfolding" in time, a sensible location in the flow of things. Both the manic and the depressive have lost their rootedness in time. The sense of order and security that an integrated experience of time provides is missing.

These results, scientific and clinical, indicate significant differences between personal experiences of time and the measurement of time by clocks. In general, the tendency is to be surprised that personal experience is so out of synchrony with clock time. Underlying this way of thinking is an unsaid belief that clock time is more "real" than its psychological counterpart. Is it not just a little odd that we never consider it the other way around, that clock time is so out of synchrony with temporal experiences of everyday life? Measuring something always seems to make it more significant than living it.

TIME AS A SYSTEM IN ADULT LIFE

The clock, including all of the units that derive from it, ranging from pico-seconds to millennia, is not the only way human beings are aware of time—at least in Western culture. There is also the calendar, and much may be learned about the systemic meaning of time by considering the structure of the calendar. On most calendars, each month has its own name and the year at the top, a series of seven day-names just underneath, and a set of 28 to 31 numbers usually arranged in rows and columns so that each number is lined up with a specific day of the week. If we move to the next page, a similar arrangement is noted, with two exceptions: the name of the month changes and (usually) there are changes in specific pairing of days and dates. Over the course of a calendar year, similar changes take place until January, at which time the year number changes. Unlike the days of the week and the months of the year, this number never comes back—once it changes from 2002 to 2003, 2002 will never again appear except on an "out-dated" calendar.

The impression conveyed by calendars is that time is both repetitive (months, days, seasons) and non-repetitive (years). These two properties suggest that time may be described either as a repeating circle or as an open-ended line, and these two properties give rise to two different types of temporal systems: a circular (or closed) one and a linear (or open) one. Although Western culture attempts to capture aspects of both in its calendar, it is clear that cyclic events are subordinate to the linear pattern.

Not all cultures choose the "openness" of an open system. If a culture prefers the regularity of a cyclic system, "accurate" records of time and age are rarely kept, and no one is ever early or late for an appointment. Obviously, our Western world could not exist without the order and structure provided by a linear time system composed of equal units. The price for such precision is that we often feel coerced by time (what nurse doesn't know where she or he is supposed to be every minute of the shift?), and we are left with an uncomfortable concern for the "beginning" and "end" of time. It is here that two social institutions—religion and science—move in to provide their separate answers. Whether we consider Big Bangs, Genesis, or Armageddon as the preferred understanding, it remains true that both hypotheses are necessitated by an open, or linear, system of time.

One consequence of a linear system of time—and one that applies with less significance in more cyclic systems of time—is the idea of a past, a present, and a future. While clock and calendar time quantify past, present, and future in quite specific numerical terms, other cultures may express similar phenomena in terms of the vividness of an event (see Whorf, 1956, for a description of time concepts in certain Native-American cultures). In the English language, we frequently capture experiences of time by the use of two different verbs: "flows" and "passes." Whenever time is said to "flow," it is assumed to be a moving substance, such as a river, that flows with us from past to future. According to this conceptualization of time, the past anticipates the future and allows us to predict some future present. In domains such as "scientific" prediction, we are able to do an extremely accurate job; in other domains, such as history or the stock market, precise predictions are seldom possible.

When time is said to "pass," it is thought to go from some source in the future and pass by us in the present. In fact, Heidegger (1927/1962) suggested that time can only be experienced "as future lapses into past by coming into present." Unlike scientific or historical time, the future retrospectively defines what will be seen as significant in the past, not vice versa. A final piece to Heidegger's approach to the meaning of time is his contention that the only certainty I have of the future is that I will die there. Only by accepting death, not as an abstract possibility that happens to other people but as *my* death ("I will die"), does it become possible for me to face and claim my life as a being-toward-death in which my accomplishments (past) and projects (future) reveal themselves as uniquely mine.

Gadamer (1966) has noted that it is sometimes difficult to see how the future and past influence each other in a non-causal way. In discussing this issue, he asserts that "there can be no doubt that the great horizon of the past . . . influences us in every-thing we want, hope for, or fear *in the future*. History is only present to us in light of our futurity" (pp. 8–9). What Gadamer suggests is that the future continuously makes relevant what is significant about our past and our present. It is not that the past con-trols the future (as scientific thinking has it), but that the future continuously reorga-nizes which aspect of the past is relevant. Hence, our projects are as important as our history and serve to select what now shapes us from the past. Becoming is more impor-tant than having been.

A different view of time is presented by Merleau-Ponty (1962) who is considerably more concerned with the way in which we experience time. Time, in our direct expe-rience, is not a system of objective positions through which we pass but a mobile set-ting that moves toward and away from us. The key concept here is what he calls the "bursting forth" of time—by analogy with a flowering plant bursting from its pod. In using this metaphor, Merleau-Ponty means to point out that it is only in the present that consciousness and time coincide. While it is true that we can grasp time through thinking about the past or in some expectation of the future, it is also true that we only do so in some present situation. Unlike Heidegger, death does not assume a critical role for Merleau-Ponty; in fact, at one point he says, "I live then, not in order to die, but forever;" in this quote, "forever" means in some present situation in this world. Just as our experiences of an object depend on the specific perspectives from which we view it, so too do experiences of time involve constantly changing perspectives between us and the specific aspects of time we experience. Because we are always in some present situation, events experienced as relating to time constantly change our relationship to what went before and what is to come. The present is the point on which past, future, and present turn; it is that moment in which we glimpse time past and time future as these emerge in time present.

THEMES IN THE HUMAN EXPERIENCE OF TIME: FINDINGS FROM PHENOMENOLOGICAL RESEARCH

As we have seen, Merleau-Ponty contended that the human experience of time depends upon moments that burst forth, uniquely revealing time to the person. It was largely for this reason that Marilyn Dapkus (1985) asked 20 adult participants to "think about an experience . . . when you were particularly aware of time," and then used these answers to develop a thematic description of what time means to contemporary adults. The average age of her participants was 43, and the majority were college-educated. Half were men, half women. On the basis of her interviews, Dapkus concluded that there were four interrelated meanings to the human experience of time: **Change and Continuity, Limits and Choices, Now or Never,** and **Fast and Slow.**

Themes of the Human Experience of Time

The first of these four themes, **Change and Continuity**, is meant to capture experiences of things changing yet remaining the same. On a personal level, this theme concerns being particularly attuned to changes in one's friends, children, and parents. As one participant put it: "Since I've had children, I've been more aware of time because you see them grow up; you see them change from year to year. My daughter—who I can look to eyeball-to-eyeball now—it seemed like yesterday I was cradling her in my arms."

The second major theme, **Limits and Choices**, is meant to capture the experience of doing things in time; in doing things, we make choices and accept limits. Most participants experienced themselves as not having enough time to do everything they wanted to do. One participant noted: "I'm most aware of time at work—not having enough time to do everything, and to do everything well, and that's a real frustration. I make lists of things I need to do . . . and if I get interrupted, . . . I get tense and frustrated 'cause I feel I'm not doing as good a job as I should."

The third theme, **Now or Never**, represents an attempt to capture our most basic experience of time, going after things we want or feel we need in life. This theme relates to our earliest experiences of time and an urgency to get what we want, lest we never get it. One dieting participant noted, "I'm very aware of time—time has gone very, very slowly—on diets, in the past. When you're waiting from meal to meal, living for the moment you eat the next time, time seems to drag."

The final theme, **Fast and Slow**, pertains to experiences of tempo. This theme emerged as a thread that ran through each of the other themes and describes the rate at which events take place. One participant noted: "I'm afraid that as I get older, time will seem like it's running away, going faster, getting away from me faster than I want it to."

Speaking about their experiences of time seemed to lead most participants to touch on its larger role in their lives and of the role of death in providing a structure to their lives: "Since my father's death, I'm more aware that time has a limit . . . I still tend to think that I have many more years, which is probably why I'm not motivated to make some changes now. A person diagnosed as having a terminal disease will immediately set some new priorities, make some changes. If you're not hit over the head, it's easy to keep doing it the old way."

The issue of death, consistent with Heidegger's view, seems to bring about a different understanding of time. As some of the older study participants noted, time becomes a precious possession, especially when they become aware of a dwindling supply. When this happens, the object of our experience becomes time itself. Milestones such as midlife crises, retirement, and the death of parents, among others, promote a greater awareness of how we have spent the hours of our lives and of what is yet to come. Awareness of death is often a catalyst for re-examining the choices already made in life and for deciding anew what we will try to do with the time remaining. In the following chapters, we examine first-person accounts of disruptive events that broke into the ordinary flow of time. Patients who faced death and struggled to recover from severe psychological and/or physical health crises tell us their stories and, in so doing, fill in some of the specific details concerning the experience of time when we are either just past or in the midst of life-threatening situations.

11*

"One Day You're Working and the Next Day You're an Invalid": Recovering After a Stroke

"And sometimes they don't understand, you know . . . they don't understand stroke or don't understand aphasia. . . . And and so, so, and also I guess, 'cause I talk but I can't, so I say, you know, 'Forget it, I'll go sit in my room' or whatever. And it's, that is hard I think because lonely, you know?"

—an aphasic stroke survivor interviewed for the present study

Stroke is a common cause of disability, with an annual incidence in the United States of 500,000 and a prevalence of approximately 3,000,000 (Noll & Roth, 1994; Sacco, 1995). Stroke is most common in older individuals (73% of strokes occurring in those 65 years or older), and, as the population is aging, the incidence is not likely to decline (Kuhlemeier & Stiens, 1994). Of those who survive their stroke, 40% have a mild disability and 40% have a moderate to severe disability (Cifu & Lorish, 1994). Most survivors have comorbidities such as hypertension, diabetes, and cardiac disease (Sacco, 1995). Neurological improvements following a stroke may continue for up to a year, but the rate of change after six months is limited, and improvement in cognitive function is less likely after three months (Gresham et al., 1995). Not surprisingly, stroke survivors heavily populate American rehabilitation units where nurses have an essential role in the rehabilitation process. In such units, the articulated goal is improving patients' quality of life (QOL). In reality, the focus is on impairments resulting from the stroke, and most treatment goals concern functional outcomes. Thus,

* This chapter is based on a doctoral dissertation, "Quality of Life Following Stroke: The Survivors' Perspective," by Janet A. Secrest, the University of Tennessee, Knoxville, 1997. An earlier report of this research appeared in *Rehabilitation Nursing*, 1999, Vol.24, No. 6, pp. 240–246. Reprinted by permission of the Association of Rehabilitation Nurses, Glenview, IL.

quality of a stroke survivor's life is seemingly equated with improved functional outcomes. This value is reflected in the many studies with functional outcomes as the criteria for success of rehabilitation. It is questionable, however, whether such outcomes are suitable as measures for the patients' quality of life. QOL measurements invoke predetermined categories or dimensions that cannot adequately capture what the quality of life is for individual stroke survivors. The determination of quality of life "should be left to the competent patients themselves" according to Hayry (1991).

RELATED LITERATURE

Doolittle (1990) conducted an ethnographic study demonstrating the inadequacy of present views of stroke recovery. While the patients viewed recovery as the ability to return to previously valued activities, i.e., meaningful activities that "gave them identity" (p. 238), their care providers valued the aforementioned functional abilities. Goals of care providers took precedence over those of patients. Study participants perceived care providers to be focused on neurological impairments, and not on their experience, thereby suggesting that empathy for the patients' total experience was lacking.

In a study of problems faced by stroke survivors following a course of inpatient rehabilitation, nearly half reported being dissatisfied because there was insufficient consideration of their prestroke lifestyle and "real goals" (Davidson & Young, 1985). Among participant comments were the following: "did not have enough say about when and where I did things" (p. 126) and "I never did that before the stroke and I certainly don't want to do it now, so why did I have to learn how?" (p. 127). These findings indicate that perceptions of needs were incongruent between provider and patient.

That QOL following stroke involves more than just functional abilities was also demonstrated by DeHaan, Horn, Limburg, Van Der Meulen, and Bossuyt (1993) who correlated stroke severity with disability, handicap, and QOL. Although there were high correlations among stroke severity, disability, and handicap, correlations were low with respect to quality of life. In addition, Ahlsio, Britton, Murray and Theorell (1984) found that even with a significant improvement in activities of daily living (ADL), an indicator of functional outcomes, an individual's quality of life did not necessarily improve. The latter finding, in a sample with a mean age of 71.9, was replicated in a younger sample of stroke survivors (mean age 48) by Niemi, Laaksonen, Kotila, & Waltimo (1988). "Good recovery in terms of discharge from the hospital, ADL, and return to work" (p. 1105) did *not* restore an individual's QOL.

The effects of stroke extend beyond physical limitations. Depression is a very common consequence (Dromerick & Reding, 1994), and emotional instability, in which the person cries easily in response to discussions of sad situations, is seen in as many as 21% of survivors (Sandin, Cifu, & Noll, 1994). In one study of stroke survivors, depression was the strongest predictor of QOL, whereas functional status was a weak predictor (King, 1990). There is some debate in the literature as to whether the psychological consequences of stroke are a direct result of the lesions or a reaction to them.

Because the lives of stroke victims have been profoundly disrupted, it is understandable that hospital and rehabilitation unit personnel set initial treatment goals. Stroke survivors may not be able to participate fully in this process in the early days following the ischemia or hemorrhage. But on what do nurses and other providers base their guidance of the recovery process? Studies have provided information on particular aspects of stroke survivors' lives, but this information is decontextualized and compartmentalized. A sense of the whole person in his or her context is missing. Without a fuller understanding of survivors' experiences, it is difficult for nurses to have an empathic understanding of what lies ahead. Thus, guidance provided to stroke survivors derives from the nurses' perspective—which research indicates may be inadequate. The purpose of this study was to investigate the quality of life as experienced by stroke survivors themselves following rehabilitation. Survivors were invited to describe specific experiences which stood out for them since their strokes.

THE PRESENT PROGRAM OF RESEARCH

Fourteen stroke survivors (seven men, seven women) were recruited through personal contacts and "snowballing," in which participants referred others. The criteria for an individual's inclusion in the sample were: (1) willing and able to articulate the experience; (2) had been hospitalized for a primary diagnosis of stroke; (3) had completed inpatient rehabilitation; and (4) at least six months from time of stroke. Participants ranged in age from 40 to 93; length of time since the stroke ranged from nine months to 23 years. The majority of participants had suffered a left hemisphere stroke (10 of the 14). One reported a right hemisphere stroke, and three participants' strokes occurred in either the brainstem or cerebellum. All lived at home, 10 with spouses and four living alone. Although most had achieved independence in activities of daily living, all still experienced neurological deficits at the time of the interview, with various combinations of aphasia, memory loss, hemiparesis/plegia, and sensory changes. Three of the participants had marked aphasia, using various strategies to convey their experiences to the researcher. These three made extensive use of gestures and repeated attempts to say words that were initially not understood by the researcher. Luke, in talking about his neighborhood and an assisted living center under construction, walked fingers over a coffee table to represent people, places, and relationships. Calvin was able to write some words he was unable to say. The researcher frequently sought clarification and consensual validation of her understanding of what was being communicated. Although the interview proved to be emotional for several participants, they seemed pleased to have been able to participate and thanked the researcher. One participant expressed some feelings of hopelessness and helplessness, although he denied suicidal thoughts at the time of the interview. He was under the supervision of a psychiatrist and taking antidepressants. He was advised to recontact his psychiatrist which, in a subsequent call, he indicated he had.

Bracketing Interview

The bracketing interview, conducted prior to beginning the study, revealed a number of surprises and revelations. Prior to the interview, I (Secrest) had matter-of-factly decided to study stroke survivors because I thought they would be an easy population to access for studying quality of life in people with neurological dysfunction. My background included 10 years of experience with neurologically impaired individuals, mainly in acute care with a neurosurgical population, although I had worked more recently in a rehabilitation unit. As the interview progressed, I remembered experiences with stroke survivors and with my own family that I'd forgotten. These were emotional experiences that I'd not ever fully explored. My choice of patient population clearly came from motivations other than convenience!

In my bracketing interview, the life of the stroke survivor was described in negative, bleak terms. For example, the stroke survivors whom I subsequently interviewed talked to me about experiences of being **in control/out of control**, but at the time of bracketing I saw only **out of control**. I was imagining that the survivors' quality of life was significantly and irrevocably diminished, characterized by profound losses and a foreclosure of future possibilities. I was extremely sad during the interview, crying at one point. The overlay of my negative perspective could have been a threat to the credibility of my study findings had I not had the assistance of the interpretive group in becoming aware of my own suppositions about quality of life after stroke.

FINDINGS

The world of a person who has had a stroke is experienced as one of **loss and effort**. This overall theme appears most directly to the stroke survivor in terms of **connection and disconnection with others, independence-ability and dependence-disability,** and feelings of being **in or out of control** in certain aspects of life. The stroke survivor experiences a **continuity of self over time**, while simultaneously experiencing a **discontinuity of self**. The person is both the same and not the same as before the stroke. While each theme will be described separately, all are interrelated. Time, others, and the importance of present situational contexts modulate the meaning of the experience for the stroke survivor.

Loss/Effort

Loss and effort are inextricably connected and permeate each of the other themes: loss/effort of control, loss/effort of independence, loss/effort of connections with others, and loss/effort in the continuity and discontinuity of the self. **Loss** is described in terms of many experiences, with different meanings for participants. Over half the participants described a loss of memory: "I used to remember streets . . . but certain streets and stuff I can't remember" "I can't remember places and dates as quick." An emotional quality to loss weaves through several of the interview transcripts. For Mary, "it hurts to not be able to remember." Loss is sometimes expressed in terms of what has been regained. Luke says of his speech, "at first, nothing" but gradually, "better, better, better." Rob gives a clear, vivid description of a time when he grieved his losses:

> It was probably a full year after my stroke that [wife] and I were riding home one day in the early fall in [mountains], that I looked out [at the] really sunny day, a fall day. The colors were out and bright. I looked over at the mountains there, and I realized for the first time that I could no longer walk those mountains. And that got to me and still does. And I started weeping that day and finally had to pull over and let her drive and continued for about three hours crying, just grieving, and . . . letting those emotions out.

Accommodation to losses involves **effort**, and the effortfulness of everyday life is echoed throughout the transcripts. Effort was felt in the interviews as participants struggled to move about, find words, or recall events. For many, the unreflected, taken-for-granted way of being in the world now becomes a conscious effort. Rob, left-handed before his stroke, had to learn to use his right hand to write with. Walking was "real hard work" for Nell. Mary had to expend considerable effort to relearn street names in order to resume her sales business. Rose, whom you met in Chapter 1, provided many examples of efforts to accommodate her losses, including innovative modifications in once-simple kitchen tasks such as chopping okra and making jello:

> I make jello and I couldn't get it from the sink to the refrigerator without spilling it. So I'd put the dish—you know I had put it in a big dish—and put the dish in the refrigerator, then going to pour it in the refrigerator, you know, in the dish. So there's several ways of doing things.

In Control/Out of Control

The sense of being in or out of control emerged in many experiences across transcripts. The first thing that stood out to Harry was a specific time when he was **out of control**. One of his early experiences with his scooter, a means of greater independence, resulted in a frightening accident when a neighborhood dog "came after me and I was trying to get away and I turned over on the scooter." The stroke itself was seen by several participants as something over which they had no control. The bewildering and sudden loss of control at the time of the stroke was described by one woman as "[It] just hit me like lightning." Julie was particularly bewildered since she had always taken good care of herself to minimize (control) health risks: "I didn't know what happened. But I have never had high blood pressure, I've always eaten right, kept my weight under control, so a stroke was the furthest thing from my mind. . . . It never entered my mind." For many of the stroke survivors, the unpredictability of their bodies was an aspect of being out of control. Instances of unpredictability also related to memory, emotions, and speech. Lack of control of speech included not only an inability to say something but also unacceptable profanity. As Bob related:

> I talk to him [8 year old son], but I use the wrong words. . . . I don't want to use them. I don't know why it does that. . . . I know not to use it and I've even caught myself in church saying it. And I know and still can't . . . and you try to stop it and it don't get stopped.

Another participant described a time when he became "shut down . . . when I say shut down, I mean I just can't think, I can't work, I can't function, I can't do things." He illustrated this with a story about a time his wife required medical attention and he was unable to fulfill his caretaking responsibilities as a husband and a man: "My mind shut down . . . it was kind of scary . . . you feel helpless . . . I was frozen, couldn't function. That makes you feel very vulnerable, especially with a man, I think." This man had once been responsible for a large dental practice.

Being out of control is experienced by some stroke survivors through a tempo that seems dysynchronous with those around them. Julie has to wait for her husband to do things for her, such as putting on her makeup or clearing the table, but she has no control over when and how he does these things. Mary loses control over her speech when her husband does not give her enough time: "It bothers him 'cause I'm not saying it right. But if he'd give me a little time, I'll correct myself."

As if to balance this loss of control, participants also spoke of experiences in which they were **in control**. These included mastering new skills, adapting old skills, and changing their environment. Nell keeps telephones in every room in addition to a cellular phone in her wheelchair. She uses plastic dishes, although she hates them, to avoid additional breakage. John exercises daily at the YMCA, determined to "beat this thing" through "hard work and perseverance." Howard, who has difficulty with numbers and money, always gives the cashier a twenty-dollar bill when getting gas for the car because that way he knows he will get change back.

The strategies used by participants to maintain control serve to enhance continuity with their pre-stroke selves. For example, Nell was always very involved with her family and friends. John was a hardworking engineer who solved problems. Maintaining control was important in the sense of continuity of themselves, while being out of control was a challenge to independence and relationships with others.

Connection with Others/Disconnection with Others

Connections with other people meant reciprocity, being with and understood by someone, and experiencing help from others. Relationships helped bridge the schism in the continuity of their lives. John plainly said, "The thing that kept me going was this contact with the other person . . . you have to have another person . . . you have to have another person to help you get through the first year anyway." For Nell, maintaining **connections** was paramount. Her entire interview focused on interactions with family and friends. While keeping multiple telephones reflects a strategy for control, it also ensures that she is always able to connect with others. During the interview, Rob emphasized his newfound, post-stroke connections with God and his second wife, which he described as part of a "fulfilled" and "satisfied" life, but these connections came at a cost of broken connections with his ex-wife, children, and brother. Harry's relationship with a young man in his neighborhood is one of reciprocity which gives him pleasure:

> One of my . . . favorite things to do, and always has been, is I like to fish. And I have found out that I'm still able to go fishing. As a matter of fact, another fellow that lives here in the subdivision . . . he also likes to fish. And I have a fishing boat and he doesn't have, so he comes down, and he'll get the boat in the water for us and things like that, which I'm not able to drive a vehicle . . . Unfortunately for him, his stepfather doesn't enjoy anything like that at all. And so I think he's trying to learn things from me. . . . And I think it's working out really well. . . . He's only an 18 year old fellow. So I'm three times his age. But the age difference doesn't seem to matter. We get along just fine. . . . If you don't catch anything it's still a good time to me. And I think he feels the same way about it. . . . I think it's working out well for both of us.

When connections are broken, the experience was described as particularly painful. Bob relates a sense of **disconnectedness** when he says, "I guess I want to be a part of somebody's life." His unpredictable profanity with his children and at church distances him from others ("makes things awful"), and his difficulty with memory interferes with relationships as well: "I will remember I played with him [son] or maybe I won't." Calvin's sense of disconnection with others is profound. His relationship with his wife is altered by fatigue, aphasia, and lack of sexual intimacy. He can't even remember friends' names, and he goes to bed at 8:30 P.M. instead of his usual 10 P.M. because he has difficulty understanding the television.

Aphasia isolates Luke from others. He speaks of his "lonely house" and neighbors who "don't understand stroke or don't understand aphasia or anything like that. And and so, so, and also I guess, 'cause I talk but I can't, so I say, you know, 'Forget it, I'll go sit in my room' or whatever. And it's, that is hard I think because lonely, you know. . . . It's, it's you know, like they try and help but they don't understand, you know?" For Luke, his computer is a "Godsend" (a term he mentions several times) because "just talk, me and computer and sometimes listen and talk and then back." With the computer, at least, he is able to achieve some symmetry in dialogue. He looks to the future for connections, imagining easy camaraderie in a community center for disabilities which is under construction.

Most of the participants related times when they have received help. However, connections with others are interfered with when the other person offers help that is experienced as unhelpful. Luke talks about the frustrations when he first came home after the stroke and his parents tried to help: "They try to help, but it's no good, 'cause I say 'Look, wait, how about you, say, slow down, hold and time out.'" Nell, describing a time when she was crying and couldn't stop, was told by her son, "Mother, it's nothing to cry about" and by her grandchildren, "Grandmother, we don't want to see you cry." For Mary, her husband's frequent correcting of her speech interferes with her sense of connectedness with him. Several times she expresses her irritation at his corrections but acknowledges her dependence upon him.

Stories were told of connectedness and disconnectedness with physicians, physical therapists, and other health care providers. Mary felt betrayed because she had never been told that a stroke could follow her cardiac bypass surgery: "They should tell people when they're going to operate on them that they may have a stroke or something." Julie's experience of rehabilitation was "terrible" in several respects: "I supposed to had therapy . . . the woman was supposed to be my head therapist wasn't even there. And they said I was so much percent bathtub ready. Couldn't get in and out. And I didn't know they even had a bathtub. So everything they did was wrong . . . [treating me] like an invalid or somebody lesser than a whole person. . . . I didn't feel that way myself. They made me feel that way." Harry felt information was withheld from him:

> But they told me I had reached a plateau and there really wasn't much else they could do at that time. So that's when they released me. . . . One thing I still don't—I really can't figure out for myself is why those people didn't tell me that I wasn't going to get any better. . . . I suppose the possibility that if they told people that, people might get into a depressed state over it. But on the other hand, the more I think about that, that doesn't make a heck of a lot of sense because sooner or later somebody's going to figure it out anyway—so, same boat . . . I just, I kind of felt like they held information from me that I had the right to know.

Independence-Ability/Dependence-Disability

Independence-ability and dependence-disability are considered here as different aspects of the same theme. Participants spoke in terms of what they could and could not do, thereby relating to their pre-stroke life and to the kind of person they were and are. Participants wanted to maintain independence. A loss of independence challenged their sense of themselves. The loss of ability to drive was particularly difficult, forcing them to depend on someone else to transport them for routine errands. Disability often became apparent through interaction with others: "She tells me I got the wrong number." "I don't even know what I'm saying. . . . My wife will begin to point out that I do that." Pride was evident in recitations of recent accomplishments such as doing housework, gardening, making a quilt, painting, cutting the grass, and making a three-layer cake.

What independence-ability meant to each participant was individual. Although Nell and Harry had similar physical limitations, the meanings for them were vastly different. To Nell, who was wheelchair bound, what was figural was her **ability** to manage her, albeit different, household. She adapted her routine to her changed abilities and did not find it bothersome to depend upon others' help with shopping and cleaning. Harry, on the other hand, found his **inability** to return to paid employment figural in feeling disabled. He was able to engage in many activities independently, but they were merely "things to keep occupied," a lesser substitute for what was really important to him.

Continuity and Discontinuity in the Experience of Self

The experience of self as continuous from the time before the stroke, while simultaneously discontinuous, was described by each study participant. This theme derives from the sense of sameness and disruption experienced in terms of the other themes. While all participants reported experiencing both aspects of this theme, some experienced more **continuity** than **discontinuity** whereas for others the reverse was true. The degree to which the various themes were figural indicates essentials aspects of the self for that individual; in other words, the themes serve to define the self. Mary's loss of ability to recite the scriptures was a distressing disruption in her sense of continuity. Howard's identity was integrally tied to his ability to work; for him, recovery meant returning to work. The longest passage in his interview concerned different jobs he had over the years and his increasing responsibilities. The inability to work left him feeling diminished. Rose experienced a profound disruption in her identity at the time of the stroke, which brought tears to her eyes as she described it three years later:

> One day you're working and the next day you're an invalid . . . you think you're through . . . you think you'll just never be a whole person again when you realize you're paralyzed . . . it was devastating. One day you're who I was, you know. You're in business . . . and you're a grandmother and a wife and you drive, you go anywhere you want to, write a check, buy groceries or whatever. And the next day you're flat in bed, helpless. . . . I couldn't do my hair properly, and being a beautician, that was degrading . . . and you're stuck in the hospital with a lot of depressed looking people. And you go to breakfast and they're sitting around, you know, depressing. And some of them have been in wrecks, with tubes in their nose and all this. It's not the atmosphere that you're used to. And you're one of them. That's the bad part.

Discontinuity in the experience of the body was frequently expressed by participants. Among the anomalies that they mentioned were numbness, loss of taste, and mistrust of the functioning of one's hand. Ida's vivid description comprised five pages of transcript. Eating was "like trying to swallow a bowling ball" and her entire left side felt like she had been "scalded." More than one participant said their brains did not work as well although some, like Sally, were adamant that "I still had my mind. I just couldn't think lots of times." Some of the changes were located in the natural flow, or continuity, of their lives: "I'm 72 years old . . . you don't expect that your golfing, you're golfer that you were before. Or dancer that you were before." "I've been awfully hard of hearing since [the stroke]. But I think I was beginning to have it anyway, hard of hearing, you know."

Some changes brought about by the stroke were viewed as beneficial. For example, Mary says that her pre-stroke life was a cycle of ups and downs in energy and emotion, but after the stroke, her life was on a more even keel. Another participant lost 60 pounds and became more extroverted. Rob felt that his stroke "set me free" from a bad marriage:

> [I had] a Damascus Road experience, like Paul did, going to Damascus. . . . I was radically saved, radically changed . . . for the first time, I think, really had hope in my life. And I guess the whole of my soul was filled up. . . . I don't have to be the macho man I used to be. I don't have to prove myself . . . and here I am today, 14 years later, living a life that is very satisfying.

While disruption was seen in all of the transcripts, so too was a sense of continuity: "I have always enjoyed cooking, so I fix dinner for all of us every night and it's ready when they get home." "I'm computer expertise . . . but this is, I can type and stuff like that." "I've always been kind of a knot head . . . pretty stubborn." Mary's sense of continuity was bridged to her post-stroke life through her ongoing relationship with her husband. Although correcting her speech sometimes breaks the connection between them, paradoxically it also maintains the continuity: "Oh honey, he's always told me what to do." Although unable to return to work, Harry was pleased that people from his place of employment still valued his expertise and called him at home to ask him questions.

The tension between experiencing a sense of personal continuity while at the same time a discontinuity was most poignantly expressed by Bob:

> You, you look around, see all you are to different people. And that's good. Then just turn around and you've lost part of what you are . . . and really you haven't lost it. We're the same people . . . yeah, you're not missing but you are. And I don't know how it is. Cause you—I just now notice but you, I don't know, it's hard, especially now. 'Cause I'm feel like I'm missing a bunch, but I'm not . . . I just hadn't really set down and thought out how that was different but is all same. It's, it kind of, it kind of different but all the same.

DISCUSSION AND CONCLUSIONS

While most previous studies have examined quality of life in stroke survivors from a purely mechanistic, functional perspective, the present study demonstrates that functional abilities have meaning only within the context of an individual life. Taken out of this context, it is not surprising that DeHaan et al. (1993) found only a weak correlation between QOL and stroke severity, disability, and handicap, although the latter three variables were highly intercorrelated. Similarly, it is not surprising that Ahlsio et al. (1984) found little improvement in QOL in stroke survivors whose functional abilities improved. The quality of one's life following stroke, as shown in the present study, depends upon a continuity in the sense of one's self over time.

Erikson (1980) views identity as a reassuring continuity in the face of change. The consequences of a stroke can disrupt the person's sense of control, connections with others, and independence-abilities. The degree to which these themes are figural to the person will influence his or her sense of continuity and discontinuity. The experience of both continuity and discontinuity was bewildering for some participants, as Bob's words so movingly expressed. The person who experienced the greatest discontinuity was Calvin whose stroke was most recent. He was fully functional in activities of daily living, but his speech and short-term memory were impaired, and he had altered body sensations. This so affected his sense of himself that he had considered suicide.

As noted in Chapter 3, Merleau-Ponty (1962) points to the difference between the lived body, or the first-person experience of it, and a third-person view of the body as an object. The experience of the body as lived is not separate from one's experience of self, and, as stroke survivors experience their bodies differently, it changes them. The rehabilitation view derives largely from a third-person perspective, in which the body (object) of the stroke survivor is either functional or nonfunctional. Bodies such as Julie's were termed "bathtub ready" in the way that you might speak of putting objects in a laundry. The rehabilitation emphasis is on "fixing" or adapting to the nonfunctional. While these adaptations may improve an individual's functional abilities, his or her sense of discontinuity may not be lessened.

A striking omission in participants' narratives was nursing care. Nurses were barely mentioned, although all participants had been hospitalized at some time during their stroke experience. Participants who did mention nurses described situations in which they felt estranged from the caregiver. Mary said it was a nurse who told her husband to correct her speech and this advice was apparently taken to heart by him, serving to break Mary's sense of connectedness with him. She also mentions briefly a nurse trying to remove sutures and the doctor taking over in a rough manner. The nurse apparently made no effort to intervene on her behalf when the doctor was rough. Beth recalled a time prior to the stroke when she was trying to leave the hospital after two weeks of studies about which she received no information from her doctor. She remembers a nurse with a clipboard demanding that she sign "against medical advice." In none of these instances did the participant report feeling supported by nurses.

Encounters in rehabilitation were figural for only three participants. Sally thought everything was "wonderful," but she was referring to camaraderie with the other patients. Rose initially thought that the physical therapists were "cruel" but came to understand "there's a reason." Julie thought going to rehabilitation was the worst mistake she ever made. Mistrust and betrayal were evident in some experiences with physicians. What seemed to be missing in participant accounts was an overall sense of connectedness with health care providers. Considering the amount of contact they had with professionals whose presumed intent is to support them, this finding is disturbing.

IMPLICATIONS OF THE STUDY FINDINGS FOR NURSING PRACTICE

The results of this study have a number of important implications for the role of nurses in rehabilitation of stroke survivors. While other disciplines involved in rehabilitation, such as physical therapy and occupational therapy, have clearly defined boundaries, the role for nurses has been less clear. In this study, nurses were not experienced as positive forces in rehabilitation. They did not connect in a meaningful way with these participants, and perhaps contributed to their sense of discontinuity by not understanding the individual meaning of the changes heralded by the stroke. The virtual absence of nurses in participants' narratives suggests, at best, a peripheral, if not invisible, role. Yet nursing, as one discipline having prolonged interaction with patients across a variety of acute care and community settings, has much to offer.

The current focus in rehabilitation often decontextualizes or disembodies the impairment from the person, thus neglecting the fundamental interrelatedness of human experience. All nursing theorists, from Nightingale forward, have emphasized holistic care of the person. Such an approach to care seems particularly important in rehabilitation where patients are learning how to reintegrate their lives after an often-catastrophic, life-changing event. Lydia Hall, a visionary nursing theorist and pioneer in rehabilitation, saw what nursing could bring to a person's rehabilitation experience. She brought her ideas of patient-centered care to life in the Loeb Center, a nurse-run rehabilitation unit in which nurses facilitated patient decisions and goals (Loose, 1994). Unfortunately, she has not received much attention in the last few decades and was not even mentioned in a recent review of nursing's role in rehabilitation (Kirkevold, 1997).

Hall's ideas are especially relevant today in a health care system which divides a patient's care among multiple specialties and facilities. Advanced practice nurses are in a position to cross health care boundaries in creative ways, following patients throughout the illness experience. In a study of individuals with chronic illness, being "known" by the caregiver, in this case nurses, fostered self-confidence (McWilliam, Stewart, Brown, Desai, & Coderre, 1996). Coming to know the person over time could provide consistency in helping the person regain a sense of continuity of self after surviving a stroke. Goals that enhance continuity of self could be mutually developed by nurse and patient. Specific strategies would be selected based on what is important to the patient, not on a predetermined schedule based on generalizations about type and location of stroke. As other rehabilitation disciplines teach specific motor and linguistic skills, nursing can help integrate these skills into meaningful experiences.

Nurses could also play a substantial role in reconnecting stroke survivors with other people. The disconnection from others described by these study participants was not because of lack of contact; rather, it concerned a lack of understanding. Unhelpful "help" from others was described by several participants. Corrective help, for example with speech, was particularly unhelpful. Assisting families to understand socially inappropriate behavior caused by the stroke, such as profane outbursts and heightened emotionality, may mitigate the shame and confusion expressed by some participants. Significant others need to learn how to adjust the tempo of conversation and family activities to accommodate the slower pace of the stroke survivor. With a bit of patience on the part of listeners, even patients with nonfluent aphasia can make themselves understood. Interviews with aphasic patients in this study resulted in meaningful dialogue despite the slower tempo and occasional necessity of relying on gestures or writing words on paper. Computer discussion groups could provide stroke survivors with a means to connect with others without time constraints or correction.

As recovery from stroke evolves over time, so too do figural events and their meanings. Goal setting cannot be a one-time, fixed event but rather ongoing as the meaning of life experiences following stroke unfurls. Dialogue must be ongoing, and continuity of care must become more than a much-touted phrase.

POST-STUDY REFLECTIONS FROM JANET SECREST

Phenomenological research has deeply affected the way I teach and the way I practice nursing. My focus with both students and patients is now on connection and the meaning of experience—a shift for me which has resulted in more satisfying and holistic practice. As a former ICU nurse, being with patients meant "doing for." I've learned that "being with" in and of itself is therapeutic in a much deeper sense, and I try to convey this to students.

I have learned from personal experience that being open and listening to someone else's perspectives is a skill that can be taught. The "Foundations" course at our school of nursing was a predominantly psychomotor skills course. Now, I focus it more on connections with others—the skills now providing the entree to connection. Students begin the course by exploring health and illness experiences of each other, and then with well, elderly individuals using the same questions (e.g., "Think of a time when you were in pain [were ill, etc.]. Can you describe that for me?") Students have reported how connected they feel with those they have interviewed. With students in clinical sites, I find myself asking more: "What was it like for Mrs. B.?" rather than: "What did her x-ray show?" In post-clinical conferences, students are asked how the experience was for them, what stood out. Our post-conferences, as a result, have become much richer, with students exploring their own reactions and the perspectives of others. Similarly, clinical evaluations focus on what the experience meant to students.

When once taken-for-granted perspectives are revealed to be more than or different from what was expected, I can no longer assume that I know what is true—I want to understand how others perceive experiences. Phenomenology has made me more curious! Most importantly, though, phenomenology has brought more humanism and art into my education and nursing practice.

12

"The Point of No Return": Formerly Abused Women's Experience of Staying Out of the Abusive Relationship

"I knew if my little girl could be so brave and strong, I had to get out. I felt so empowered. I broke free and ran. I slammed both doors behind me."

—words of an abused woman interviewed for the present study

A bused women often leave their partners. In fact, many women leave seven or eight times before they leave for good, decide to stay, or are killed in the process of leaving (Hilberman, 1980; Ulrich, 1991). There is an extensive literature in nursing and other disciplines on abused women, providing information to increase awareness of abuse and to guide professionals in identifying it and intervening (Campbell & Humphreys, 1993; Hotaling, Finkelhor, Kirkpatrick, & Straus, 1988; King & Ryan, 1989). Relatively few studies, however, have explored the factors that enable women to leave the abusive relationship. Still fewer have examined the experience of formerly abused women *staying out* of the relationship. This is a significant gap in the literature, prompting the present phenomenological investigation.

* This chapter is based on an unpublished doctoral dissertation, "The Point of No Return: Formerly Abused Women's Experience of Staying Out of the Abusive Relationship," by Karen S. Reesman, the University of Tennessee, Knoxville, 2000.

RELATED LITERATURE

Vavaro (1989) defines an abused woman as "one who has been deliberately and repeatedly physically, emotionally, or sexually abused in her home by an intimate male such as husband, ex-husband, boyfriend, ex-boyfriend, or lover" (p. 1). Another frequently used term is "domestic violence," but its use is not confined to female victims of male attacks. Many myths and misconceptions surround the abuse of women, and its shame and stigma prevent many victims from reporting injuries to health care providers. When they do summon the courage to report abuse, only one in 10 victims is officially identified as an abused woman by nurses and physicians (Henderson, 1992). The name of Nicole Brown Simpson became a household term in 1995, galvanizing national attention and heightening awareness of millions of people about the nature and frequency of abuse of women. Every nine seconds a woman is the victim of abuse in the United States (Federal Bureau of Investigation, 1995). Any woman, regardless of her social, racial, ethnic, or personal characteristics, can be a victim. Men's violence toward women is reported to be directly experienced by one in three women throughout the Western world; one in 10 women is physically abused by an intimate male partner (Sampselle et al., 1992).

Research on violence in families is just a little more than 30 years old. No research articles with the term "violence" in the title were published in *The Journal of Marriage and Family* (a major source of family research) prior to 1970. Some feminist researchers (Dobash & Dobash, 1988; Martin, 1988) hold that a patriarchal society has had a strong impact on research questions and methodologies, preventing women's voices from being heard. Feminist critiques have brought about an increase, particularly in qualitative studies, in recent years (Reinharz, 1992).

A variety of explanations for woman abuse have been advanced. According to sociologist Murray Straus (1976), it is sexist attitudes and practices that condone woman abuse for the following reasons: (1) stress and frustration cause some men to resort to violence in order to reinforce their position as head of the family; (2) antagonism between men and women may occur because of gender-role stereotypes and inequality; (3) it is difficult for many women to escape violent partners due to the lack of alternative roles for women and family pressures to remain in the relationship "for better or worse;" and (4) it is exceedingly difficult for women to obtain legal protection from abusive partners in a male-oriented criminal justice system.

Some researchers have proposed that a family systems perspective is useful in understanding partner abuse (cf. Shupe, Stacey, & Hazlewood, 1987). Feminists, however, have opposed viewing partner abuse from a family systems perspective because it focuses on a "dysfunctional" family or couple rather than on male violence and the societal influences reinforcing male domination and control. Nursing scholars Campbell, Harris, and Lee (1995) review four theoretical models: one depicting the abuser as mentally ill, chemically dependent, and/or disabled, a second maintaining that the abuser learned the use of violence in childhood (often by being a recipient of it), a third attributing an abuser's violence to lack of skills for dealing with stress, and the fourth explaining the violence in terms of the male's need to control the female. Gelles and Cornell (1990) advocated a combination of social control and exchange theory, within which they put forth three propositions regarding family violence: (1) family members are more likely to use violence in the home when they expect the costs of being violent to be less than the rewards; (2) in the absence of effective social controls (e.g., police intervention), the costs of one family member being violent toward another are decreased; and (3) certain social and family structures reduce social control in family relations, therefore reducing the costs and increasing the rewards of being violent.

Learned helplessness theory, developed by Seligman, has been used by psychologist Lenore Walker (1979) to explain women's response to abuse. Learned helplessness results when one begins to realize that random painful experiences cannot be stopped or circumvented. The person experiencing the pain becomes less inclined to try to avoid it. Eventually, there is a perception that there is no solution (Campbell & Humphreys, 1993).

Leaving, mistakenly considered by the general public as the simplest solution, is fraught with many difficult issues. As Ulrich notes, "being beaten is not the only issue, or at least not the critical one" (1991, p. 471). Safety of self or children, economic factors, and availability of a support system are among the important considerations of a woman preparing to leave an abusive relationship. Research shows that homicides increase when battered women threaten to leave or actually do so (Campbell, 1986), and many women are hunted or stalked by their abusers after they leave. Newman (1993) interviewed abused women who had escaped to a shelter, discovering many of the reasons why "it was easier to give up and return to the relationship than to seek alternatives" (p. 110). The majority of the women she interviewed had made previous attempts to leave but returned due to lack of resources and feelings of isolation and loneliness. They spoke of the difficulty in getting health care workers to identify them as having been abused and of the complexities of obtaining various types of aid from social agencies. In a study conducted by Mills (1985), women justified staying in an abusive relationship by minimizing the violence, focusing on their own strengths, and making excuses for the partner. The women told the researcher they did not feel victimized, they felt loved. Before women are able to extricate themselves successfully from such relationships, it is clear that disengagement must take place. Disengaging was the third phase in a process described by Landenburger (1989), of binding, enduring, disengaging, and recovering. Landenburger's data illuminate both intra- and interpersonal processes with respect to being in an abusive relationship, getting ready to leave, and leaving.

Although researchers have viewed leaving as an event, a study by Ulrich (1991) showed that leaving is a process, not a discrete event. She recommended further study of this process, a recommendation acted upon by Merritt-Gray and Wuest in two grounded theory studies (Merritt-Gray & Wuest, 1995; Wuest & Merritt-Gray, 1999). Survivors of abuse described a complex process of "counteracting abuse" and "breaking free" which spanned between one and 10 years. "Not going back" was the third stage in the process of leaving, followed by a final stage of "reclaiming the self."

THE PRESENT PROGRAM OF RESEARCH

While research has revealed important aspects of a woman's exodus from an abusive relationship, no study has examined what she experiences once she has left. Phenomenological interviewing provides these women the opportunity to tell their stories of staying out of abusive relationships. Nine volunteers were interviewed for the study, recruited using a network or snowball approach. Access to participants was facilitated by a personal friend and colleague who is a survivor of abuse and the director of an abuse shelter. All participants were female, 21 years of age or older, and out of the abusive situation for at least two years. In addition to the usual measures taken to preserve participant confidentiality, human rights, and safety, the researcher was prepared to make a referral to a counselor and/or the local mental health center, should a participant become distressed while revealing emotion-laden information. No referrals were necessary. Prior to undertaking interviews with the participants, the researcher was interviewed by another member of the interdisciplinary phenomenology group.

Bracketing Interview

The thought of the interview was intimidating. I (Reesman) remember thinking how little I knew about violence and abuse, and I wondered what George would think of me for attempting to engage in this type of research. I chose George to do the interview because I thought of him as kind, gentle, astute, and insightful. So I assumed it would be easy for me to talk with him. As I told George when he interviewed me, I have not been abused; I have not personally experienced that type of relationship. But George got me talking about my childhood and what it was like for me growing up. I recalled an incident when I *was* abused by other children. I had been playing with some older children whom I was not allowed to play with. I was about four years old and they were perhaps seven or eight. They wanted to play "doctor" and I was to be "the patient." I was somewhat apprehensive but I played anyway because I wanted to be included. At some point in the game I was up against the house facing the wall and surrounded by four or five children . . . one or more of whom stuck a pin or two in my bottom. I remember it hurt and wanting to leave but being afraid to do so. Finally, I got up the nerve and broke free, ran home, and told my mother. I never went back. George asked me if I thought about going back and I told him, "Oh no, I'd *never* go back." In reflecting on my bracketing interview, I realized that, actually, part of me did want to go back. It was important for me to realize that I had feelings of wanting to be included, to fit in . . . much like the women in my study.

I also told George about experiences I had while observing violent situations. One such experience happened more than 20 years ago when I witnessed a New York City policeman using a night-stick on a woman in a subway station. He wanted her to leave the station believing her to be a prostitute. I was appalled and interceded. As a woman and a visiting nurse I felt compelled to intervene. The telling of this situation brought to my mind how much I abhor violence. It also made me realize that I have felt this way for many, many years. This bracketing interview taught me a lot about how I think and feel about abuse. I realized that I do have some understanding of how the person being interviewed might feel, and hopefully, this awareness made me a better interviewer.

FINDINGS

The experience of formerly abused women staying out of the abusive relationship was described by participants in the context of time. All participants spoke of a temporal sequence of their experiences. First, there is the violent time before the woman leaves the abuser, then the time when she leaves (which is called "the point of no return"), the recovery period, and the "now," when the narrative is being told. Other people are also important, because the woman's experiences are viewed against the background of her relationship with the abusive partner(s) and, to some extent, other people in her world. The major themes that emerge from these existential grounds were: (1) self and others experienced as good/bad, (2) self and others experienced as stable/unstable, (3) self experienced as empowered/helpless, and (4) others experienced as contributing to self's feeling of being empowered or helpless.

The Violent Time

Participants began by talking of times when they met the abuser, at a dance or party; they also talked about events leading up to the first occurrence of abuse. Some described the tempo at which the relationship developed: "He moved in on me really fast. Before I knew it, he had moved in." Specific events were named by some women in connection with the first abuse ("It all started when he came back from Vietnam. He was a changed man;" "The first time was after the birth of our first child"), while the beginning was a fuzzier memory to other women ("I can't even remember when it all started. I can't remember a time when he didn't abuse me. It seems to me that for as long as I was associated with him, he abused me.")

Participants went on to describe the frequency and duration of the abuse: "He beat me every weekend; it was like clockwork. Oh, he beat me other times too, but I could count on every Friday after work and it lasting through the weekend;" "When he'd be beating me . . . it seemed like forever . . . even though it may only be 20 or 30 minutes, it seemed like it lasted forever—and sometimes it did . . . last all night." Most of the women cited a specific number of years of abuse (e.g., 9, 17, 27), but time also became distorted. This woman's confusion was not atypical: "It was January, no February, no January, no—maybe it was March . . . Oh, I can't remember, but I *think* it was winter." Metaphors were used to describe that time in the abused woman's life: "It was the winter of my life;" "The abuse I took, what I endured . . . it was the dark before the dawn." Death threats from the abusive partner were common, creating fear that the woman would not live to see another dawn.

Despite the degrading and injurious treatment, making the decision to leave nonetheless took a long time for some of the women: "It seemed like I could *never* make up my mind; it took the longest time;" ". . . it took me forever. Well, nine years anyway." In some cases, once the decision was made, the action was swift: "It seemed like years and years and years, but once I finally, actually, decided, it was like I decided in a split-second, and picked up and left." In discussing the actual leaving, all of the women precisely identified a time: "I left on the 4th of July;" "I waited until summer vacation when my kids would be out of school." Repeated departures and returns were described: "I left twice before I left for good;" "It seemed like I left a hundred times, but it was probably three or four." Eventually, the women reached a point in time when leaving was imperative; this was described as "the point of no return."

The Point of No Return

The women described how they knew the time was right to leave. A particularly severe beating served as the impetus for several. The following exemplar is illustrative:

> He was just whaling on me and I started to pray. I prayed for all I was worth. I asked God to make it stop; make him stop. . . . He just kept at it, and I couldn't seem to get away, and nothing I did would make him stop so I kept praying, asking God to make it stop and I'd leave for good. I promised I'd leave for good. All of a sudden he just fell over . . . it all just stopped.

The interviewer asked, "Was he dead?"

The participant chuckled and smiled and said, "No, honey. He was drunk and wore out from beating on me and I guess he just went unconscious." This woman believed God had answered her prayer, compelling her to keep her promise to leave.

Two of the women actually used the phrase *"I had reached the point of no return,"* which was chosen as the title of the study because all of the women described such a point. Powerful metaphors were used to describe the time of leaving, such as "spring following a hard winter." Other examples of metaphors follow: "It was like being sprung from prison. My time was up. I did my time;" "It was like closing a door. When I left, that was all behind me . . . in the past;" "It was . . . the dawn in my life."

The Time of Recovery

The third stage, after the women left the abusive relationship, was also contextualized in time. Women named the number of years they had been "out" and also named the number of years they had been involved with subsequent non-abusive partners. Women often compared the amount of time in the abusive relationship with the amount or length of time out of it: "I can finally say I've been out as long as I was in;" "I've been out for 11 years and that's almost as many years as I was with that sicko."

The "Now"

In discussing the fourth period or present phase, the now, participants most often summed up their entire experience. The woman who had used the seasons of the year as her metaphor described her "now" as the summer of her life. Another woman spoke of abuse as the wake-up call when she started her metaphorical day, "then the time after I left, that's like the afternoon, and now, now I have the whole evening to enjoy." A final example refers to developmental stages:

> Before, during all the time I was taking the abuse, I felt like a child. Like it was in my childhood. Kids are always being told what to do, how to do it, when to do it, and not doing it right. When I couldn't stand it anymore, when I just knew I had to leave or else, when I had reached that point of no return, I felt like a rebellious teenager. . . . Once I left, in the beginning, I felt . . . like a young adult. . . . Now I feel like an adult. . . . Oh, don't get me wrong, I still need to make my way, but it's different. Now, I'm more mature in the whole process.

FIGURAL THEMES

Over time, the women described changes in themselves and in their relationships. The first theme, **good/bad**, was present throughout each of the four periods, but in different ways. The women described feeling good about themselves and their abusers in the beginning. Attention from the men (who were often described as handsome or charming) was flattering. Feeling chosen by such a man made them feel special; this relationship was often the first enduring relationship the woman had experienced. The following transcript excerpt is representative:

> When I first met him, I was so amazed that he'd be interested in me. Here he was this big, important pro ballplayer from ___. The best thing I'd ever seen . . . really fine, tall, good looking. Yep, he was good. We were at a party I was invited [to] by a friend who also worked at the bank. I was pretty plain; I don't wear makeup.

Oh, I'm slim and all, and decent looking, but there were all these women there who were dressed up, makeup on, big hair, you know . . . drop dead gorgeous type . . . and then there was me . . . and he singled me out . . . me.

Once the egregious abuse began, the women had drastically altered their perceptions of their partners, seeing them as "bad," "evil," or "a devil." As one woman described, "You can't even imagine how bad he was. Bad. Bad. Bad. I woke up to him burning me with cigarettes. When he wasn't doing that he was slicing me . . . little slits . . . with a razor, real small, like paper cuts. It was hard for me to believe at one time I thought he was so good [that] I questioned if I was good enough for him."

In the leaving stage, participants often described a "good" rescuer who enabled them to escape the "bad" abuser. The rescuer is called a "guardian angel" or "savior" who helps the women to begin feeling better about themselves, once again more **good** than **bad**. During the recovery period, the women begin to think less of their former partner. Now, at the time of the interview, the women seem to be more differentiated and independent of others, feeling good about their new-found strength and their ability to begin helping other women.

The second theme of **stable/unstable** was also present across the complete trajectory of the abusive relationship and recovery. The partnership initially brought security and stability to the woman's life, which quickly degenerated into chaos, with the ups and downs of the turbulent relationship combined with multiple moves and crises. The instability of her home life carried over to work, preventing the woman from concentrating on her work. There were periods of unemployment for both the women and their abusive partners. At times, the women turned to friends and family for help or temporary lodging, but found such hospitality and tolerance were limited. Staying a whole week with relatives was considered an unusually generous respite from a "couch to couch" existence. Exemplars of this theme follow:

It wasn't just that my home life was unstable . . . I was unstable. Sometimes I didn't know . . . or couldn't think of . . . or couldn't remember my own schedule. That may sound dumb, but . . . when you can't even remember which place you're living in that day; when your life is so unstable . . . you're moving from place to place—sometimes one place in the morning, go to work, and go home to a different place that night—it's hard to think of much else. You're just trying to find some stability.

. . . one couch to the next; that's how I judged how stable my life was . . . whether my kids and I had a couch to go to . . . to sleep on that night. Basically we went couch to couch; pretty, ironic, don't you think? Some people are what they call couch potatoes . . . living on the couch all day. You'd just hope they'd be ready to get off by the time you were ready to settle the kids for the night.

During the leaving stage, the partner becomes extremely **unstable** and out of control. One woman succinctly captured the instability by saying "He was off his rocker most of the time." Verbatim descriptions from the data reveal the nature of the cruel, extreme measures he takes to tighten his control of the woman: "He took me for a drive and put me in the middle. He knew he was going to beat me. He put our son next to the door and the rest of the kids in the back. And he, he, he just started beating me so bad that, finally, I reached over and opened the door and my son and I rolled out onto the highway;" "He had me spread-eagle on the bed, tied to the bedpost for three days. He didn't let me up to use the bathroom; I didn't have anything to eat or drink. He kept playing heavy metal [music], blaring it as loud as it would go, and he'd keep waking me up all night long when I finally could go to sleep from sheer exhaustion."

During the recovery period, women began to regain **stability**: "I can't believe how much more stable my life became . . . right off the bat; it was unbelievable [that] I had people who cared and who were *there* for me." Specific indications of greater stability were mentioned. For example, a woman who formerly took four or five Valiums a day spoke of cutting her dosage down to half a Valium. Another woman who had constantly moved from place to place was able to remain in the same place for four years. Increasingly, the participants felt empowered to make choices about their lives, which brings us to the third theme.

As with the previous two themes, **empowered/helpless** was manifested in all stages, albeit in different forms. Initially, before the abuse, the women felt empowered by their affectionate and solicitous partners: "Honey, I thought I had the tiger by the tail. He sweet-talked me and in the beginning he acted like I couldn't do anything wrong. He made me feel great and . . . like I could do anything." The same woman later noted, "All that sweet-talking didn't last too long. He started putting me down all the time 'til I got to the point I felt I couldn't do anything." Another contrasted her partner's "Honey this or honey that" during their courtship with: "Pretty soon, it became 'Honey *do* this' and 'Honey do that' and 'Honey wash the car' and 'Honey get your fat ass home.' I couldn't do anything on my own or by myself, he saw to that." The women described increasing helplessness and constraints on their freedom. In some cases women were confined to certain rooms of the house or physically restrained.

Eventually, the women were able to make a triumphant escape, empowered by rescuers who gave advice or aid. In the following example, a safety plan created with the staff of a women's shelter was crucial. Perhaps even more instrumental in the success of the plan, however, was the inspiring courage of a seven-year-old girl. The participant who had been tied spread-eagle in bed for three days related, "When the kids were in bed, he started choking me with a belt. My daughter came in and saw what was happening (she was seven) and she got her brother and, just like in the safety plan we practiced that the staff told us to do, she went out and got the two of them in the truck and started it up. I knew what they were doing; I don't think he had a clue. Each time I'd black out and start to come to, I'd hear the truck . . . I thought to myself, I didn't have much time. I felt so good all at once. I felt like I could do this. I didn't feel helpless anymore. I knew if my little girl could be so brave and strong, I had to get out. I felt so empowered. I broke free and ran. I slammed both doors behind me. My daughter had put the lock on both so when they closed, they locked. It was just enough time . . .

those few split seconds he had to fumble with the locks . . . for me to hop in the truck and drive down the hill to the gas station. . . . The police were there. I felt so good knowing he couldn't do a thing." Note the woman's satisfaction that her partner is now the helpless one.

Oftentimes the people who help these women escape were perceived as magically coming out of nowhere. One woman, appearing in court before a judge, was asked if she had an attorney. When she replied that she could not afford one, the judge recommended that she "better just go home." At that moment, a woman attorney who was present in the courtroom walked up and said, "I'll take your case for $10.00 a month." Another woman, hidden from visitors in the bedroom while her partner entertained guests, told about one of the female guests accidentally entering that bedroom while looking for a bathroom. Appalled when she saw the woman's bruises, the guest helped her escape:

> She told me we were leaving, and she went out and talked with _____ [the partner]. She told him she had to go back to her house, which was not very far away, and wanted to take me with her. She made up some excuse about needing my help for something, and he bought it, but told her not to be gone long. . . . As soon as we got to her place, she called 911. The police came and took me and busted him at the same time. I felt so empowered. I had tried to escape several times before that, completely on my own, and never made it. This time was different. . . . I had someone helping me.

During the recovery stage, women made temporal references such as "going slowly" and "taking it one day at a time" as they described the process. Even in the "now," as the narrative was being told to the interviewer, participants did not think in terms of having completed their growth. As one woman put it, "It's not as if I think I have arrived." Another said, "I know I am still becoming." What helped them to stay out of the abusive relationship? Participants described concrete assistance from others (for example, from friends who helped them find jobs) as well as empowerment through prayer. Although women also mentioned meditation, relaxation techniques, and reading, the power of God and prayer gave them the strength that enabled them to stay out of the abusive relationship. Here are just two of many examples:

> I'd pray for all I was worth. I knew it was gonna get me through. I prayed all the time. I'd pray in the car, I'd pray fixing dinner . . . it didn't matter. I knew it helped me.

> I once read about a man who was a prisoner of war. He was in a cell all by himself; he had very little food—just barely enough to keep him alive—and he was cramped. He always had to sit down or lie down because the cell was too small for him to stand in. There were other prisoners but he couldn't talk to them and they couldn't talk to him. He didn't even have a pot to pee in—he just had to do that in the corner into the dirt. Anyway, no matter what happened the one thing

that kept him going, and kept him from going nuts, was he'd say the rosary. . . . So that's what I'd do. It may sound kinda crazy. You'd think I'd just think my life was wonderful, not being beat anymore, but it was real hard, especially at first. I kinda felt like that man [the POW]. I felt alone and even tho' there were people around me, I didn't feel like I could talk to them. So I'd pray. He made it. He always had the hope he'd be outta there one day and have a new life. Well, I had a new life and I wanted it to continue . . . so I'd pray.

DISCUSSION AND CONCLUSIONS

The women in this study see themselves and others as good/bad, stable/unstable, and empowered/helpless against the ground of time. Time was divided into four stages or phases: the violent abusive phase, the phase of leaving (when the women reach the point of no return), the recovery phase, and the time at which the narrative was told, the "now." Temporal references abound throughout the interviews. The women talked about the frequency and duration of the abuse, specific events that prompted abusive treatment (pregnancy, childbirth, attempts to leave), and that moment when a magical rescuer empowered them to escape their living hell. Day by day, they grow stronger during the recovery period. All of the themes are summarized in the following examplar:

Before my life was hell. My husband was the devil and I was his toy. He had a stronghold on me and I felt like I couldn't do anything. I felt helpless to do anything about it. I was abused in every way. Then, the one time I was able to get to a friend's house, there was a nurse there and she helped me. She told me I could get away and how to do it. She told me I could call and get help 24 hours a day. I wasn't alone. . . . She gave me strength to leave. It wasn't easy, and I'm glad I'll never have to do it again. I talked to that nurse a lot, before I left and after I left. She was there for me. I prayed a lot too. Now I have a good partner and friends and a stable relationship. I have a nice place to live. These are the things that help me every day to put the past behind me and go on.

Themes of this phenomenological investigation are consistent in several respects with previously conducted grounded theory studies (Merritt-Gray & Wuest, 1995; Wuest & Merritt-Gray, 1999) as well as with Landenburger's ethnographic study (1989), although the role of the rescuer is perhaps more prominent in accounts given by the present group of participants. The rescuer is instrumental in helping the abused woman leave and to stay out of the relationship as well. Throughout the extant literature, leaving is a process described as taking place in stages and over time. The women in the present study had moved beyond the stage of minimizing their partners' violence (as described by Mills, 1985) and were in the process of "reclaiming the self" (as described by Merritt-Gray and Wuest, 1995)—although a more appropriate title for the latter stage is "becoming an empowered self." Unique to the present study is the emphasis of the present sample of women on their relationship with God. They did not describe involvement in organized religion; however, all of them did describe the strength they gained from "talking to God" and praying. They also made specific reference to reading inspirational material and meditating. Yet to be discovered in future studies are the best ways for helping professionals to obtain disclosure of abuse, to mentor individuals who are recovering, and to reduce the recidivism rate of women repeatedly returning to abusive relationships.

IMPLICATIONS OF THE STUDY FINDINGS FOR NURSING PRACTICE

Talking with abused women who have experienced atrocities, degradation, and humiliation can be very uncomfortable. It can be difficult to begin an interaction that will elicit the grueling details of an abusive relationship. However, nurses must accept the challenge of listening to, and helping, these women. From this study, it is clear that the empowering actions of one person can enable these women to flee and begin the process of regaining a safe and stable existence. In the final exemplar cited above, the empowering person was a nurse. Who better to work with these women than nurses? Nurses must be prepared to give them direct care, anticipatory guidance, and education. As nurses, we have access to women everywhere: at work, in hospitals and clinics, in the community, at health fairs and health screening events. We can judge when it is appropriate to exclude a significant other from the examining room in order to have a private conversation. We are educated to know when to intervene or intercede.

Every nurse should know the telephone numbers of 24-hour abuse hot-lines, shelters, and other resources in his or her community. Nurses can not only recommend and/or refer women to support groups but also become support group facilitators. In-shelter groups are useful for women in the throes of making a break from their partners, whereas groups in the community can help women who have already left. When confronted with women who have left abusive relationships, nurses can share some of the strategies that have proved helpful to other survivors. When women tell us they are thinking about going back or longing to be with their partners again, it is up to us to ask them what it is they are remembering or thinking about. As they begin to tell their stories, they will begin to situate themselves in the time of violence once again, and we can help them to recall that the good times "did not last very long" and were "few and far between," in the words of one participant in this study. Much like recovering alcoholics attending Alcoholics Anonymous meetings, these women benefit from repeatedly telling their stories because it is the remembering that will help them to stay out of the abusive relationship.

Knowing that women are at their greatest risk of homicide when leaving the abuser (Campbell, 1986), we must be forceful in our conviction that they should not return. We must capitalize on the fact that they are out of the relationship and help guide them through the transition process, which takes time. Some helping professionals become discouraged when women return to their abusers, eventually developing a cynical attitude toward intervening. As Ulrich (1991) has pointed out, however, intervention should never be viewed as meaningless even when women go back to the abuser. There is always reason to hope that the next time will be the "point of no return."

POST-STUDY REFLECTIONS FROM KAREN REESMAN

I came to this study from a feminist perspective with a belief that no woman should ever be intentionally hurt. Through my clinical experience as a nurse and my volunteer work in the community, I have come in contact with women in all phases of abuse and those having experienced many types of egregious abuse. I have seen how the experience of abuse impacts on the individual, her perception of herself and her world, and her interactions with other people. But I did not know, until I conducted this study, how a woman reached the "point of no return" and what survival skills enabled her to stay out of the abusive relationship. Listening to the stories of my study participants permitted me to discover important elements of surviving abusive experiences. The stories of these empowered survivors have inspired me and helped intensify my resolve to continue advocacy efforts on behalf of all who remain silent victims of domestic violence.

13

"It Was the Dark Night of the Soul": Wresting Meaning From a Time of Spiritual Distress

"It causes me to question God's sanity in a sense. What's go'n on, God? Can't you intervene? You did it in the Old Testament. You did it in the New Testament. Where are you right now?"

—questions posed by a participant in the present study of spiritual distress

Although nursing education ostensibly prepares practitioners to recognize and intervene in the physical, psychological, social, and spiritual concerns of human beings, spiritual concerns remain most difficult for many nurses to recognize and treat (Burkhardt, 1991). More than half of nurse practitioners participating in a recent survey said they rarely or never provided spiritual care (Stranahan, 2001). Oncology nurses queried by Taylor, Highfield, and Amenta (1994) also reported rarely providing direct spiritual care, although they prayed privately and made referrals to clergy. These studies support earlier findings of Granstrom (1985) and Piles (1990).

Hesitant and uncertain, many nurses avoid patients who say they are angry at God or losing their faith in God's presence and power. Yet, spiritual distress is a common phenomenon nurses cannot successfully avoid. Remen (1988), a physician, believes that unrecognized spiritual distress may be at the root of much illness. Illness, of course, can also be a source of spiritual distress. During an illness, many people struggle with its meaning.

* This chapter is based on a doctoral dissertation, "The Wonder of Meaning: A Phenomenological Understanding of Spiritual Distress," by Carol J. Smucker, the University of Tennessee, Knoxville, 1993. An earlier version of this paper appeared in *Nursing Diagnosis,* 7(2), 81–91. Reprinted by permission of Nursecom, Inc.

The uncertainty that nurses experience in recognizing spiritual distress and giving spiritual care can be attributed to several causes. For early nurses who were educated within religious orders, attending to spiritual needs was second nature. Often, hygiene and prayers were all these nurses had to offer those in their care, but most contemporary nurses are not educated in and do not practice in religious settings. Moreover, they tend to receive limited content on spirituality in their nursing programs. Additionally, care priorities in many facilities revolve around technology, allowing little time for nurses to address needs other than the physical ones. Research-based literature, although burgeoning, is still scarce in comparison to the vast literature on physical and psychosocial caregiving.

RELATED LITERATURE

Prior to adopting a holistic health paradigm in the 1970s, many nurses were taught that spiritual care primarily related to a patient's religious preferences and practices (Piles, 1990). Nursing literature after 1970 reflects a broadened understanding of human spirituality and an increased interest in the nurse's role in spiritual care. While religion refers to a specific set of beliefs held in common by a group, spirituality refers to "any attempt to approach or attend to the invisible factors in life and to transcend the personal, concrete, finite particulars of this world" (Moore, 1992). Thus, all persons exhibit spirituality when they feel connected to the universe or ponder the ultimate questions: "What is the meaning of life?" or "What happens when I die?" Spirituality, like holism, is considered an integrative concept—one which emphasizes the unity or wholeness of the human being.

The nursing diagnosis movement stimulated an interest in the spiritual dimension of nursing (Fehring & Rantz, 1991) and gave impetus to research on spirituality. The diagnostic label *spiritual distress* had its origins in the First National Classification Conference of the North American Nursing Diagnosis Association (NANDA) in 1973 and was refined at the 1980 NANDA meeting. For the diagnosis of spiritual distress, there are 13 defining characteristics: 1) expresses concern with the meaning of life/death and/or belief system; 2) describes anger toward God; 3) questions the meaning of suffering; 4) verbalizes inner conflict about beliefs; 5) verbalizes concern about relationship with deity; 6) questions meaning of own existence; 7) is unable to participate in usual religious practices; 8) seeks spiritual assistance; 9) questions moral/ethical implications of therapeutic regimen; 10) displays gallows humor; 11) displaces anger toward religious representatives; 12) has nightmares/sleep disturbances; and 13) exhibits alterations in behavior/mood evidenced by anger, crying, withdrawal, preoccupation, anxiety, hostility, apathy, etc. Of these 13 characteristics, the first one is considered to be the "key defining characteristic" which must be present before labeling a patient's response as spiritual distress (Hurley, 1986). Credibility is a problem in the acceptance and revision of this diagnosis, and the other NANDA diagnostic categories as well, because they are based on opinion of clinicians rather than on research.

Only two studies have been performed to evaluate the diagnosis of spiritual distress, and the purpose of these studies was to validate the defining characteristics of the diagnosis. In the first study, Weatherall and Creason (1987) identified cues of spiritual distress from the literature as found in the Cumulative Index to Nursing and Allied Health Literature (CINAHL) and from the NANDA bibliography on spiritual distress (Kim, McFarland, & McLane, 1984). These cues from 34 nursing articles were compared with assessment data on spiritual distress obtained from 13 patient records. Results suggested that five characteristics were the most valid and clinically useful. The three that were included in the NANDA characteristics were "questions meaning of suffering," "verbalizes concern about relationship with deity," and "verbalizes inner conflict about beliefs." The other two, "hopelessness" and "cues having to do with relationships with others," were not added to the list of defining characteristics. The study's usefulness, however, was limited by the small sample (13 patient records) and by the variability in nurses' charting.

The second study was a descriptive one by McHolm (1991). A random sample of oncology nurses was asked to identify defining characteristics used in clinical practice when diagnosing spiritual distress. From a list of 41 defining characteristics provided by the researcher, the nurses primarily selected items pertaining to mood alterations (e.g., depression, crying). The one defining characteristic specifically related to spiritual concerns was "cues that religious/spiritual needs are important." This study suggested that nurses have difficulty differentiating spiritual from psychosocial distress. Only a small percentage (28.9%) of the nurses actually used the nursing diagnosis of spiritual distress in their practice.

These two studies highlight two important issues in research on spiritual distress. One of these is the continuing confusion over the definition of the term *spiritual*; the other is that religious, spiritual, and psychosocial needs overlap. There has been no research on spiritual distress using dialogical methods such as are used in phenomenological studies.

THE PRESENT PROGRAM OF RESEARCH

The purpose of this study was to describe spiritual distress as it is experienced by adults in the general population. The study focused on the "key" aspect of spiritual distress—concern about the meaning of life/death and/or beliefs. Participants were sought who: (1) had experienced spiritual distress; (2) were able and willing to articulate this experience; (3) felt free enough to express inner feelings; and (4) were adults (persons older than age 18) and not nurses. Nurses were not asked to be in the sample because of the likelihood that their familiarity with the nursing diagnosis of spiritual distress might bias their description of personal experiences related to this domain. Five women and five men from the researcher's church, neighborhood, and community took part in the study. The researcher had known nine of the participants for three years. The tenth participant and the researcher had talked only during brief periods for several months prior to the study. Over time, the researcher became aware of events in these persons' lives that suggested that they might have experienced spiritual distress. Because a trusting relationship had been established with these individuals, it was thought that they might be likely to agree to be interviewed and willing to share thoughts and feelings at a deeper level than they would with a stranger. Ages ranged from 33 to 66, and education ranged from tenth grade to a doctoral degree, with most participants having graduate preparation. All participants were affiliated with Protestant religious denominations. Before proceeding with the study, the researcher was interviewed by a fellow research group member using the same interview question developed for use with participants.

Bracketing Interview

I (Smucker) learned from the bracketing interview that some research participants might be quite nervous, initially, about being interviewed and would need encouragement and support from the interviewer. Based on my own experience, however, I had greater confidence that participants would likely find sharing their stories fairly easy to do, given an empathic interviewer. I suspected that research participants, knowing the nature of the question ahead of time, would probably give much thought to what they were going to share, would do so in some detail, and would find the experience quite emotional. I anticipated that being concerned about meaning would encompass more than personal concerns/life experiences, but would extend to concerns of world injustice and suffering. The themes that emerged from my bracketing interview were similar to those that later emerged from the complete set of 10 interviews. Because of the importance of some of these themes to my own personal experience, it was evident in the first couple of interviews that I was attempting to have the participant focus on these themes. Thus, I continually re-bracketed throughout the 10 interviews to keep from imposing my personal values and interpretations.

FINDINGS

The experience of spiritual distress presents itself as having two clear phases. The metaphor, "web of life," was taken from the words of a participant named Jean, who used it to describe both phases of the experience:

> And one does wonder on the death of a child . . . what (sighs) . . . that's very difficult . . . it's very difficult. Parents, you know, it's going to happen and one way or another they get less able and less enjoying of life and that isn't . . . it isn't the

same . . . they break your web of life and you obviously have to rebuild around it and put the scar tissue around it to make it work and you . . . you kind of encapsulate them and all their memories in your life . . . in the way you operate. But it's . . . but a child . . . it's much harder. I find it that way. And it took a lot longer to get over that than the parents.

Based on these words, the first phase of spiritual distress was termed **Breaking the Web**. This aspect of the phenomenon begins when an event suddenly or unexpectedly breaks into one's life, ripping or tearing the fabric of life and interrupting the continuity of time. A second phase follows the first and was named **Rebuilding the Web**. In this phase, the person comes to some acceptance of the event and is able to find meaning in it through positive actions in the world. Figural to the phase of Breaking the Web were the following themes and subthemes: *falling apart* (pain and instability), *wondering* (questioning), and *something beyond* (feeling, presence, mystery). Themes of Rebuilding the Web included *stability* (strength and security), *change and growth* (self and beliefs), and *wondering* (no answers and accepting limits to knowing). The movement experienced by participants between the phases is a rebuilding process that occurs over time and varies across individuals. While phase one represents spiritual distress, phase two is characterized by spiritual growth. There is a sense in which the restructuring is never fully completed. As was evident throughout the interviews, when a participant recalled and discussed an event that had once been distressful, there was a reexperiencing of the distressful elements to some degree. Coming to terms with some events is a life-long process.

The experience of being concerned about the meaning of life, death, and/or beliefs takes place within the context of time. Examples of time as ground were present in all of the transcripts. One dimension of time that participants talked about was the time that is measured in man-made units, such as hours, days, weeks, or years. For instance, the specific date or precise time was sometimes given for a traumatic event that broke into the ordinary flow of time, or specific times were mentioned by participants as reference points for when they became concerned about the meaning of life. Jean, whose words about the death of a child were cited above, stated, "But certainly one significant point at which I was concerned with this was when my niece was killed in a . . . was run over by a truck. On April 30." Because the year of this event was not given, the interviewer asked if the death had happened this year, to which Jean replied, "No. It was 20 years ago." One man began his interview by saying, "On March 29, 1988 my wife and I awoke one morning and discovered that our three-month-old daughter had died during the night of Sudden Infant Death Syndrome." Another dimension of time described by participants was a feeling of time without bounds, when feeling *something beyond*. There was also the sense of time passing when participants talked about the changes that had taken place over time. We turn now to the thematic elements which emerged against the ground of time.

Phase One: Breaking the Web

Events which "broke the web" included divorce, illnesses, accidents, and deaths of significant others. Catastrophic world events or the awareness of the paradoxical elements of nature could also jolt individuals out of their ordinary unreflected existence. However, being in a crisis situation did not necessarily catapult a person into thinking about the meaning of life. Conversely, reflection on the meaning of life/death and/or beliefs occurred during happy or quiet times as well as during times of tragedy. Thirty-four of the 54 events which prompted participants to ponder the meaning of life/death and/or beliefs did *not* involve spiritual distress, while 20 of the experiences did.

Whether an event was experienced as distressful seemed to depend on the participant's perception of the event. For example, a parent's death may or may not be a time of spiritual distress or trigger a concern about the meaning of the event. The wide diversity of experiences in which spiritual distress occurred makes it clear that a prediction of spiritual distress cannot be based on the type of event alone. One man's story of a Christmas Eve during the Vietnam War is a good example of an experience which sounds, on the surface, pleasant, but unexpectedly produced disturbing emotions and spiritual distress:

> I was off-duty and . . . I was just sitting on the steps of the barracks where I was quartered and it was right along the perimeter of the base where I was stationed and . . . the base . . . was inside a suburb of Danang . . . and so . . . the community was right up around it. . . . There was next door to where we were a little school . . . an orphanage, actually, that was operated by a group of French nuns . . . and on Christmas Eve they gathered there along the fence and sang Christmas carols and . . . that meant a great deal to me in 'What's it all about?' Here are these children . . . their lives have been wrecked by war. . . . Here we were . . . several of us American military personnel there hearing them. Here we were for God only knows what reason and yet something good and beautiful was happening in spite of the sounds of war that were going off in the hills beyond us there . . . the ugly fireworks of war. So, you know, there it was, peace and war going on at the same time. And in situations like that I think questions about the meaningfulness or meaninglessness, whatever, of life . . . come to mind. . . . I guess the frightening thing about that is that if something so beautiful can come out of ugliness, can beautiful things turn ugly too?

A broad range of feelings was elicited by distressful events. Rarely was the same word used by any two people to describe their feelings. Despite differences, however, feeling words could be clustered into three main categories: falling apart, pain, and instability.

Falling apart

The words participants used to describe this aspect of their experience communicate a sense of disconnectedness, separateness, coming apart, and sometimes total destruction. Illustrative are the following verbatim quotes: ". . . emotionally you crash." "It's like being in a war. When you're hit by the bomb and it just sort of explodes." "I was a basket case." "It was the dark night of the soul for me and I thought . . . 'Well, now's the time for God to pull a miracle here and show up'. . . . But God did not show up and I was a wreck."

Pain

Words grouped in this category represented different levels of pain, ranging from being uncomfortable to hurt or agony. Pain was evident not only in the words people used to describe how they felt during these times of distress but also during the interview itself. Most of the women were able to describe their emotions using feeling words and cried openly. The men in this study had more difficulty talking about and showing their emotions. The researcher came to realize, after it happened several times, that when men stopped talking, cleared their throats, or lowered their voices, their emotions were very close to the surface. At these times, the researcher acknowledged the difficulty of talking about emotional events and waited before continuing the interview. Some men then attempted to put words to their feelings whereas others were not able to continue and changed the subject.

Instability

While there were a variety of descriptive words within this category, all conveyed a sense of becoming unstable, losing control or hold of something, or being insecure. The first example of instability occurred during one man's experience of discussing religion with another man who considered himself an atheist. As a result of this encounter, the participant "lost" the "shallow" faith that he said he had "taken on" as a church member. Other selections from the transcripts depict the instability experienced during this phase of spiritual distress: "I literally was out on a limb and I went to live with my parents that summer. It was the worst summer—in terms of anxiety—I ever had in my entire life." ". . . you're really adrift. I just remember the very feeling . . . that I had to hang on to some feeling of a center post because of the fact that I had these two small children who looked up to me."

Wondering

"Wondering" was the word used by several people to indicate a period of questioning and trying to make sense out of what was happening to them. Participants wondered: Why me? Why this? Why now? Many of the participants' questions addressed a deity:

"Why should God kill a baby? These questions come through your head." In searching for a reason for some events, a few participants asked if they were to blame: "Why,
being 15, why do I have to go without a dad? I'm a good guy. I didn't do anything
wrong. Why am I being punished for that?" Questions arise when one is aware of both
the order and disorder present in the natural world: "The evidence that we see in this
world is absolutely contradictory. We see nature with immense order and structure and
grandeur and beauty and at the same time tornados and hurricanes and earthquakes
and forest fires and pestilence and plague and starvation . . . just absolutely contradictory from the scientific perspective."

As shown in these exemplars from the data, God's action and presence were not
beyond questioning. Questioning God seemed to lead participants to experience God
in new ways during times of distress. Crises were described as making people more
open to experiencing God emotionally rather than on the basis of rational thought or
argument. Participants identified this feeling of God's presence through the use of the
words "something beyond."

Something beyond

Seven of the 10 men and women in this study used the specific term "something
beyond," while two used the term "God." When they talked about something beyond,
they referred to that experience as a feeling, supportive presence, or a mystery. These
differences were not always clear-cut, and no attempt was made to categorize statements. God and "something beyond" were often talked about at the same time. Trying
to reach something beyond was an act of despair in some instances, as in the narrative
of a woman who asked for a "sign" that her husband would live following a car accident in which his neck was broken. Experiencing something beyond did not occur in
all distress situations described by participants. Sometimes, experiencing something
beyond occurred only when reflecting on the meaning of an event, not during the event
itself. For one man, there was no sense of a comforting presence in his time of distress; confidence that there was something beyond gradually evolved over many years.
Illustrative interview segments follow: "I suppose I am trying to talk . . . and it's not
even to someone. It's to something beyond what I can understand." ". . . there is some
incredible something out there that comes to people's aid when they need it and I did-
n't sense that in my dark night."

Phase Two: Rebuilding the Web

The second phase of spiritual distress was characterized as a time of rebuilding the web
of life. This phase of rebuilding involved a change in feelings and beliefs about self and
the world; in general, participants perceived these changes as positive. During this period,
the event that caused the break was incorporated into life, just as the scar from a wound
gradually recedes in prominence. The web is rewoven, thereby encapsulating the break
and making the web intact and functional once again.

Stability

In contrast to the sense of falling apart expressed in phase one, participants talked about things becoming stable, stronger, and more secure. Participants used the word *strength* to refer to changes in themselves and their beliefs: "The death of my daughter caused me to even feel better about . . . doubts because it was very healthy . . . it made me a stronger Christian to be able to question." "His illness made us stronger, better people. And here's what his death gave me: the courage to face my own death." The experience of *security* in this phase was not the same kind of false sense of security that participants had experienced before their world had fallen apart. They now knew that no matter how "good" they were, this did not protect them from being hurt: "What I'm secure in is that I will be okay." "For awhile, before my daughter died, there was this false sense of security in the world, that bad things just happen to other people . . . not to me, and that God's got a good grip on my life. So, if there was one thing that really changed for me was not really my view that chance happened, but that all of a sudden I was included in how I viewed the world."

Change and growth

Participants talked about growth in the self and beliefs, as time passed. But growth was not attributable solely to the passage of time; they purposefully chose to pursue it. All participants gave examples of the ways they had chosen to give meaning to the distressful events in their lives; finding meaning in the events involved hard work. Participants voiced gratitude for the way their lives had unfolded, despite all the difficulties that had come their way. Each person identified positive things that had come out of what initially looked like a negative circumstance. For example, one woman asserted that she was a better mother to her other two children because of her handicapped child. Actions were taken to turn bad into good for themselves and others. These actions were described within the framework of responsibility: "I've tried to help several close friends through that process since my mother died and I've had relatives of those people tell me that I was very attuned to how to go through that with another person." "I had called the hospital and said that I would be . . . that I had been trained to visit newly diagnosed families in the hospital . . . and that I'd be happy to do that here."

Wondering

Rather than continually questioning the "why" of distressful events, participants described the wondering of the second phase as more of a sense of awe at the mystery of life. Although questioning did not completely cease, there was an acceptance that there need not be any answers: "There really are no answers in the area of death for me." ". . . I liked answers. . . . I wanted black and white. Well, I've discovered that is not possible and that's the part for me to deal with in terms of my belief system and the Bible and all of that because I didn't like all those inconsistencies that I kept running up against." "I don't have the answers. But I still continually search for these answers, hoping in some small way. Then . . . when my time comes, I want to feel that I have accomplished something and that's all we can do."

There also is a realization of the limits to human knowing. Rather than expressing frustration at this turn of events, participants reported reaching a new level of faith or trust. Participants concluded that the ways of God are unfathomable and, in the end, one must stand in awe and wonder at the great mystery that is life: "I mean it's not given to understand the nature of the creation. We're stuck with accepting it and having the faith that it makes some sense."

Something beyond

Helping participants to live without answers to their questions was their belief in "something beyond." The experience of something beyond was present in the rebuilding phase for all 10 participants. The man who had not experienced something beyond in his time of distress said it took him twenty years to rebuild his shattered faith. Now his renewed faith is not a fragile belief system that he just "took on" from others.

DISCUSSION AND CONCLUSIONS

The experience of spiritual distress, as described in the present study, involves both the breaking of the web of life, and eventually, the reweaving of that web through gradual changes, over time, in feelings and beliefs. The word *wonder* frequently appeared in the transcripts, conveying a sense of puzzlement, doubt, and curiosity. Wondering was evident in both phases of the spiritual distress experience. First, through asking questions or wondering, a person attempts to figure out a rationale for the disruptive event. Later, in the second phase, the questioning appears to continue at a lesser intensity even when answers are not forthcoming. Belief in "something beyond" seemed to be the force vital to the rebuilding process. Participants in this study had not become bitter because of the things that had happened to them. Similar to Frankl's (1946/1959) attitude during his imprisonment in concentration camps, they had chosen to take a constructive stance toward the events that ripped the fabric of their existence, eventually wresting meaning from their spiritual distress. They discussed a sense of responsibility to help others in crisis, adopting a new mode of being similar to the self-transcendent commitment that Frankl talked about. The transformational change and growth described by the men and women in this study is consistent with Prigogine's theory of dissipative structures, in which physical systems driven away from stability regain it at a higher level of organization (Prigogine, cited in Schorr & Schroeder, 1989).

Findings of the study suggest a new definition of spiritual distress. The current NANDA definition is "a disruption in the life principle which pervades a person's entire being and which integrates and transcends biopsychosocial nature" (Hurley, 1986, p. 543). This definition does not include the inherent potential for growth and change. A proposed new definition of spiritual distress might read as follows: an uncomfortable experience of spiritual and/or existential struggle within which there is potential for growth. Of the current defining characteristics for the diagnosis, the majority were validated in this study. The characteristic "unable to participate in usual religious practices," however, is probably an antecedent to the diagnosis, and it is recommended that it be removed from the list.

The characteristics of the rebuilding phase of spiritual distress found in the present study may be a result of the uniqueness of the sample, 10 healthy people to whom religious and/or spiritual beliefs are very important. Many nurses will encounter people at times of crisis who do not have spiritual resources to draw upon. How these people would describe spiritual distress might be quite different. In future investigations, interviews should be conducted with patients in various health care settings who have been formally diagnosed by nurses as spiritually distressed. To see if a similar thematic structure would emerge from asking other individuals the same question, future studies should include persons with more diverse religious views as well as persons having no denominational allegiances or interest.

Congruence of this study's findings with Seidner's (1987) study of "falling apart" provides some reassurance regarding universality of the experience. In the Seidner study, participants described threatened or actual loss of the familiar world of people, places, and relationships and an alteration in the continuity of time. Similar words were used in both studies to describe feelings of hanging on, questioning faith, being isolated, disconnected, and disoriented. Themes of the resolution phase described by Seidner's sample are consistent with aspects of "rebuilding the web" in the present study in which reconnections were made with familiar people, places, and things. Feelings of order, security, and resilience ensued. How can nurses help their patients to achieve this state of resolution?

IMPLICATIONS OF THE STUDY FINDINGS FOR NURSING PRACTICE

Based on the findings of this study, it is likely that the first indication a nurse may have of a patient's spiritual distress is when he or she verbalizes feelings. Dugan (1987/88) points out that the spirit speaks through the partly conscious and partly unconscious phenomena of emotions and dreams. The nurse must be very observant of non-verbal behavior and listen carefully to what is often symbolic language. If the nurse is comfortable being with the patient and indicates a willingness to listen, the patient may eventually disclose his or her doubts and anguish. A participant cautioned that "I might not be inclined to tell her unless she establishes some trust and I don't know exactly how you do that 'cause I've seen enough nurses to know that some nurses could and others would never get it done . . . that's getting pretty close to stuff you don't talk to strangers about."

In the first phase of spiritual distress, patients may be expected to report feeling hurt, scared, or anxious. Dialogue was mentioned as the intervention most helpful to participants when they experienced their world as falling apart. Phrases such as "instability" and "falling apart" indicate a need for support. The nurse can ask the person to think of people and things that proved supportive to them in the past. Pastors, chaplains, and visits from church members may bring great comfort. If prayer is important to a person, the nurse can ask the patient how he or she usually prays and if prayer by the nurse is desired. Prayers can be brief and simple, including patient requests, or reciting a favorite prayer with someone.

In giving spiritual care, the nurse must be exquisitely sensitive to and respectful of a patient's cultural and religious beliefs. It is always best to ask patients how you can assist them. At the height of the crisis when emotions are intense, nurses should bear in mind that patients and their families may try to protect themselves from these emotions by keeping busy or trying not to think. They may view an exploration of their feelings, excessive questioning, or provision of too much information, as insensitive and intrusive. For example, a nurse had told one study participant "blow by blow" what happened when her husband had a respiratory arrest, which the participant tried not to think about because it was too painful. This woman's experience reminds us that distressed individuals may not want to know clinical details of a family member's deterioration or death.

Patients in spiritual distress may have many "why" questions concerning either religious or philosophical issues. The results of this study may help nurses to know when patients are struggling with finding meaning. The nurse's role is to encourage the patient to be open to new ways of thinking, to not be afraid of the questions, and to look ahead to the new meaning that is possible as a result of the event. Nurses can tell patients that questioning—even of God—is a natural part of being human and trying to make sense out of the world. Making meaning in life is an ongoing process. Participants in this study saw more meaning in events at the time they were interviewed than when the events originally took place.

Some patients may become stuck in phase one of spiritual distress, either because they have not come to terms with the reality of there not being answers to everything and/or they have not been able to experience "something beyond." Growth would seem possible only when pain is acknowledged, when one is open to the transcendent dimension, and when limits to knowing are accepted (Trice, 1990). One of nursing's roles has always been to create a healing environment. An environment that is conducive to finding meaning may be one that allows the patient some time in solitude. Steeves and Kahn (1987), in a study of the experience of meaning in suffering, describe a phenomenon frequently observed by nurses in hospice settings. In this study, individuals talked about various kinds of transcendent experiences in which their suffering was temporarily lifted. Simply working in the garden or listening to music provided some patients an opportunity to access something beyond the self. The researchers viewed such experiences as beneficial to patients' well-being and suggested that nurses create times of solitude in which such helpful phenomena could occur.

Ashurst and Hall (1989) compared a therapist to a sherpa or mountain guide. By substituting the word "nurse" for "therapist," their words seem to provide a fitting conclusion to this study:

> "The nurse is like a sherpa or mountain guide who knows something of the terrain and is more familiar with it than the person he or she is guiding. The sherpa cannot, however, take the steps for the traveler or stop him from experiencing some further pain on the way: but can, by his or her presence, support and reassure and take away the loneliness and terror of the journey" (p. 10).

It is hoped that this study will help the nurse to be a good guide for patients experiencing spiritual distress.

POST-STUDY REFLECTIONS FROM CAROL SMUCKER

My examination of the phenomenon of spiritual distress did not end with the study reported here. In 1995 and 1996, I interviewed 10 more people. Findings from this study, which included a more diverse sample, produced the same model for the two phases of the spiritual distress experience. However, three female participants did not experience spiritual distress despite experiencing a variety of events that are usually distressful. Two women attributed their lack of distress to their strong religious belief system, while the other woman, who experienced the "killing fields" of Cambodia as a child, said she had focused only on survival.

Through the years, I have learned to be a good phenomenological interviewer and also a better listener. I have learned ways to help men articulate/express their emotions. I have a new appreciation for the continuing freshness and emotional power of past emotionally charged life events. I recognize the universality of patterns in similar life experiences. I understand how important meaning is to health and healing. I am convinced that nurses must learn to provide basic spiritual care to their patients. The importance of prayer to people in crisis has been affirmed in my parish nurse work. Often, people have told me that they were too ill and did not have the strength to pray and welcomed someone praying on their behalf. When I made rounds to patients the evening before their surgeries and asked if they would like me to pray, no one refused.

From my research I obtained a clearer definition of spiritual distress and developed a model of how it is often resolved. I have communicated my understanding through journal articles and lectures to diverse audiences of nurses. The study findings helped me formulate a spiritual well-being tool and a spiritual assessment form for use by the parish nurses in a program I founded after receiving my doctoral degree. My interest in spiritual care has deepened, leading me to pursue a course of study in lay ministry.

V

Nursing and the Human Experience of the World

The nurse is still here. Then
She is not here. You
Are here but are not sure
It is you in the sudden darkness. No matter.
A damned nuisance, but trivial—
The surgeon has just said that. A dress rehearsal,
You tell yourself, for
The real thing. Later. Ten years? Fifteen?
Tomorrow, only a dry run. At
5 A.M. they will come. Your hand reaches out in darkness
To the TV button. It is an old-fashioned western.
Winchester fire flicks white in the dream-night.
It has something to do with vice and virtue, and the vastness
Of moonlit desert. A stallion, white and flashing, slips,
Like spilled quicksilver, across
The vastness of moonlight. Black
Stalks of cacti, like remnants of forgotten nightmares, loom
Near at hand. Action fades into distance, but
You are sure that virtue will triumph. Far beyond
All the world, the mountains lift. The snow peaks
Float into moonlight. They float
In that unnamable altitude of white light. God
Loves the world. For what it is.

—Robert Penn Warren, excerpted from "Three Darknesses" taken from
New and Selected Poems 1923–1985.

Reprinted by permission of William Morris Agency.

14

The Human Experience of the Non-Human World

Any approach to human life that concerns itself with being-in-the-world must have something to say about the physical world. The word "world" itself is composed of two parts—*were* and *aeld*—both of which are recognizable in other words: *were* as in werewolf (man-wolf) and *aeld* as in old. Adding these two together gives *world* a meaning something like "in the time or age of man" or, more generally, "in the era of human life," as contrasted with a more spiritual world neither of this time nor of this life. Initially, the word "world" did not mean, as it now does, the earth or physical environment; this meaning only emerged in the tenth century (Ayto, 1990).

But we still do use the word "world" to capture certain aspects of its initial human and time-related meanings. So it is possible to speak of the (human) "world of the theater" or "of medicine" as well as the more (time-oriented) "biblical" or "medieval" worlds. Basically, "world" has meant, and continues to mean, any organized totality concerning people or time. The philosopher John MacQuarrie (1973) points out that the word "world" always includes "the point of view of the person who is talking about the world. [It] does not stand for something independent of those who talk about it. . . . This is not to be taken . . . (to mean that) . . . the material universe depends for its existence on the minds that perceive it . . . When I say that there is no world apart from man . . . I am making a linguistic point: Whenever we talk of world, we talk at the same time of man, for the expression *world* implies a human standpoint from which everything is seen" (pp. 79–80).

Despite these connotations, we usually take the word "world" to mean the physical world independent of human presence. From this perspective, a number of different scientific disciplines claim one or another topic as their domain. If we talk about the earth, we have geology; if we talk about abstract space, we have geometry; if we talk about locations and places we have geography; if we talk about matter, either on earth or elsewhere in the universe, we have physics; if we talk about animals and plants, we have biology, and so on. Since, with Heidegger, we have learned to look at the history of words to provide a new perspective on human life, consider the following three words: *"nature," "physics,"* and *"matter."* "Nature" comes from a root word meaning to be born, "physics" from a root word meaning to give birth, and "matter" is a variation on the word *mater* (mother.) Moving on to geometry, geology, and geography, the *geo* part invokes the name of Ge (mother earth) and *metry* means to measure, *ology* to study, and *graphy* to write about. Whether natural scientists like it or not, the idea of the physical world as initially dealing with mother and/or birth is too obvious to miss. It also seems clear that biology comes from *bios*, meaning life, and that many sciences have been named in view of the world's likeness to some maternal or life-giving figure such as "Mother Earth."

Geology, geography, geometry, physics, and biology are all concerned with an objective, or third-person, understanding of the world. Such an approach is to be contrasted with a more first-person one in which human experiences of the world must be included. In this regard, the empty space of geometry becomes the lived space of human movement; the maps of geography become places invested with meaning, such as "my home" or "my country"; the anonymous formations of geology become the religious and cultural meanings of nature in which rocks are sacred and forests foreboding; and, finally, the physical matter of natural science becomes the special possessions and objects of some specific human life. No less than the domains of body, time, and others, the domain of world may be considered either from an objective point of view or from that of a being whose destiny is to be found and understood only as meaningful being-in-the-world.

THE MEANINGS OF SPACE AND PLACE

The classical statement about the lived meanings of *space* and *place* is eloquently presented in a book by phenomenological geographer Yi-Fu Tuan (1977). As one aspect of his concern with lived space, Tuan offers an analysis of the space surrounding the human body. As he notes, there are clearly different experiences and meanings attached to the space in front of and behind, to the right or left, and above and below the person. Because each person experiences him or herself as "the center of his or her world," the idea of center has a further meaning and significance in human life. Using the body as center, and the upright, waking position as a point of reference, Tuan points out that space "projected from the body is biased toward front and right. The future is ahead and up. The past is behind and below."

The meanings of right and left are clearly different, as any lefthanded student sitting in a lecture hall will tell you: the writing surfaces of desks are always on the right side of the chair. Even the word "right" in English means not only power but also correctness (do it right), freedom from guilt (righteousness), and law (Bill of Rights). Then too, we have phrases such as "right of way" and "left behind." The Italian word for left is *sinestra* (sinister) and in pictures of the "Last Supper," Christ is often painted with his right hand toward heaven and his left toward hell. The right-left orientation of the body is every bit as differentiated as that of front and back, and both make the same point: lived space, unlike the empty and abstract space of geometry, is never equal in significance in all directions from some neutral origin.

Generalizing this type of spatial analysis, the French philosopher Gaston Bachelard (1969) discussed brick and mortar houses in terms of different meanings and experiences associated with attics and basements, front and back porches, passages and thresholds, central hearths and cooking areas. He was especially mindful of the meanings of inside and outside, particularly as these are defined by windows and doors. In the case of "above" and "below," Bachelard notes that we usually go down to the basement and up to the attic, suggesting the attic as a more pleasant and anticipated location and the basement as a more negative and avoided one.

Extending the meaning of bodily space to cities, Tuan notes that "people everywhere . . . regard their own homeland as the middle place or center of the world." In fact, certain traditional Chinese cities have a clear front and back, with the front oriented toward the south (and the male or yang principle) and the back oriented toward the north (and the female or ying principle). This usage overrides the usual dominance of right (east) and left (west), since facing south makes left the preferred direction. The more general point, however, remains the same: lived space is not homogeneous and some directions are more significant than others.

With this move from bodily space to houses and cities, the topic of space has subtly changed into that of *place*. Although geographers may list and locate the places of the world on charts and maps, the human experience of place seems much more intimate and personal. Working on the assumption that each of us has, or had, some special places in life, Peacher (1996) asked adult participants to talk about "places that were special" to them. On the basis of her analysis, five themes were found to describe participant experiences of special places. The first of these themes, **Identity**, concerned the way in which special places strengthen a person's sense of who he or she is, provide continuity across life, and evoke poignant memories from earlier times. The loss of a special place invariably is described as emotionally devastating. The second theme, **Connection**, concerned place-based relationships to loved ones, some of whom may be deceased, as well as to something larger than oneself such as a university or city. Many participants expressed comfort in knowing that their special place might endure after their death. **Security**, the third theme, embraced the ability of a special place to provide a sense of permanence and tradition, to ensure familiarity and safety, and to afford moments of escape from life's ongoing problems. The fourth theme, **Possibilities**, encompassed the ways in which participants experienced a particular place as challenging their abilities and affording opportunities for change and growth. The final theme, **Beauty and Awe**, concerned feelings of appreciation for the beauty of one's own special place as well as for a spiritual oneness with the universe when in that place.

It is interesting to consider how places get their names. Take the case of Jacob, one of the more prolific biblical travelers, who named places such as Beth El, Galeed and Pineal. The first name means "house of God" and concerns Jacob's dream of the ladder. Galeed is composed of the word "ed" meaning witness and "gal" meaning a pile of stones; hence, Galeed denotes the pile of rocks placed by Jacob to witness the end of bad feelings between him and his tricky father-in-law, Laban. Jacob gave the name Pineal, meaning "the face of God," to the place where he wrestled an angel (or God). In considering these place names we can imagine Jacob looking out over the vast expanse of desert and perhaps feeling daunted by a lack of signs to guide his journey. By naming places he specified unique areas in which something important happened to him. Thus, *place* serves to define a center of significance or meaning that may be used as a guide for oneself and/or other travelers. Tuan (1977) describes place as space "made into an object;" Merleau-Ponty talks about it as a "thickening of the spatial medium." Both stress the same point: place emerges whenever the homogeneity of space takes on a bit of renewable definition capable of offering direction to travelers.

While not as grand as Jacob's namings, contemporary place names also express unique meanings. New York, New Jersey, New Orleans, and New England all invoke a nostalgic connection to a previous home. The cities of Lincoln, Washington, and Columbus refer to heroes of our country. Many place names in North America, such as Tallahassee and Mississippi, reflect the earliest inhabitants of our country. Religious figures are honored in names such as San Francisco and St. Louis. Other bases for naming also come to mind, and all lead to exactly the same conclusion: geographical places invariably describe something of importance to the namers, whether this something is religious, historical, or personal. Place, then, is never without meaning.

Objects and Things

A similar analysis may be applied to objects and things. Heidegger (1927/1962) felt that the relationship between the world and human life often was disclosed quite powerfully in terms of such items. According to Heidegger, objects bear at least two different relationships to human being: *Zuhand* (at hand, useful to our projects) and *Vorhand* (on hand, something understood in terms of properties such as weight, density, or substance). The first of these relationships refers to objects and things of concern to our life; the second refers to a more intellectual or reflected understanding of them. We live our lives in terms of *Zuhand*, and objects of this type permit us to work at our jobs (tools), succeed at play (toys), decorate our homes and our bodies (with works of art or jewelry), offer security when frightened (teddy bears and blankets), and remind us of earlier days and relationships (mementoes and souvenirs).

We humanize our environment "by coating it with dimensions of ourselves" (Merleau-Ponty, 1962)— "things" that make a house a home or a sterile cubicle into "my office." To appreciate the significant role "things" play in human life, all we need to do is remember the case of Rose who became lonely and confused when "her things" were taken away from her at the hospital. On this basis, many of the same themes capturing the meaning of special places—identity, possibility, connection, beauty, and security—also seem to define special objects and possessions. The implications for nursing practice, in both cases, seem relatively clear: security and relationship are diminished in the hospital setting, and it is our task to find ways of providing these meanings for patients who no longer have their special possessions nor access to their special places.

Special possessions, like special places, ultimately concern issues of safety and security. Tuan (1977) has applied these concerns to the geographical environment so as to yield a simple but elegant characterization of the difference between space and place: "Place is security, space is freedom." Whether we consider space in terms of outer space, Jacob's desert, or the vastness of the American frontier, feelings of freedom are clearly expressed by phrases such as "don't fence me in" or "the sky's the limit." Whether we consider place in terms of neighborhoods or more specific, special places, the feeling is one of security: "Home is where they have to take you in."

Although the contrast between space and place, between security and freedom, is a significant one, there are counter-examples where place is not security (the operating room) and space is not freedom (the space beneath an airplane). The most significant counter-examples, however, concerns a pair of psychiatric conditions, claustrophobia and agoraphobia. Claustrophobia, a fear of small places or of being enclosed, offers a meaning for place that is not one of security but of fearful constraint (or non-freedom). Agoraphobia, a fear of open spaces, suggests that being in some uncharted outside may provide an experience of fearful paralysis quite at odds with Tuan's formula. Place, which on most occasions and for most people may be said to provide a situation of security, may at times provide an experience of coercion and unfreedom. Space, which for most people on most occasions, may provide an experience of freedom, sometimes provides an experience of a fearful lack of support. Considered in this way, Tuan's "formula" must be extended to recognize that the major themes defining space and place are bipolar: freedom vs. constraint and security vs. fear.

Being Lost

Issues of fear and security also emerge in regard to the special person-world condition known as "lost." Being lost has a number of different connotations in addition to its literal environmental one. For example, when Michael Thweatt (2000) asked college students to talk about situations in which they experienced themselves as lost, they described three different types of situations: (1) those in which the person was spatially disoriented, as in a fog or snowstorm, the usual meaning of lost; (2) those in which the person was lost in terms of interpersonal dislocation, perhaps at the end of a significant relationship or the death of a relative or friend; and (3) those in which the person experienced being lost in a spiritual sense. When Thweatt arrived at a thematic meaning of "lost," he discovered that three themes captured the pattern, such that the person who is lost, in any sense of the term, feels disconnected, isolated, and lonely (theme 1); helpless, afraid, and in despair (theme 2); and uncertain and confused (theme 3). All three themes were summed up by a participant in the study in the following terms: "being lost means being someplace where nothing stands out to give you any direction to go in." Although it may be going too far to describe the people we see in our day-to-day clinical practice as lost, they too report that they do not know which way to go, and, like a lost child or traveler, could use someone to provide direction, connection, and/or purpose.

THE MEANING OF NATURE

Concern with place and space relates most directly to geometry and geography. What about geology, physics, and biology? Although differences between third- and first-person perspectives could be discussed on a discipline-by-discipline basis, it seems better to consider a single domain such as nature that relates to all three to some degree. For natural science the question always seems to be: "How does it work?" and the problem is to understand nature on the basis of some theory. For more humanistic, or first-person, perspectives, the question is always: "What does it mean?" The task is to describe human reactions to nature either in terms of phenomenological descriptions or specific works of art. In the case of art, nature may serve as a setting for some novel, play, or movie or may itself become the focus as in landscape painting or architecture. To discover what nature means when it serves as a setting or ground, Pollio, Levasseur, Anderson, and Thweatt (2001) asked a large number of participants to think of movies in which nature played a significant role and then describe how it related to the film's major theme or themes. On the basis of these descriptions, Pollio et al. concluded that nature, as represented in films, is defined by five major themes: **Power and Scale, Danger and Safety, Change and Permanence, Beauty**, and **Connection and Alienation**. Although these themes do not exhaust contemporary meanings for nature, they do provide a reasonable initial set.

In a different, but related, study Pollio and Thweatt (2000) selected 10 famous landscape paintings and asked participants to imagine themselves in the environment portrayed. Although there was a clear preference for some landscapes over others, most participants were able to create narratives concerning their reactions to the landscape. When these narratives were analyzed, many of the same themes emerged as were true for movies: Power, Safety/Danger, Predictability/Change, Beauty, and Light/Dark. The last theme obviously relates to the realm of painting, per se. Considered together, results of both studies suggest that concerns with power, danger, predictability, and beauty define a general set of meanings for the human experience of nature.

Present ideas about the possible ways in which human beings think about nature, either as figure or ground, are strongly influenced by landscape architecture of the late eighteenth and early nineteenth century. It was during this period that a controversy arose as to whether the precise geometric gardens at Versailles were to be the standard of beauty or if gardens that were less controlled and more picturesque would define the ideal landscape. At issue was not an aesthetic controversy but a more general concern over the way human beings ought to think about nature. For the formalist, the landscape architect was to bring nature under the control of rigid geometrical precision; for the naturalist, nature and the landscape architect were to respect one another, with nature always free to change what the architect developed. This controversy also related to more than just landscape, in fact, it concerned nothing less than defining an ideal human being either as a product of control, education, and logic (wild, until civilized) or as one needing only a bit of "taming" to develop his or her natural goodness (good, unless corrupted by a malicious and manipulative society).

A different aspect of nature in which a contrast between rationalism (defined as predictability, control, and safety) and romanticism (defined as unpredictability, freedom, and danger) took place concerned the topic of weather. The very word used to describe the scientific study of weather—"meteorology"—gives some hint as to the flavor of the historical controversy. Although we may think of meteors as solid bits of matter from outer space, their original meaning was something like "things on high," implying "unpredictable things" such as shooting stars or weather. The unpredictability of weather-related phenomena, in fact, proved to be somewhat of an embarrassment for the neat analyses of early enlightenment and scientific thinkers who felt that rational thought ought to be able to predict and control the natural world. It was for this reason that English poets such as Shelley and Keats took delight in the unpredictability of the weather, describing it in terms such as "delightful terror."

The weather, however, had, and continues to have, other connotations. Words relating to weather, or climate more generally, often are used to describe human emotion and temperament. For example, consider the pairs hot/cold and sunny/stormy. To say that someone is "hot" is to imply passion and excitement; to call someone "cold" is to imply an aloof and unfriendly person. A "sunny" person is quite different from a "stormy" person, and both are quite different from a "fair-weather" friend.

Perhaps the major issue in regard to the human response to nature (weather included) pertains to power and control. The anthropologist Florence Kluckhon (1953) long ago suggested that human societies may be categorized in terms of three different attitudes they hold toward the relationship between people and nature: (1) people are less than nature, and therefore, always at its mercy; (2) people are greater than nature, and therefore, should attempt to dominate it for the human good; (3) people and nature are in harmony, and therefore, should seek a balance with one another. Theoretically speaking, what is at issue is whether nature and people are to be in harmony or conflict, and who is to have control: us, nature, neither, both.

NURSING AND THE MEANINGS OF NATURE

While a concern for the meanings of nature may seem far removed from the nurse's day-to-day concerns, there are a number of different lines of evidence to suggest that patient experiences of the non-human world have significant implications for health. First of all, there is the case of pets. Companion animals provide a number of health benefits to individuals of all ages (Baun, Oetting, & Bergstrom, 1991). There is a substantial amount of research on the elderly, including those with Alzheimer's disease (Churchill, Safaoui, McCabe, & Baun, 1999). Pets reduce loneliness in older adults, reduce systolic blood pressure and plasma triglycerides, and serve to relieve stress, thereby reducing visits to physicians for stress-related concerns (Jennings et al., 1998; Keil, 1998). Although these effects are not large, they suggest that lonely individuals might improve their health by sharing their lives with a pet. Obviously, if a person is afraid of animals or feels no connection to them, having an animal would not reduce stress or loneliness. The crucial issue is whether the person and the animal form a bond with one another.

Probably the one aspect of the natural world that hospital nurses are quite used to seeing in patient rooms are plants and flowers. Although the sensual and aesthetic properties of flowers and plants are obvious, what is somewhat less obvious are their symbolic meanings. When Csikszentmahalyi and Rochberg-Halton (1981) asked respondents about cherished objects in their homes, plants were among the top 10 items mentioned. When participants were asked why plants were so significant, most spoke of them as a source of living companionship. They also mentioned plants' decorative function and ability to purify indoor air and make a room feel alive. People talked about liking to take care of plants. As the researchers noted: "A house that contains plants [is] pretty and full of life; a person who tends flowers gets in touch with nature, grows as a person and helps make the world healthier; a person who gives plants . . . is sensitive [and] communicates an appreciation for beauty and the life process" (Csikszentmahalyi & Rochberg-Halton, p. 82).

Almost all of these themes make plants an ideal expression of concern for a sick person, either at home or in the hospital. Perhaps the major themes of the human experience of plants and/or flowers concern their ability to evoke meanings of care and being cared for, combined with those of life (and death). Within the Christian tradition, themes of rebirth also are implied; the daffodil bulb that is in the winter's ground will, in the spring, break free from the earth and become a blooming plant. The natural re-emergence of plants and flowers would seem to provide hope and the possibility of growth and change for most patients. For a few patients, however, the death motif may be more powerful and frightening, and, here, flowers are not appropriate.

A final way in which patients may be helped by feeling connected to nature concerns the seemingly simple case of what the patient can or cannot see when looking out the window. Research has shown that patients assigned to rooms overlooking a park or garden have shorter postoperative stays and use fewer medications than patients assigned to rooms overlooking another building or a brick wall (Ulrich, 1984; Verdeber, 1986). In a case reported by Baird and Bell (1995), a young leukemia patient even preferred a room with windows facing a cemetery to one with no view of the outside world at all.

Perhaps the most dramatic example of the positive effects of nature on the quality of human life is captured in the following story told by Frankl (1946/1959) about a dying young woman incarcerated in a concentration camp hospital:

> This young woman knew that she would die in the next few days. . . . Pointing through the window she said, "This tree here is the only friend I have in my loneliness." Through that window she could see just one branch of a chestnut tree, and on the branch were two blossoms. "I often talk to this tree," she said to me. I was startled and didn't quite know how to take her words. . . . Anxiously I asked her if the tree replied. "Yes." What did it say to her? She answered, "It said to me, 'I am here—I am here—I am life, eternal life'" (Frankl, 1946/1959, pp. 109–110).

> Although this may be an extreme case, the more general point seems to be that our patients' experiences of the non-human world are never irrelevant to the quality of their life nor to the speed and extent of their recoveries. Considered in this light, it seems quite reasonable that a person who feels a kinship to pets, flowers, or the world beyond his or her sick bed will be more likely to recover than one who feels distant and alienated from nature.

In the next two chapters, we present the findings of phenomenological studies explicitly designed to discover significant elements of the world of the patient. In nursing's metaparadigm, four core concepts have been identified as the phenomena of concern for the discipline of nursing: *person, health, nursing*, and *environment* (Fawcett, 2000). While a substantial amount of research has been conducted regarding three of the metaparadigm concepts (*person, health*, and *nursing*), the fourth concept, *environment*, is seldom studied. Environment, as defined by Fawcett, includes the physical setting in which nursing occurs—sometimes the home, most often a hospital or clinical agency. Little is actually known about patients' perceptions of hospital and clinic environments because researchers simply have not asked them. We turn first, in Chapter 15, to stories about the world of the hospital; in the following chapter, we will examine patients' experiences of the outpatient world.

15

"Eventually It'll Be Over": The Dialectic Between Confinement and Freedom in the World of the Hospitalized Patient

"You have to be in the hospital so you have to be in the hospital. Eventually it'll be over . . . I just thought, endure this, we'll get through it."

—words of a patient interviewed for the present study

The word "hospital" comes from the Latin term, *hospes*, meaning guest or host. Established with a benevolent intent, hospitals in some historical eras became places of horror. People who entered did not come out alive. To this day, many people are almost phobic about visiting a hospital and have an even stronger dread of being admitted to one as an inpatient. Perhaps it is time to return to the original connotation of hospitality, thinking of patients as "guests" and ascertaining what would help to create a more hospitable environment for them when they arrive for treatments or surgeries. Unfortunately, little is known about particular aspects of the world of the hospital that may (or may not) matter to patients. Aspects of the environment such as "pleasantness and appeal of the hospital room," "availability of visitor parking," and "professional appearance of hospital staff" are often included on questionnaires used to measure patient satisfaction. But are these environmental variables, assessed by rat-

* This chapter is based on a study conducted by Mona Shattell at the University of Tennessee, Knoxville. Contributions of the following members of the research team are gratefully acknowledged: Tracey Martin, Alison Hicks, and Kathy Smith.

ing scales, actually tapping what matters? As long ago as 1972, Ronco pointed out that the patient has "been ignored if not forgotten in the [hospital] design process," and the hospital environment still remains the least studied attribute of patient satisfaction and service quality (Hutton & Richardson, 1995). Because patients seldom have been invited to describe their experience of the hospital, the purpose of the present study was to elicit such a description. First, however, it may be useful to review a bit of history.

RELATED LITERATURE

A Brief History of Hospitals

In his book on the history of hospitals, Risse (1999) details their transformation from "houses of mercy" in the Byzantine period to "houses of rehabilitation" in the Renaissance era to "houses of dissection and cure" in the eighteenth and nineteenth centuries, to the "houses of high technology" in which contemporary nurses practice. This thumbnail sketch provides us with an understanding of the way in which hospitals reflected, and continue to reflect, societal values in different historical eras.

Sloane and Sloane's (1992) review of hospital history provides a different perspective, emphasizing religious and military influences on their purpose and construction. In fact, the first hospitals they discuss were grand marble temples, built several centuries before Christ in honor of the Greek physician Aesculapius. These temples were lavishly decorated with statuary and other art works. Patients who visited these temples brought gifts and worshipped with the hope of being healed by the spirit of Aesculapius. Upon admission, patients were bathed and clad in white garments, and their care involved plenty of sunshine, fresh air, exercise, and entertainment (Jamieson, Sewall, & Suhrie, 1969).

During the Roman Empire, the first army hospitals were developed. After the fall of the Roman Empire, the Catholic Church took over the responsibility for caring for the sick. During early Christianity, people were cared for in churches in which beds were set up in vestibules and along aisles (Sloane & Sloane, 1992). Later, during the Middle Ages, the church promoted hospital construction (Jamieson et al., 1969). In these hospitals, nuns nursed female patients and monks cared for male patients. It was believed that God would cure and faith would heal. Specialty hospitals came into existence during this time and persons with leprosy, the elderly, and the poor were housed in such hospitals. Conditions in early hospitals were variable, ranging from horrendous to tolerable. One medieval hospital, built to accommodate nearly 1,000 patients, has been described as having "fortress-like characteristics. . . . Windows, small and narrow, were sunk deep and high in thick stone walls. The patient . . . saw nothing of the world outside [and] was also deprived of fresh air. Tapestry or wall hangings helped to take the chill from bare, cold walls in wintertime. . . . To prevent drafts and ensure privacy, each bed was enclosed in a tentlike curtain" (Jamieson et al., 1969, pp. 118–119). Patients in institutions such as this were segregated according to their status as members of religious groups, pilgrims, or laity.

During the Renaissance and Reformation, the Catholic Church's control over hospitals declined. King Henry VIII originated a network of non-profit, private voluntary hospitals, among them St. Bartholomew's in London (Sloane & Sloane, 1992). The unsanitary conditions of these hospitals, however, soon made them breeding grounds for epidemics. As many as 100 patients were crowded together in huge wards. Nursing care was provided by untrained women, younger ones being employed for the day shift and "old women" for night duty (Jamieson et al., 1969). Because of the deplorable conditions, hospitals were places to be avoided if at all possible. Incurable patients whom the hospitals refused to treat were sent to prisons and asylums (Sloane & Sloane, 1992).

During the Crimean War, Florence Nightingale (1820–1910) cared for British soldiers in Scutari, Turkey, and had a profound impact on the nature of the hospital environment. She was charged with providing skilled nursing care to soldiers, but "to achieve this mission . . . she needed to address the environmental problems that existed, including the lack of sanitation and the presence of filth (few chamber pots, contaminated water, contaminated sheets and blankets, overflowing cesspools)" (Pfettscher, de Graff, Tomey, Mossman, & Slebodnik, 1998, p. 70). When the British people learned that the mortality rate of soldiers at Scutari declined from more than 40% to 2.2%, Nightingale's radical transformation of hospital care was acclaimed. After the war, she was instrumental in improving conditions in other military and civilian hospitals, and she disseminated her ideas across the globe in voluminous publications.

In the United States, hospital conditions improved during World War I and World War II through advances in nursing, science, and medicine. Facilities built during the modern era aimed for a "clean sterile look—an efficient functional block appearance of sameness and anonymity" (Watson, 2001, p. 299). But there is growing recognition that bland sterility promotes neither patient comfort nor healing. Marck (2000) has expressed concern about the dominance of high technology in hospitals, observing that many nurses seem to be watching monitors and machines more than patients. She wonders, "do modern hospitals still aim to heal?" (p. 75). Some contemporary architects are seeking to create more hospitable institutions with greater integration of nature and aesthetically pleasing features into their designs, Based on this review of history, however, it appears that hospital architecture has yet to match the beauty and elegance of the healing temples of the ancient Greeks.

Studies on the World of the Hospitalized Patient

Florence Nightingale (1860/1969) is considered the first researcher of the hospitalized patient's environment. She wrote extensively about aspects of the environment such as ventilation, light, noise, variety, bed and bedding, and cleanliness (George, 1995). Since her pioneering work, however, few researchers have sought to expand the knowledge base. A review of contemporary nursing research revealed a tendency to focus on selected aspects of the environment such as noise, light, music, and environmental factors theorized to correlate with sleep disturbances (Baker, 1992; Biley, 1996; Holmberg & Coon, 1999; Lai, 1999; Redeker, 2000). Stress or stimulus-response theoretical frameworks served as the basis for studies examining hospital sound levels, which, not surprisingly, showed that increased environmental sound caused increases in patients' physiological measurements such as heart rate and blood pressure (cf. Baker, 1992; Holmberg & Coon, 1999). While studies such as these shed light on discrete aspects of the hospital environment, this body of literature contributes little to an understanding of the entirety of that world as the patient in the sickbed experiences it.

In a 1993 study conducted at Beth Israel Hospital in Boston by the Picker/Commonwealth Program for Patient-Centered Care (Gerteis, Edgman-Levitan, Daley & Delbanco, 1993), patients met with researchers in focus groups to discuss their health care experience. In response to structured interview questions about the physical environment, they voiced complaints about cramped spaces, inadequate privacy, uncomfortable "institutional" seating, harsh bright lights, noise, stark walls, and the lack of soothing wall decor. Cleanliness of the hospital environment was a high priority for Beth Israel patients who found piles of soiled laundry, used bandages, and other evidence of dirt disconcerting. In a qualitative study about patient perceptions of inpatient mental health care, the environment emerged as a subtheme to the more general theme of quantity and quality of care (Wallace, Robertson, Millar, & Frisch, 1999). Wallace et al. found that the environment where care took place "did not facilitate recovery . . . the wards were dirty, dark, depressing, bland, and generally a downer" (p. 1148).

Although minimal, research on the hospital environment can be found in environmental psychology, health care marketing, and health care administration literature. Studies in health care marketing and health care administration have explored the relationship of environment variables to service quality and patient satisfaction (Bitner, 1990; Bitner, Booms, & Tetreault, 1990; Reidenbach & Sandifer-Smallwood, 1990; Woodside, Nielsen, Walters, & Muller, 1988). For example, a telephone survey of recently discharged patients showed that one of seven factors significantly related to patient satisfaction was a "physical appearance" factor that included items about the hospital room (Reidenbach & Sandifer-Smallwood, 1990). The patients were not questioned, however, regarding any specific features of the hospital room that were appealing.

Several lines of research have examined patient or consumer behavior in response to the environment. Environmental psychology studies of hospital settings investigated the effect of the environment on patient behaviors such as social interaction (Ittelson, Proshansky, & Rivlin, 1970). Marketing research has focused on environmental factors that induce consumers to purchase certain products. The term *atmospherics* was coined by Kotler (1973) to describe "the physical and controllable environmental components affecting the buyer's 'purchasing propensity' to consummate a marketing exchange" (Hutton & Richardson, 1995, p. 49). *Servicescapes* (Bitner, 1992) is another term used to describe the environment's effect on "purchasing propensity" in service organizations. A theoretical model developed by Hutton and Richardson (1995) combines the previous two conceptualizations to form the concept *healthscapes*, defined as "the emotional, affective, cognitive, and physiological influence on patient-customer and staff-provider behaviors and outcomes caused by elements of the physical health care environment, including facility and tangible elements of the service encounter" (Hutton & Richardson, 1995, p. 52).

This theoretical model is, in part, based on research findings from studies in airports (Bitner, 1990) and retail stores (Harrell, Hunt, & Anderson, 1980). Its propositions are based on premises that (a) patients are customers and (b) health care settings are similar to retail settings in their impact on behavior. This conceptualization, therefore, fails to consider how radically different hospitals are from retail establishments which customers visit voluntarily—to transact everyday business of far less importance than the crucial life-and-death matters that bring them to hospital doors. Clearly, it is time to ask patients about their perceptions of the hospital environment, without imposing inappropriate theoretical models or structured interview questions.

THE PRESENT PROGRAM OF RESEARCH

The purpose of this study was to explore the patient's experience of the phenomenal world of the hospital. Nine patients were interviewed from three large metropolitan hospitals. Researchers met with unit charge nurses to discuss the purpose of the study and to solicit participants. Unit charge nurses then recommended patients who met inclusion criteria: at least 21 years of age, not seriously ill or acutely distressed at the time of the interview, and willing to talk to researchers about their experiences. Researchers targeted a range of hospital units in an attempt to gain a wide variation of experience. Oncology, labor and delivery, coronary care, transitional care, and psychiatry were represented in the sample. See Table 15.1 for a demographic summary of the participants.

Written informed consent was obtained from each study participant. Most participants were interviewed in their hospital rooms. One participant was interviewed in her home after discharge from the hospital. The duration of each interview was approximately one hour and there were no incentives for participation. Interviews were audiotaped, transcribed verbatim, and analyzed on the basis of the interpretive procedures described in Chapter 2.

Bracketing Interview

Prior to conducting interviews, I (Shattell) was interviewed about my experience of the hospital environment. The interview was transcribed and analyzed by the interpretive research group. Themes that emerged illuminated the essence of my experience of

TABLE 15.1 Demographics of Study Sample

Gender	Age	Occupation	Education	Reason for Hospitalization
Male	48	Plumber	High School	Suicide attempt
Female	34	Disabled	Some College	Suicidal thoughts
Female	62	Retired RN	College Graduate	Cancer and atrial fibrillation
Female	57	RN	College Graduate	Cancer
Female	28	Teacher	College Graduate	Childbirth
Male	58	Disabled	Less than High School	Substance Abuse
Male	39	Welder	High School	Substance Abuse
Female	82	Retired	Unknown	Stroke, Transitional Care
Female	86	Retired	Unknown	Fractured Pelvis, Transitional Care

hospital and clinic environments. An understanding of my experience enabled me to interview participants without imposing my presuppositions on them. One of the themes that emerged from my bracketing interview was my need for order and efficiency in the health care environment. For me, the manner is which physical surroundings are maintained is a direct reflection of the care that is rendered.

I was also aware of the use of time, specifically what I called "wasting time." In the outpatient health care environment, I felt that extended waiting time prior to being seen by my health care provider was an imposition and showed a lack of consideration. Prolonged waiting time also implied inefficiency, a characteristic that was thematic in my bracketing interview.

In addition to the theme of efficiency/inefficiency, I also became aware of my own spatial orientation to the world. I realized that what was figural in the health care environment was how physical "things" in the environment were arranged, all in relation to me. I was attuned to the designs of the setting and the detail of how chairs were arranged in a primary care setting. If the chairs were arranged so that none of them faced the receptionist's area, that told me that the office staff were often behind schedule and didn't want patients peering at them—as if to say, "When are you going to call me back? How much longer do I have to wait?"

A final theme in my awareness of outpatient health care practices concerned relevance and was particularly manifest in the reading material available to me in the waiting room. Most often the magazines were not of interest to me; for example, in the office of my gynecologist, every magazine is related to parenting. The reading material available, therefore, is entirely geared toward obstetrical patients of the OB/GYN practice and not toward the gynecological, non-childbearing, non child-rearing patients.

FINDINGS

Hospitalized patients spoke of the world of the hospital in terms of a constant dialectic between confinement and freedom. Unexpectedly, the thematic structure of the experience of the hospital environment for medical patients emerged, in many respects, as diametrically opposite to that of psychiatric patients. The overarching theme for medical patients, weary of confinement and longing to be free, was: "Eventually it'll be over." In contrast, the dominant image in psychiatric patient narratives was the hospital as a "refuge from my self-destructiveness." The environment was described as restraining them from substance abuse or suicide attempts, but at the same time granting freedom: to rest, to be nurtured, to connect with other patients. In some respects, the thematic structures for medical and psychiatric patients were mirror images of one another. For example, identity was stripped from medical patients but affirmed for psychiatric patients. Elaboration on the two structures follows, with delineation of the themes that were figural in each.

OVERVIEW OF THEMATIC STRUCTURES

Medical Patients

For the hospitalized medical patients, the hospital was a place where they "had to be." Participants reported having no choice but to be in the hospital, and they saw the environment as confining. The environment was viewed as a dangerous place where they were disconnected from others and the outside world. The hospital environment was described as a hindrance to participants' individual identities, stripping them of their distinctiveness. The predominant theme was **"Eventually it'll be over."** The remaining themes were: **No possibilities/Possibilities, Not me/Me, Insecurity/Security**, and **Disconnection/Connection**.

Eventually it'll be over

Participants disliked being inpatients and longed to leave the hospital behind. They reported reminding themselves, "You have to be in the hospital so you have to be in the hospital. Eventually it'll be over;" "I just thought, endure this, we'll get through it." One participant, acknowledging that the inevitability of hospitalization at some point in her disease trajectory, stated, "I knew I would have to go some time. But you know, you're always thinking it's some other time."

Participants frequently spoke of getting out of the hospital and going home. Although well aware that they "had to be in the hospital," they simultaneously wanted to go home as soon as possible. Even before participants were officially "patients," while waiting in the admissions area, they were already expressing a desire to go home: "I wanted to get up and walk out." "Just take me home, take me home." A laboring mother, waiting to be admitted to the hospital, enjoyed her husband's future-oriented projection regarding their yet-to-be-born baby's discharge: ". . . the thing that ended up being the most fun about it was, Joe would say 'she's going home.' And it was kind of a thing that could make us feel lighter, just the comparison, oh my goodness . . . she's going home."

Some participants were fearful of not being able to go home. Death and long-term care were two dreaded alternatives. One elderly patient on a transitional care unit said this of her urge to go home:

Time doesn't pass very fast. It would if you were laying down or sleeping or something, but I decided that [since] I'm this close to going home, I'm not going to lay down and sleep in the daytime. I went next door somewhere and another man [told me that] their 'transitional' is not just from here to home. It's some-where else. I don't want to do that if I can help it. I don't know how much good I can be, but if I can help it, I don't want to do that.

The hospital was experienced as confined and encased: "You're . . . shut up in here"—especially for patients who were unable to move their bodies in space. Immobile patients were more dependent on nursing staff and experienced the environment as a small nonnegotiable space. Relative positions of exits, number and location of windows and doors, and the unit's height from the ground floor all were of interest to patients in terms of how readily they could get out. Although she had a window view, one participant expressed discontent because "You can't see a road from here as far as I know. The fact of the matter is, I think we're enclosed almost around." In a descrip-tion of the hospital room, one participant seemed to derive reassurance from the fact that "it has more than one way to exit." Participants were keenly aware, both literally and figuratively, of how to get out of the hospital, how to escape the confinement in order to be free. They described biding their time by doing what was expected of them, believing this would lead to quicker release.

Physical movement helped ease the experience of confinement in the hospital environment. Freedom to move one's body through space allowed some patients to feel less confined. Participants who were unable to move experienced the world as more confining and more insecure. Although movement was often physically painful, participants reported that they would rather feel pain in freedom than distress in confinement, as depicted by the following exemplars from the data:

I'm trying to do all the exercise where I can walk. See it hurts to move my pelvis and my side. And it's hard to walk." "I could walk the halls if I wanted to . . . I didn't want an epidural in the first place because I wanted the option of walking." "I wasn't feeling too stupendous yet and I went for a walk . . . when I started, I just felt hunched over . . . I could barely move my legs . . . As I was walking, I started to be able to stand up taller." "I can't get around and go up and down the halls or anything . . . I am shut up right now . . . later I can open the door and take a walk down the hall so I won't feel quite so bad . . . if it wasn't for that window I probably would go home.

All participants discussed the importance of being able to view the outside world. Having a window enabled them to look out and experience, from time to time, the freedom that the outside world seemed to grant. In this way, they could continue to participate vicariously in the ongoing stream of life. They described what they could see from the windows in their longing to be out of the hospital. One participant said,

We have a nice view . . . I've watched boats go up and down and there's people skiing. And you know, [on] the other side you have nothing to look at but cars going by and horns honking. . . . It's pleasant and peaceful . . . I'm just, you know, wishing that I was out there on the boat instead of in here.

A participant who didn't have a window view said, "I can't see out. . . . They come in and tell you the sun is shining, but . . . you can't tell. . . . It would be nice to have a room that you could see out of and know what's going on."

No possibilities/possibilities

Participants described themselves as being at the whim of an environment where they did not even have control over things that were done to their bodies. The environment was experienced as unsupportive of individual efficacy and personal control. Being-in-the-world, in which power and control were taken by that world, created a perception of no possibilities. Family members had coerced one participant to go to the hospital where she experienced even greater powerlessness: "I figured I didn't need it . . . they haven't convinced me yet that I had a stroke. They talk about it all the time but they haven't convinced me."

The hospital environment also was described as taking away the possibility of restful sleep: "They come in at night and wake you up. You can be sound asleep and they wake you up . . . and they expect you to go right back to sleep and you can't." "I understand why people don't want to be near the nurses' station, you know. . . . It is noisy. But you know, I'm a nurse and I work, and I know . . . but it is noisy and you do hear people laughing and carrying on and everything."

One possibility presented by the hospital environment was death. A participant described her hospital birthing room in this way: "[There was] a lot of space for like the flowers . . . and then there was like this big weird fluorescent light thing behind me in case something weird happened."

Not me/me

Participants consistently compared facets of the hospital environment to those of their homes. In the hospital, aspects of home that help mirror identity and create comfort were not present. Most often, the hospital was seen as "not me." Patients experienced their personal identities as stripped from them and their existence as becoming homogenized. The comfort and identity that came from food, clothing, and personal objects was missing. Typical comments follow:

"They give you a lot of variety of food that I wouldn't eat at home. . . . I don't care much about grits . . . I'm not a Southerner."

"I don't like the [remote] control [for the TV] because I can't go forward or backward, I have to go all the way around. . . . Mine at home isn't like that."

"Being the kind of person I am, I like company, [but] they said they're all private rooms."

"There was not a shower in the room. I enjoyed my shower at home very much."

Another aspect of identity that was not supported by the hospital environment involved the patient's ability to function in his or her customary social roles. Roles that were significant to patients outside the hospital were meaningless in this environment. Such concerns were particularly confusing for patients who were also nurses. For nurse-participants, the environment created conflict and confusion in their identities. For example, one nurse-participant spoke of impulses to react when she heard the sounds of beepers and IV pumps, but then she reminded herself "I'm a patient." Another nurse-participant remarked, "It's different from the other side. On the other side."

Insecurity/security

The hospital environment was experienced as insecure and created feelings of danger. Physical symptoms of illness, side effects from medications, and unfamiliar noises at night contributed to patients' experience of the environment as insecure. Body position in space also had an impact on the precariousness of insecurity/security. While in the hospital, one female participant would not lie supine, experiencing the world as more dangerous than in either sitting or prone positions. Participants who had limited mobility felt especially vulnerable. Insecurity in the environment for this immobile participant was fostered by an experience with an inattentive nurse:

> One of the RNs . . . came in, introduced himself and then I don't remember seeing him the rest of the night. He could have been. All I know is the next morning at 5:00 he came and asked me . . . if I could estimate how many times I had been up to the bathroom that night. And I thought 'you haven't taken care of me all night long. You don't have a clue what's wrong with me. You don't have a clue that I can't move, that I cannot get up or anything, that I have a Foley catheter in' . . . it was a horrible experience.

Physical distance between participants and their caregivers was related to the degree of feeling secure or insecure. The environment was perceived as more secure when nurses and doctors were in proximity. One participant, describing the multiple monitors in the labor room, said, "I was aware that the nurse could be somewhere else and know what was going on with me. Or, she could know that something was going on with somebody else and that they needed her more." The nearness of supplies and equipment such as medications, phones (to call for help if needed), and gloves also helped participants feel more secure in the environment.

Some participants actively sought ways to increase their experience of security of the environment. Increased mobility helped improve feelings of security and freedom. Participants who had family members stay with them experienced the environment as more secure: "My family has been here and they do a good job of taking care of me." The presence of family not only produced comfort and security but also supported identity and connection.

Disconnection/connection

Medical patients talked of boredom and loneliness; the hospital was described as an environment in which they felt disconnected from others. Participants longed to relate to others: "I like having the company. I don't like to be alone . . . it's [the television] on now, without sound, because it's just company." One participant described why she wanted a semi-private room versus a private room, "I thought it would be . . . time would pass better if there was somebody with me." The theme of disconnection/connection is illustrated in the words of another participant:

> It's just so boring. The only time it's not boring is when I have plenty of company. That helps. I've noticed that the nurses are very, very, they're just really nice to you. Most of them are really, really pleasant. They seem to care, and housekeeping comes in (or whatever they're called nowadays) and they're always

pleasant. So, it's pleasant people to be around. So that takes up part of your day, keeps you from being so bored.

Patients in the hospital reported wanting to experience connections with other people such as family, nurses, doctors, and other patients. They wanted to see "their own" doctor each day, not one of many physician partners in the practice. Inconsistency and discontinuity in their medical care provider created feelings of disconnection: "I don't see my doctor as much as I'd like to. There are several doctors in there and it seems like the other ones have been in more than he has . . . but they're all in the same office, but you know, when you get a doctor you like, you go to him."

Comparisons to other patients were commonplace. For example, in response to the research question as to what was noticed in the hospital environment, one participant replied,

Nothing, only just being sociable and being together down at the exercise place. It's wonderful to be down here and just look at all of them, and see how bad you could be, like that, and they're worse off and you feel a lot better.

Another participant compared herself to others while waiting to be admitted to the hospital, "I saw a number of people come in and, although there were a number in the waiting room too, I thought they were worse off than I was." Participants could measure their progress towards freedom by comparing themselves to others in the environment.

There were times that participants reported feeling that they needed more from the hospital staff than they were getting. In these cases, the hospital environment was experienced as disconnecting. A woman with a radium implant was keenly aware that "everybody's afraid of you . . . dietary would bring the tray, but then they wouldn't come pick it up and here was this food [left in the room]. . . . The night nurse acted like she was terrified out of her mind . . . slid my pills around on the tray . . . And one little nursing assistant was afraid to come out from behind the shield. . . . They didn't clean me . . . you feel nasty."

Another participant commented on the timing and irrelevance of questions by a nurse when she was in active labor. The nurse did not seem to be attuned to the patient's intense focus on her contractions:

She stood on that side at one point during my labor and was asking me questions. And it was like, 'Have you had any stress in your life?' I'm having a baby! I think she meant have you moved recently or changed jobs, blah, blah, blah. It was funny, she would ask me questions, and I would be in the middle of a contraction and I'd say 'Can I answer that in a minute?'. . . . I knew she had to do it, but it felt ridiculous.

In describing an interchange with a nurse anesthetist who was preparing her for an epidural, this same participant said, "He wanted me to get into a ball, which is ridiculous, but okay, I tried." Another participant seemed resigned in her summary of nursing care: "They look in on you and they give you a bath every day and they throw a pill down your throat. After all, I guess you can't get well without medicine. I wouldn't say it's a pleasant experience but I knew before it happened that there would be a time when I would have to go [to the hospital]."

Some participants described "good" or "nice" nurses and other hospital staff. Positive statements about nurses and other hospital staff included the following quotations: "I got good care. Caring people." "It [the hospital] is wonderful. Because the girls are so good and they're well-trained and they know how to treat you when you come in. That's the main thing. Don't be afraid to say 'hi' to somebody. The patient loves that better than anything." "They take all the pains in the world out at that recreation center . . . and that means a lot." "They [the nurses] do everything in the world to make you happy. Those girls are wonderful." "They were very responsive to what I wanted."

Psychiatric Patients

"Home is my Bethlehem, my succoring shelter, my mental hospital, my wife, my dam, my husband, my sir, my womb, my skull. Never leave it. Never leave it."

—Anne Sexton (1981)

Unlike medical patients, who experienced the hospital environment as confining, psychiatric patients experienced it as freeing. Paradoxically, they reported feeling safely grounded and unconstrained within the confinement of the locked psychiatric unit. The meaning of the hospital to psychiatric patients was *a refuge from self-destructiveness.* The remaining themes that emerged from analysis of their interviews were the same as those emerging from medical patients—with the notable exception of a change in emphasis. Whereas medical patients emphasized no possibilities, psychiatric patients emphasized possibilities. In the same way, each of the remaining themes also received an opposite emphasis. The figural themes of the hospital environment for psychiatric patients were: possibilities/no possibilities, security/insecurity, me/not me, and connection/disconnection.

Refuge from self-destructiveness

Each of the participants described his or her experience of the hospital as a refuge from the chaos of the outside world. The hospital was portrayed as "neutral territory" and "a cooling place." Being hospitalized on an inpatient unit provided a calming respite from their daily struggle against self-destructive impulses (substance abuse and suicide attempts). Metaphorically they described admission as being "received" by a caring surrogate family. The hospital was a place where "you could cool your head and mind," "just become limp," and "be subdued by the environment." One participant described a cocoon-like experience: "The first two or three days I just laid in here [patient's room]. Couldn't sleep, depressed, and couldn't sleep, just depressed. Just laid, kept the drapes shut and the lights off and just stayed by myself for two days. And finally I just got to feeling better."

All participants described the hospital environment as protective against, in the words of one participant, "my own vices." One participant described his hospitalization as an "interlude between my self-destructiveness." The environment afforded security. In addition to a break from self, participants also described the experience as a break from others: "I don't have to worry about anybody that don't like me or anything. Or come down here and try to cause trouble for me. I just feel very safe here." "There's a lot of things going on outside of this place that I've got to deal with when I get out of here, so. But I've told myself not to even worry about it. I've got to concentrate on staying sober and drug-free. Stay away from some people that's bad." "You know that the papers that I signed when I came in, say I have the right to refuse visitors. If I didn't want to see certain people, and the fact that we're behind, in a locked up unit, makes me feel comforted." This theme is consistent with first-person accounts of the psychiatric hospitalization experience found in popular literature. The hospital is described as a refuge from the demands and expectations of the outside world—as a place where you can be free from work, school, people or anything "except eating or taking your medication" (Kaysen, 1993, p. 94).

In the world of the psychiatric patient, there was a specific "inner sanctuary," a world within a world. This inner world was the unit smoking room. The smoking room was described as "very therapeutic," because "people will sit in there and talk and get some things off your mind that you don't feel comfortable doing in a big group, you know, like in group therapy." Even non-smoking participants spoke positively of the smoking room: "And I don't smoke, but I go down there every now and then, to talk to people." One participant related a fear of losing the smoking room followed by a plea stressing its importance:

> Honest to God, I believe if they took that away, I think it would, oh Lord, I don't know whether you could stand it or not. I'd beg, I'd advise anybody, don't take that away. Because . . . what happens up there is we get to talk to each other, about maybe what happened in class. And sometimes we can help each other . . . with no teacher or person around. So I would[n't] dare to think that they would get rid of the smoke room.

The smoking room provided a sense of freedom and privacy within the confinement of locked psychiatric unit. In describing the privacy provided by the smoking room, one participant stated, "It doesn't seem like there's any cameras on you or anything in there, or any kind of intercom system that people could listen to you while you're talking about private things. That's why I like it. It's, it's private." Another description presented benefits of the social element of this inner sanctuary:

It gives smokers somewhat of a little more freedom than say someone who is not smoking, because you can go in there and sit when you're not in groups, and you can just sit in there and talk or you can smoke, or you know, just cut up and kid around. You can talk maybe more about deeper issues with people there because it's more private, because you've got the two doors there and you can see when somebody's coming in and you can stop talking and maybe when they leave you can continue. I like that. That's a real big benefit for us. For smokers anyway.

Participants described viewing the outside world by looking out of the windows. One participant said, "When I look out the window there in the smoke room and see the water out there, that's very soothing." This "vicarious consumption of free places" (Goffman, 1961, p. 237) was described by most of the participants. One participant described how she liked to look out the window and "daydream at little." The benefit of observing others through the smoking room window is illustrated by this quote:

The paint in there is kind of gloomy looking, but it has a good view of the river down there and at night you can see the lights down there on the river . . . it is so beautiful and so soothing. That's another thing I found out about that room. I like to go in there at night and watch the lights and stuff and during the day you can sit there and watch people going by on their boats and pulling their little kids on the skis or little inner-tubes and things, and that's a lot of fun.

Kaysen (1993) refers to this as a "parallel universe," invisible to the outside world. People on the outside cannot look in; however, once in, the outside world is clearly visible. In the words of Kaysen (1993), "every window on Alcatraz has a view of San Francisco" (p. 6).

Possibilities/no possibilities

The world of the hospitalized psychiatric patient was seen to render future possibilities. Medication provided a sense of new life for some patients. An orientation towards the future was noted in statements such as these: "I haven't had a goal in years, you know. Since I've been up here and gotten this new medicine I feel . . . more goal-oriented, and the groups have helped me too with that, to take a look at myself and think, 'what am I doing with my life?'" "I came into the room and it was purple . . . I said, 'this is so pretty' . . . the color of love and it's also to me the color of passion, like the passion to live again, you know, to live. And I like that."

The hospital environment created the possibility of goals after discharge: "I'm looking forward to getting out and going home. And I'll try to work the 12-Step Program" and "I'll be getting out tomorrow, sometime tomorrow . . . and follow up with rehab." In another participant's description of his plans for outpatient treatment after discharge, he reiterated:

"I'm going . . . I am really determined. I am really determined." Despite such optimistic statements, most psychiatric patients were nervous about getting out of the hospital. In contrast to medical patients who eagerly anticipated discharge, psychiatric patients reported being afraid of what might happen when they were released from the safe hospital environment: "You can be up here and be joyous, and five minutes after you're out the door, you go right back into your anxiety and fears."

Some patients were unable to envision future possibilities. Continued existence was itself in doubt. With foreboding of death, one chronically suicidal patient said:

So many years ago . . . I had what could have been small problems, but now I've come to seeing [them] to be a matter of death or life, and it's an inescapable feeling that I feel now. It's progressive. My sickness has progressed to an extreme height . . . it makes you feel like there's no hope . . . It's like the only thing left for me is the box [coffin]. . . . I doubt I'll see the year 2001. I brought 2000 in in a coma this year, and that's quite an easy way to kill yourself, by the way . . . tastes sweet, antifreeze, tastes sweet.

Security/insecurity

Safety and security were experienced in the environment of the psychiatric unit. Study participants pointed out that "the fact that we're in a locked up unit, makes me feel comforted that I don't have to worry about me trying to run away." "When I'm left alone or when I'm on my own, then I can do as I please, but here I can't and I know that I could do myself great damage if I were outside." The inpatient unit was described as a "safe house" where "they keep a good eye on you." This metaphor describes the security experienced in the hospital:

I'm down 24 feet in the dirt in a ditch. I'm drilling and shooting the rocks, and I've got my rock drill going and I can feel the bank shake, you know. That environment is rather frightening. I'm in a trench box and it's been handmade, it's been hand welded. You don't know how strong the welds are, and it doesn't take a lot of dirt to make a ton. When you're down 24 feet, if it collapses you're going to be crushed into a pancake. And I've been in those environments and felt safe. And I've been in this environment [the inpatient unit] and felt safe.

This same participant acknowledged that the security of the unit was tenuous, however: "So on the one hand you feel more safe here, but on the other hand you're aware that you're left on your own an awful lot and there are less staff than there was."

Me/not me

Like medical patients, psychiatric patients also compared the hospital environment to home, but in a more positive identity-affirming way. In the psychiatric unit, identity was affirmed as "me" versus the "not me" experienced by patients on medical units. Participants described the environment of the psychiatric unit as like home for them, "a close-knit adopted family" where a personal sense of identity was experienced as mirrored by the environment. Some patients described important roles they filled within their "adopted family" such as the comedian or the greeter of new admissions. Like surrogate parents, staff met patients' needs for food, comfort, and structure. Participants commented approvingly on well-stocked refrigerators and snack cabinets. Pride was evident in one patient's description of the hospital's cleanliness: "The hospital is always clean, and up here, there's one thing about us drunks, we try to keep it that way."

The me/not me theme was also evident in the social comparisons made between participants and others in the environment. Looking toward others for similarities and differences shaped participants' judgments of self. These judgments often had a positive effect either by normalizing events, thoughts, or feelings, or by lessening the severity of the illness experience: "Other people tell you their stories and yours in some cases seem insignificant compared to what happened to them." "Most of them have experienced some of the things that I have, and most of them have experienced suicidal thoughts or even suicide attempts." "It's easier for me to focus on other people because I look at other people, and as many times as I have been hospitalized for psychiatric reasons I just watch them and sort of study them, and see a picturesque view of myself, so many years ago."

One participant succinctly summarized the benefit of comparisons:

> The most help it seems like a person can get in here is usually from the other patients, when you make comparisons. . . . I was talking to a lady earlier, she was telling me that she thought she was really bad off until she got up here, and I said, 'Well, it's kind of like a man who has no shoes and feels he's got it bad until he sees someone without any feet.'

Connection/disconnection

The connection "half" of the connection/disconnection theme refers to an experience of the environment in the act of connecting with other people (family members, other patients, nurses, doctors, other hospital staff and the outside world). Most psychiatric patients expressed connection while in the hospital environment: "The staff is very supportive. Anytime you need anything, whether it's to light your cigarette or a drink of Maalox or your blow dryer or a pillowcase or anything like that, they're just very helpful." The environment created a connection to the past for one participant, wherein color of the carpet and of the bedspread caused her to be pleasantly reminiscent of her childhood. The size of the rooms where group sessions were held facilitated connection. One participant described it as "plenty big enough . . . to me, it's the closer you are the better, the better it works."

Connection with others was discussed in terms of socialization and comfort. A value for socialization was apparent in the words of these participants: "There's few people that can't get along. Matter of fact, I've not saw nobody that couldn't get along out here. And we cut up and kid, and we eat together and shoot the breeze." "At home I usually sleep till at least 9:00 you know. But over here I want to get up. I'm looking forward to it since the people, the patients are very friendly, and, you know, the staff's very friendly. And I love interacting with all of them."

While most study participants experienced the environment as creating connections, interactions were sometimes described as superficial. There was a yearning for greater closeness in interactions with professional staff rather than playing "little games" with them or attending "classes." One participant described connections with professional personnel as enormously inadequate: "I keep hoping against hope that something will be said or done for me to make a change." Another participant expressed his dissatisfaction as follows:

I don't believe that the psychiatric field is what it used to be or what it could be. I think that it could be much more, more personal, more up front, more seriously delving to find out what troubles people—and find solutions, rather than just put a pill on it or a tab on it or something, saying 'You're going to be okay now. Just hang in there.' I think we are failing and these type wards are failing.

More meaningful connections also were sought in group therapies. Occupational therapy and goal-setting were belittled as one participant pled for deeper, more substantial connections: "I think we take for granted that people are just going to get okay, that they're going to find their own ways and means to deal with things. And that's not the case. There are some of us who need much more than occupational therapy and goal-setting . . . I would like to see it more people-oriented." Another patient expressed similar perceptions:

I'm aware that this is a psychiatric ward and the dispensing of medication is probably the primary help for therapy. The doctors come by to see you once a day for a few minutes and then the rest of the time they have you scheduled for little things like occupational therapy, where you go paint or draw or do something like that. You know, like 'how was your day?' and you have goal setting . . . and at the end of the day they have you wrap up what you have done, or how you've done, as far as setting your goals. And between that, it's just boring. And it's like I'm left to my own vices like I was on the outside.

DISCUSSION AND CONCLUSIONS

At first glance, the findings of this study of the world of the hospitalized patient may seem surprising. Given the attention devoted to customer-pleasing hospital design and decor, the research team expected to hear more about the physical features of the rooms in which patients spent many long, sometimes boring, hours. Presumably, they would be aware of, and comment on, the colors, sounds, and smells present in the environment. But it was the people in the hospital environment that were most significant to patients, not the color scheme of the unit nor the voices over the intercom. Contrary to marketing theories and consumer research, responses of patients interviewed for this study suggested (by omission) that the walls, furniture, and/or flooring of the hospital were relatively unimportant. A recently hospitalized journalist, recounting her post-hysterectomy experience, wondered why patients came to be called "consumers" in the first place: "I can tell you that when you're lying there trying to remember what feeling good feels like, you're not a consumer. You are not shopping. You are spending, mostly expending, more energy than you have on things that you should not have to worry about. The crisis that brought you to the hospital is all that should be on your mind, not being safe, or clean, or ignored" (Abramson, 1996, p.29).

Findings of the present study, at first glance, also seem to be inconsistent with those obtained in the Beth Israel study (Gerteis et al., 1993). The discrepancy between our study and the one conducted at Beth Israel is perhaps attributable to differences in methodology. In the Boston study, researchers posed direct questions to the participants, eliciting detailed discussions of specific environmental features such as the wallcoverings. In contrast, phenomenological interviewing invites individuals to speak of aspects predominant to them. Such details were not predominant in the descriptions of environment obtained in the present phenomenological study. A commonality of the Boston study and this one was the high priority placed by patients on the presence of windows and views of water. Windows seem to serve several functions when people are in hospitals: they lessen the sense of confinement, admit sunlight and glimpses of nature, and allow vicarious participation in activities of passersby. Benefits of windows that permit patients to see parks or gardens were also reported in previous studies by Ulrich (1984), Verdeber (1986), and Baird and Bell (1995), mentioned in Chapter 14.

One Beth Israel participant pointed out that the severity of one's condition undoubtedly influences perceptions of the environment, a statement in clear agreement with the present sample: "When you're terribly physically sick, you want your life saved. When you're feeling better, you start caring what your environment looks like" (Walker, 1993, pp. 134–145).

Hospitalized patients in the present study spoke of their experience in the world of the hospital in terms of a constant dialectic between confinement and freedom. For medical patients, confinement was figural; they surrendered to the confinement and necessity of hospitalization, but simultaneously felt an intense desire to get out of this place that was discordant with their sense of identity ("not me") and produced feelings of disconnection. Roth (1963) found a similar theme in his study of patients in a tuberculosis hospital. Commenting on that study, Pollio (1982, p. 223) concluded that "being in a hospital is considered the same as 'doing time' in prison; in both cases the person wants to know when it will end."

For medical patients, the hospital was described as an environment of insecurity—a dangerous place they wanted to get out of—as opposed to a safe refuge for psychiatric patients who were afraid to get out. Paradoxically, within a locked unit psychiatric patients experienced greater freedom, confirmation of identity, security, and possibilities. While both groups had a keen awareness that "eventually it'll be over," the impending discharge held quite different meanings: medical/childbirth patients feared *not* getting out whereas psychiatric/substance abuse patients were fearful *of* getting out.

One's being, according to existential philosophy, is always directed towards the world, although one's awareness of that world is often not articulated. In a broad statement regarding our usual unawareness of experience, Tuan (1977) states that "blindness to experience is in fact a common human condition. We rarely attend to what we know. We attend to what we know about; we are aware of a certain kind of reality because it is the kind that we can easily show and tell. We know far more than we can tell, yet we almost come to believe that what we can tell is all we know" (p. 201). When patients were asked to describe what they noticed in the hospital environment, their descriptions focused more on connections with people than on physical features of their rooms or wards. One participant's words aptly captured this focus on people:

> I see that the environment, if you take away the people it's just empty hallways and empty rooms. . . . I think the environment is not a principal issue . . . I think the people make up the environment, and I think the process of how you work with others and how you deal with the people up here is more important than the environment that you're in, because this environment is only a fleeting moment. . . . The environment here is a very minor matter. It could be a shack with newspapers for insulation.

In addition to a strong focus on people, participants also described the hospital environment or the objects within it according to the degree of home-like qualities, such as "It's not like mine from home," or, alternatively, "It feels like home." As stated by Tuan (1977), "home is an intimate place. We think of the house as home and place, but enchanted images of the past are evoked not so much by the entire building, which can only been seen, as by its components and furnishings, which can be touched and smelled as well" (p. 144). According to Stark (1948), "This is the meaning of home—a place where every day is multiplied by all the days before it" (p. 55). Home provides a sense of identity that is taken away in the hospital environment, which is a place of "not me."

Both groups of patients described comparing themselves to others in order to feel better. Comparisons often pertained to level of illness, although patients sometimes took note of the ways in which they were the same as, or different, from others, in aspects such as degree of mobility or progression toward recovery. Camaraderie among patients was a very important aspect of hospitalization for many participants, especially for the psychiatric patients who gathered in the smoking room to share intimacies away from the watchful eyes of the staff.

Narratives of both groups revealed considerable loneliness and disconnection, punctuated by brief moments of interaction with doctors, nurses, housekeepers, and visitors. Many patients were overt in stating their expectations and wishes for something more from their care providers, especially from nurses. Similar dissatisfaction was found in a study conducted by nurses at Providence Hospital in Seattle (Storr, 1996). Concerned about reductions in nursing staff brought about by managed care cost imperatives, these nurses wondered how patients were perceiving the care they were getting. Despite intimidation from hospital security personnel, who took the names of nurse data collectors and photographed them, 70 nurses managed to hand out surveys to patients. Responses to the survey indicated that patients were not satisfied with their care on the acute care floors of the general hospital. Patients reported that the nurses appeared to be under a lot of pressure and did not have time to give them needed attention. A fruitful direction for future research would be to investigate what patients do when they want to solicit more care and attention from staff. Are there strategies that successfully draw attention to themselves and their needs? How do they create connections in an environment that works against that? From the patient's perspective, in what ways could the hospital environment be made more home-like and supportive of identity, security, and possibilities? In the words of Marck (2000, p. 63), "How do we find our way home to a deeper respect and care for hospitals and their inhabitants as healing communities in the complex health systems of our present era?"

IMPLICATIONS OF THE STUDY FINDINGS FOR NURSING PRACTICE

The findings from this phenomenological study of the world of the hospitalized patient have many implications for nursing practice, such as finding new ways to decrease the sense of confinement experienced in the hospital, creating more openness and freedom, and increasing connection between health care providers and patients. As the words of our study participants repeatedly emphasized, other people are figural in the world of the hospital patient. Consistently, participants described their experiences with nurses, doctors, and other people in their depiction of the lived experience of the hospital environment.

Nurses come into more extended contact with patients, in more intimate ways, than any other professional discipline in the hospital. With this in mind, along with what we have heard from participants in this study, the caring acts of nurses have profound effects on the experiences of hospitalized patients. We saw that patients want competent, kind, friendly, and knowledgeable nurses. They want a deeper relationship with them. As Sidney Jourard (1971, p. 201) noted, a well-nursed patient is one who "feels his nurses really care for him" and senses that the nurse "tunes in to him at regular intervals to sample his private, personal, and psychological world."

The psychiatric/substance abuse patients want individual attention from the unit staff as well as psychoeducational or therapy groups that focus on substantive issues. And they want to keep their inner sanctuary—their smoking room. From our participants we learn that they perceive the camaraderie that takes place away from staff surveillance to be very helpful. We must understand the important of patient-to-patient interaction in the therapeutic milieu. Although such "fraternization" has been discouraged in the past, our participants report that they feel something is to be gained from it.

Several other implications also emerge quite readily. When assigning rooms to new admissions, nurses should ask patients if they want to share a room. We have learned from our participants that "company" is sometimes important. Instead of assuming that a new patient would want a private room, ask what is preferred. A window view to look out at the world outside the hospital was important for participants in both groups. Think about window view when making room assignments. If there are empty rooms with a window view, use the window view room first. These are simple measures, but their importance has yet to be recognized fully. In so many ways, we are able to make all the difference in the world of the hospital patient. "Healing in a hospital community begins with committed attention to what kind of a place we think a hospital is and what kind of place we wish and will it to be" (Marck, 2000, p. 76).

POST-STUDY REFLECTIONS FROM MONA SHATTELL

Yi-Fu Tuan (1977) was right when he said, "Blindness to experience is in fact a human condition." Throughout this research, I realized how difficult it is for people (including myself) to think about, discuss, and describe the world. How can we describe that which we are surrounded by and that which we are never without? The world is probably the most obvious existential ground, yet the most difficult to articulate. When I asked participants to describe what they noticed in the world of the hospital, they most often quickly moved to tell me about the people in the hospital environment (existential ground of others), what procedures were done to them while hospitalized (existential ground of body), and aspects of hospitalization concerning the slow passage of time (existential ground of time).

In the beginning of this research, I had preconceived ideas that participants would find it easy to talk about the environment, perhaps describing physical objects such as furniture or decor. After completing my interviews and seeking to understand the meaning of the world of the hospital, I became aware of my own difficulty in thinking about the world. I repeatedly had to ask myself, "What does this say about the world?" It was challenging to examine the interviews with the world as the focus, but once I was able to do so, it was fascinating to see the themes emerge and to understand the contrasting experiences of medical and psychiatric patients. To identify confinement and freedom as the main theme in both thematic structures was intriguing, and both thematic structures appear to have wide applicability in nursing practice and research. It is truly exciting to articulate a broader understanding of "that which we know."

16

"Like a Bunch of Cattle": The Patient's Experience of the Outpatient Health Care Environment

"You're herded in like cattle and you sit there and you wait forever and there is nothing inviting about being there—there's nothing that makes you feel better to be there. . . . I spent many, many times . . . during the years in a doctor's office . . . just your normal, typical experience . . . go in and wait, hang around . . . until the doctors decide they want to see you. And then you get called back by a nurse who's never seen you before, and you go sit in a room for longer than you sat in the lobby, and then you see the doctor for 15 minutes, and you're sent on your way with five million prescriptions."

—excerpt from an interview conducted for this study

This statement was typical of the experiences reported by persons describing the world of the outpatient. Conducted concurrently with the study of hospitalized patients reported in Chapter 15, this study examined the experience of the patient who receives health care in an outpatient clinical environment—a common experience for many thousands of people each day in America. Whereas the hospital was once the primary setting for care delivery, it has been predicted that more than one-third of America's hospitals will consolidate or close in the early decades of the twenty-first century (Risse, 1999). Physicians' offices, ambulatory surgery centers, and a variety

* This chapter is based on a study conducted by Kristina Plaas at the University of Tennessee, Knoxville. Contributions of the following members of the research team are gratefully acknowledged: Bette Tedford, Tracey Martin, Gerry Molavi, Mona Shattell, and Alison Hicks.

of community-based clinics will deliver a majority of health care services. In 1995, over 29 million ambulatory surgery procedures were done in the United States during 19.4 million outpatient admissions—a profound change from the former practice of admitting patients to the hospital for two or more days to undergo these same procedures (Kaldenberg & Becker, 1999). Likewise, nursing practice is shifting from inpatient, acute care settings to outpatient, primary care settings. With this change in venue comes the need for nursing research to address the unique perspective of patients in the outpatient or clinic environment.

RELATED LITERATURE

In Webster's Dictionary (1991) "clinic" is defined as a facility for the diagnosis and treatment of outpatients, or a group practice of physicians working cooperatively. The word "clinic" comes from the Greek *klinikos*—of a bed, and *klinein*—to lean, or to rely on for support. Expanding on the original Greek meaning, Miller and Crabtree (1998) defined a clinic as a "physical and social place for those in need of support" (p. 310); in their definition, they sought to include medical, educational, legal, religious, nursing, and psychosocial means of support. They further described a clinic as "a public sanctuary for the voicing of trouble and the dispensation of relief" (p. 294). Thus, the world of the outpatient has both physical and social aspects and may be defined as a place of felt value where basic human needs are addressed.

Discussions concerning physical aspects of the outpatient health care environment can be found in the literature; however, most of this literature reflects the experience of health care providers and administrators rather than patients. Sadly, much of this literature stresses the priorities of marketing, attracting and retaining a patient clientele, reducing costs, meeting staff convenience needs, and attaining technologic efficiency instead of creating a comforting, healing environment for patients (Lindeke, Hauck, & Tanner, 1998; Mertz, 1999).

Currently, there is a boom in the construction of new ambulatory care facilities and in the remodeling of existing structures to accommodate changing health care agendas. It has been estimated that construction for health care facilities costs approximately $15 per square foot more than standard commercial office space, a significant expenditure in this era of cost-reduction in health care (Souhrada, 1990). State and federal funds for the construction and maintenance of health care facilities have been reduced as a result of the Balanced Budget Act of 1997, thereby removing a once dependable source for financing improvements. Savvy administrators and architects are, therefore, taking a new interest in expending available funds wisely. According to Frist (2000), facilities should be designed to suit the staff and the locale. He recommends focusing on the lobby decor, the first place patients see, as one place where health care administrators can get the "most bang for your bucks." In contrast,

Parimucha, Lussier, and Huelat (2000) advocate focusing on interiors, especially patient rooms, when investing in facility improvements. Unlike Frist, they advise architects to "think like a patient."

Patients do not view health care environments in the same way as staff members. Within these settings, interactions that staff may consider brisk and efficient may be considered by patients as crudely brusque and insensitive. There is a dearth of professional literature about the patient's first-person perspective on the outpatient environment. In widely circulated popular media, however, patients frequently report degrading and dehumanizing experiences while receiving diagnostic examinations and treatments. For example, the comic actress Gilda Radner described her experience of undergoing a barium enema this way:

> The technicians strapped me to a table and then put a tube in my rear end. As they poured a chalky liquid inside me and pumped gas into me so that my bowel would show up . . . they were also turning me slowly around and around on the table. . . . I had never had a photo session quite like this. . . . I felt like I was trapped on an endless Ferris wheel with someone's fist up my butt. . . . I think the word that best captures the whole event is humiliating (Radner, 1989, pp. 60–61).

Stories such as Radner's beg the question: Is such an experience common or typical? Using phenomenological interviews, the purpose of this study was to obtain descriptions of diverse patient experiences of obtaining health care in an outpatient setting.

THE PRESENT PROGRAM OF RESEARCH

Participants residing in the southeastern United States were recruited through personal contacts or referral from cooperating health care providers. Individuals were invited to participate if they: were at least 21 years of age; were not acutely ill or distressed; had recently received health care in an outpatient environment; and were willing and able to speak with the researchers about their experience. Eight participants, two men and six women, spoke with the principal investigator (Plaas) or with another interviewer about their experiences in audiotaped interviews which lasted from about 30 minutes to one hour. Table 16.1 presents demographic information about the individuals who chose to participate in the study.

All interviews were conducted in a quiet, private setting that was free from distractions, either in an office at the health care setting, the participant's home, or at another mutually agreed upon location. Informed consent was obtained prior to each interview. Participants were asked to tell what they were aware of when they obtained health care in an outpatient environment. Additional questions by the researcher sought to clarify meanings of the participants' experiences. A thematic structure was ultimately developed, following the interpretive procedure described in Chapter 2.

TABLE 16.1 Characteristics of the Sample

Gender	Age	Education	Occupation	Health Care Concern
Male	62	High school graduate	Cleaning business owner	Cancer
Female	65	College graduate	Housewife, retired RN	Appendicitis, preventive care
Female	79	High school graduate	Waitress	Cataracts, preventive care
Female	36	Some college	Computer systems	Abdominal pain
Female	19	Some college	Student	Dysmenorrhea, heavy menstrual flow
Female	26	College graduate	Business professional	Chronic illness
Female	58	Master's degree	Retired social worker	Diabetes, cardiac & renal disease, arthritis, cancer
Male	71	Some college	Insurance sales	Heart disease, post cardiac bypass surgery

Bracketing Interview

As a neonatal nurse with challenging chronic health problems of my own, I (Plaas) have spent much of the last 20 years of my life in health care environments, both in hospitals and various outpatient settings. Thus, my interest in exploring patients' experiences of obtaining health care in outpatient settings came from my own observations and experiences in these same environments. My bracketing interview revealed an intense awareness of the physical surroundings—the colors and condition of the furniture, floor, and wall coverings, ambient lighting, the type of light fixtures used, and the availability of windows. I was also aware of the space and structure of exam rooms, waiting areas, and hallways.

Many years of working in a dark, windowless neonatal intensive care unit contributed to my sense of feeling trapped when in crowded, dark, and depressing environments. Vivid language revealed my view of health care environments as unhealthy and stressful—environments in which patients are subjected to endure and relatively powerless to change. While brief mention was made of some of the people I had encountered in my experience, my focus was on what was wrong in hospitals and clinics, what I thought needed to be done to correct these problems, and the negative impact I felt from these discouraging and dehumanizing environments. The bracketing process revealed to me just how intense and negative my bias was—something that was clearly important for me to keep in mind as I proceeded to interview study participants.

FINDINGS

Participants in the present study reported having received health care in numerous outpatient settings, including physicians' offices, cancer treatment clinics, senior health centers, cardiology and cardiac rehabilitation centers, outpatient laboratories, radiology and endoscopy departments, and emergency rooms. Despite the diversity of outpatient environments, there were clear commonalities in the experiences shared by participants. While most participants noticed the physical surroundings, they were most acutely aware of the people they encountered in the environment, especially health care professionals and office staff members. They related encounters that were typical of their experiences in the outpatient health care environment, most of which they characterized as negative. Narratives often took the form of comparing two or more experiences in outpatient health settings—the "bad" experience and the "good" experience. While bad experiences predominated, participants were quick to mention good things that happened during the bad experiences. They usually contrasted a bad experience in one setting with another, more positive experience in a different environment. Thematic analysis of the transcripts revealed five interrelated themes depicting polarities of **Waiting/Immediate, Cold and Uninviting/Warm and Inviting, Object/Person, Powerless/Powerful,** and **Frightened/Cared For.**

Waiting/Immediate

For participants, the dominant theme of the outpatient environment concerned **waiting**. It was about wanting things to be done **immediately**, but having to wait instead. It was about having to wait for long periods of time without knowing why, then suddenly being rushed through a brief encounter with a physician or nurse and sent hurrying on your way with prescriptions and instructions to come back if things did not improve (see the quotation chosen to introduce the chapter). Having to wait was viewed negatively by all participants. One person identified waiting as the most frustrating aspect of the outpatient setting:

> It's very frustrating to the patient to deal with one problem for weeks and weeks and weeks on end while constantly waiting. Either you're waiting in a lobby, or you're waiting in a room, or you're waiting for test results, or you're waiting for your prescriptions to be filled, or any number of things . . . [it's] just disgusting.

Participants were keenly aware of just how long they had to wait and had definite opinions as to why they were not being attended to properly. They were critical about having to wait for a wheelchair upon arrival at the hospital or clinic and about offices and clinics that were so over-scheduled that waiting rooms were overflowing with patients sitting for extended periods of time. One participant observed: "[In a general practitioner's setting] . . . they cram so many people into their schedule that, you know, it's almost as if they don't want the environment to be inviting because they don't want you to hang around too long." Another commented: "I never understand why patients have to wait . . . like this doctor is the only one who has anything to do in this world? I mean these patients out here, they have other lives, they have things to do and places to go."

The emergency room was identified as one of the most problematic areas in which patients had to wait, particularly in large urban or teaching hospitals. Several participants used harsh words in describing having to wait for long periods, unattended to, in both the outer waiting area and in the treatment areas of the emergency room. One participant described it in the following terms: "Unless you're bleeding from a car wreck or having chest pains *at that moment* you are not a priority, so you have to sit and wait for quite a long while." Many times the long waits were attributed to inadequate staffing in the emergency department. At other times patients coming to the emergency room in the middle of the night were forced to wait to be seen until physicians arrived in the morning, as noted in the following statement:

> I went in very, very sick. I was throwing up. Well, come to find out I had appendicitis, and they stuck me in a room in a wheelchair surrounded by patients and I was totally ignored for I cannot tell you how long . . . probably 2–3 hours. And the pain was so bad I couldn't sit up. . . . I started throwing up and then I started screaming, and the only way I could get any attention was if I started screaming. . . . So finally, in the morning when the doctor came in, of course, then they were really excited and rushing around because then I was just gonna bust any minute, you know. . . . I mean I could have died and they'd probably shoved me in the corner and nobody would have found me for I don't know how long. That's how I felt.

Waiting was an important consideration for participants in judging the quality of care they received. A young woman describing an office visit for an ultrasound recounted how pleased she was when she did not have to wait long after having given her name and insurance information: "Then **immediately** after all that, this nurse came and got me." An older participant with complex health problems declared she had the "best doctor" because she never had to wait and was given 30 minute appointments instead of 15 minutes "because we need that kind of time." She credited her physician with saving her life because of the time this physician took to thoroughly consider her health problems and come up with an effective treatment plan. Conversely, another participant expressed a total lack of confidence in a physician because of a brief and inadequate visit with a physician after a lengthy wait:

> I told her what was wrong, but she was in a big hurry. She wasn't going to give me an exam at all, she was just going to talk to me and give me some pain medicine . . . and I was in there about 15 minutes and half the time she was standing in between the door and the room because she was trying to get out of there 'cause she had other people waiting. She didn't spend any time at all talking to me.

(This participant did not follow the prescribed treatment plan and found a new physician at a different health care facility).

While participants generally placed the blame squarely on the shoulders of the health care provider and the health care setting for lengthy waiting times, some also acknowledged that their perceptions of time may have been influenced by their physical condition: "When one is sick enough to be in the hospital they usually feel pretty rotten. . . . So if you wait for five minutes it feels like you've waited for 50, and when you go into the doctor's office, even though you might feel pretty bad, you don't feel bad enough to be admitted to the hospital and things are in a better perspective and more reality-based, I think."

Cold and Not Inviting/Warm and Inviting

Study participants repeatedly used terms such as cold, sterile, harsh, and not inviting to describe the outpatient health care environment. Some perceived this climate as a deliberate attempt to drive patients away from clinical facilities. They often described small, crowded spaces filled with uncomfortable furniture, and reported being distressed that their discomfort was not acknowledged. One participant confessed that she wouldn't care what colors the walls were painted, or even about having to wait, if someone, anyone, would treat her with a little love and kindness.

Dismayed by the way clinic receptionists interacted with patients, one participant remarked:

> The biggest thing is to get through those receptionists. They have a lot to learn because [they act like] they're doing you a favor by talking to you or getting you to go to the doctor or anything they do for you . . . they forget why the patient is there. They [the patients] are there for a reason, you know. They are scared . . . they are nervous . . . and most patients don't know what is going on, so they need this secure loving environment.

Speaking of an emergency room, another participant emphasized the coldness of both the temperature and the equipment, intensified by her near-nakedness in a flimsy hospital gown that opened in the back:

Everything is just real cold, and they've got all these machines and they instantly slap you on machines whether you need them or not. . . . And you walk in and they're automatically 'Get out of those clothes, strip down.'" For some participants, the temperature of the physical environment seemed to be correlated with the temperature of the emotional climate in the outpatient health care setting: "Well, you certainly don't need it cold when the person who is half undressed is freezing, especially the older folks. It's cold . . . and then they give you the little paper and it's cold . . . I mean it's **cold!** If the temperature's cold, then there's this cold feeling you're gonna feel, not a warm feeling.

Study participants had numerous thoughts about what constituted a warm and inviting outpatient environment. What they longed for was a homey feeling, conveyed by decor that was "friendly, warm, nothing pretentious." They reported liking warm colors, soothing music, warm blankets, and soft cloth sheets. They wanted big windows with lots of natural light, comfortable chairs with high, supportive backs, arranged so that patients did not have to sit in the middle of a waiting room where everyone else could stare at them. Several participants specifically expressed their displeasure at having to sit in the middle of a waiting room where others could see them suffering.

Many participants associated the state of the physical environment with the quality of care they expected to receive in that setting. They wanted facilities to be clean, but not sterile, with up-to-date equipment appropriate to the setting. Some expressed concern, however, when they perceived the equipment and other appointments to be too fancy or expensive for the setting:

"There was a whole line of these very expensive chairs and machines. . . . They were . . . the very latest, costing, oh my gracious, thousands and thousands of dollars . . . my feeling was that the bill was really going to be something else." Moreover, health care professionals were perceived to be phony and less competent when the environment was too fancy.

On the other hand, some participants associated worn carpets, nicked furniture, and damaged floors with a lack of attention to detail: "There doesn't have to be spots on the wall. There doesn't have to be nicks. . . . Chairs don't have to be worn. There's no reason for that. . . . Replace it." For one participant, such conditions indicated that the health care professional was not doing his or her job—if the condition of the environment was overlooked, the care provider was believed to be more likely to overlook something in her health as well.

Object/Person

Without fail, when study participants spoke positively about their experience of being a patient in the outpatient health care environment, it was because they felt as if they had been cared for as a human being, as a mature **person** who was valued and important, rather than as a case, a number, a child, or an **object**. Greeting the patient by her name while extending a warm handshake was described by one participant as instilling confidence that the physician had reviewed her chart and was genuinely interested in her health care concerns. Other participants also stressed the importance of being called by name and appreciated being recognized by staff members upon return visits to the same outpatient setting. Even the frustration of a long wait could be alleviated if staff took time to show concern, as this participant related: "I've actually seen a nurse come and actually bend down on their knees, to get in their face because they are sitting in a chair, and talk to them . . . pat them and walk off . . . and they'd probably wait there another two hours and be happy." The manner in which nurses and clerical staff spoke with the patient as they carried out their tasks was important to study participants. They appreciated staff "sparing a little conversation." As one participant put it, "it doesn't take much to have a friendly environment."

After a moment of thoughtful contemplation, one woman spoke about how she felt when allowed to spend the time she needed with her physician: "It lets me feel completely taken care of medically. . . . When I leave there, I never feel that I have been rushed. I never feel that I was just a number. I never felt I was just another diabetic case. I never felt that I was just a diagnosis. I . . . felt that I was an important patient to her." Individualized attention was described by another participant as giving him a psychological advantage—confidence that he was going to improve. If he adhered to the program he had been taught, he was going to get better, get well again, and not die, as he had feared.

While these positive statements about care gave reassurance that some outpatient experiences do promote health and affirm personal worth, many study participants did not report experiencing such thorough and personalized care. Rather, their experiences were described in terms of being treated like cattle or objects on an assembly line. One participant likened her experience in a particular setting to a factory: "It reminds me of a factory, like a people factory . . . and they're all working very hard and they've just got so many people to see they're not concerned about too much other than just getting right down to the basics and get you in, get you out." In this factory, she said the patients were placed in "little stalls." She concluded, "It's not a pleasant experience." Lack of privacy and ambient noise contributed to displeasure with the "factory" atmosphere: Participants spoke of diagnostic and treatment areas in which they were separated from other patients only by curtains and had no choice but to hear all the conversations and noises surrounding them.

Several participants thought they were treated more like cattle than human beings. They made specific references both to doctor's offices and to emergency rooms. The following exemplars are representative:

"You don't really want to be there anyway because you don't feel good and you've drug yourself out of bed to go [there] in the first place, and you're herded in like cattle, especially when you're dealing with these group doctor settings."

"Of course you're definitely herded in as cattle in an emergency room, and that's just the nature of that setting."

Another participant directly linked the dehumanizing care he received to the lack of professionalism in the staff members working in the setting: "Those people should receive a salary for efficiency rather than, you know, just pushing us through like a bunch of cattle. I'm paying for professionalism, at least I think I am when I see the bills that are charged here." He was distressed by disparaging remarks nurses made in his presence about other patients and by the way they treated ill adults as if they were children. After repeated instances of such unprofessional behavior, this participant found himself asking, "What the hell am I *doing* here?" His words provide an appropriate transition to the next theme of powerless/powerful.

Powerless/Powerful

This theme was evident in participant descriptions of the powerful others (They) and a powerless I. The epitome of patient powerlessness was experienced in settings, particularly the emergency room, in which health care was not provided until after all the insurance and registration forms had been completed and processed. In the meantime, the patient experienced having no choice but to sit, wait, and suffer. One participant's account is illustrative:

> I went in with a bad ankle . . . and you go in and you sit there . . . of course you're in excruciating pain, you want somebody to do **something** . . . and then you have to get back up and [give them] your preliminary information . . . and then you go back and sit and then you go see the insurance person . . . You give them your insurance card . . . and **then** at that point, and **only** at that point, will you be put on a list to be seen. And then you go back out . . . and you sit in the lobby and then they call you back again, and then at **that** point are you important. And then all of a sudden they're throwing you in wheelchairs and they're rushing you back and all of a sudden you have this really **major** problem, but only after they were **positive** they were getting paid.

Another patient declared, "Oh my gracious, the **attitude** about insurance!"

Participants spoke of barriers between staff and patient that created a power differential, such as the closed glass windows separating patients and staff in reception areas. In these settings, participants reported experiencing that staff acknowledged waiting patients only when it seemed convenient for them to do so. One participant stated: "I don't care for an office that has a sliding window . . . because they slide it in my face. They'll be busy and that window is not open and then finally they open it and it's like, 'you better hurry because we're gonna close this really quick' . . . and then they can ignore you very easily because when you come up to the window you have to knock. I don't like it!" She proceeded to question the rationale for hiding the staff behind closed windows: "Are they afraid we are going to hold them up or something or attack them?"

Participants also reported feeling powerless when phone calls to a clinic or physician's office were not returned, messages were not forwarded to the appropriate professional staff member, promised reports of test results were not mailed, staff members either did not listen to or dismissed what patients had to say, or they were left alone in examination rooms for long periods of time. One man described his frustration when no one explained the delay in performing his CAT scan: "I had a 5:00 appointment and I waited and waited and waited, and then at 6:00 they sent us down to the other end . . . making me sit there for an hour and not telling me **why**. . . . The appointment was set up days before."

While most participants described experiencing a sense of powerlessness, a few did feel they had power in certain circumstances. One woman's assertiveness resulted in her being seen before other patients who were waiting. She informed a staff member of impending hypoglycemia after an overnight NPO, and was promptly taken from the waiting room into a treatment area and given an IV. Another participant who once worked in a health-related field exercised her power to get changes made when circumstances in the environment did not meet her expectations. She maintained some measure of control as to when and where she obtained care and who provided that care. When asked if she felt like she was in an environment where she could speak up and be heard, she replied: "Oh absolutely! I'm paying for it. And you can fire doctors and you can fire nurses, maybe not from the institution but from your bedroom, and you can get somebody else in here if they're not acting right." Another study participant saw his experience in a cardiac rehabilitation program as adding to the personal power he had over his health. He felt he was in charge, and the careful attention and monitoring he received from the cardiologist, nurses, nutritionists, and exercise physiologists only served to reinforce his sense of power and control.

Frightened/Cared for

When the outpatient health care environment was perceived as comfortable, accommodating, and warm, and the care was prompt, sensitive, respectful, and personalized, study participants were generous with praise for health care providers. In such an environment, they told researchers they felt **cared for**. Having a personal relationship with her physicians was of utmost importance to one participant, in fact, she saw it as the difference between life and death. She was **frightened** and angered by the lack of continuity in caregivers at a family practice clinic, a situation which put her at risk for a limb amputation and near death. By going to another health care setting in which people knew her personally, listened, and assisted her with her needs, this participant's worry lessened and her health condition improved. Up-do-date monitoring equipment and on-site professional staff were reassuring for a male participant in a cardiac rehabilitation center, lessening his fear of dying:

When we went in . . . the first thing they did is put on a heart monitor and they monitored you as you went around. They had an RN on each monitor . . . and

[they] monitored you the whole time you were there . . . And they had a cardiologist there at all times . . . and the people . . . really had a lot of experience in cardiac rehab; [there] wasn't any of 'em that hadn't been there for several years . . . especially the nurses.

Sometimes conditions in outpatient health care environments left participants feeling alone and afraid. One participant related a terrifying experience of being very ill in a busy emergency room: "The gurney was dirty, it had all kinds of blood on it from somebody else . . . and the whole time I was in that hospital I was afraid to close my eyes because of my IV, I was afraid it would go subq. [infiltrate into the subcutaneous tissues]. I was even afraid to ask for anything to drink because every time I did, they couldn't understand why I had to have it. They were busy and had other things to do." She contrasted this experience with a visit to another emergency room which she reported as busy, but clean. In this setting, she experienced the staff as caring: "The whole time I was being cared for. I knew people were concerned . . . but I felt cared for."

When genuine caring was perceived, study participants expressed trust and confidence in health care providers, willingly accepted information given, and complied with prescribed treatments. Praise was given when care providers took the time to listen to the patient, answer questions, and allay anxieties. This participant, after a negative encounter with one provider, spoke positively about the care she received from a new provider: "She really, really talked to me and she really, really listened and she took her time . . . and I felt a lot better when I left." Without exception, sensitive and timely communication between staff and patient, regardless of the type of outpatient setting, was the key to patients' perception of being cared for.

After numerous frustrating experiences in busy primary care clinics, one participant questioned whether health care providers today really *wanted* to help patients. Patients often reported being upset by interactions with the clerical staff before they were even seen by the doctors and nurses. For example, one participant related her distress when a receptionist refused to accept the participant's long-time partner as the closest relative to be notified in case of an emergency. Superficial examinations suggested lack of caring, as exemplified in this participant's description of interaction with an office nurse:

> She didn't have me pee in a cup. She didn't take my weight. She just told me the doctor would be in to see me in a moment, and she was real giggly. I wasn't real confident with her having a great deal of knowledge or anything like that." When the doctor came in to see this same patient, the interaction was dissatisfying as well: "She was in a big hurry. She wasn't going to give me an exam at all. She was just going to talk to me and give me some pain medicine.

Being cared for meant something more than receiving prescriptions and having lab results interpreted. Patients wanted to be considered in their wholeness. As a participant explained: "You put your health and your life basically in this person's hands and they don't even take the time to care about some factors. They're looking at pure physical . . . numbers, blood counts, lab results and test results, and they're not really looking at . . . that whole mind, body, and spirit, and how they have to work together to create a whole being." A different participant describing a "good experience" of an office visit related that her physician not only queried her about her health problems but also asked "what all was going on in my life and everything." An even more significant, fundamental, meaning of "being cared for" is captured in the following participant's words: "I felt like they really cared if I lived or died."

DISCUSSION AND CONCLUSIONS

The experiential world of the patient receiving care in an outpatient setting was described as including both the physical and social environments. Outpatients reported a greater awareness of the physical environment than did hospitalized patients in a concurrent study (see Chapter 15). One participant's words suggest an explanation for this finding. She attributed her increased attentiveness to physical features of the outpatient environment to her present health status "because when one is sick enough to be in the hospital they usually feel pretty rotten"—hence, it logically follows that inpatients are less aware of the environment.

Because outpatients are more likely to pay attention to the physical environment, it behooves health care administrators and professionals, architects, and interior designers to increase input from patients when designing, building, or remodeling outpatient health care facilities. While some progress has been made, particularly within the development of the Academy of Architecture for Health within the American Institute of Architects, more research and patient input are needed to refine what constitutes an optimal outpatient health care environment. Health care professionals must give serious consideration to patient comfort when choosing furnishings for clinics and offices.

There was consensus among study participants that waiting was the most figural aspect of the outpatient health care environment, a finding congruent with extant literature (Rondeau, 1998). Participants viewed health care as an expensive service they were paying for and they expected to get their money's worth for this service. They expected to find a clean, comfortable environment with up-to-date equipment. They expected to see qualified professionals who genuinely cared about them as individuals and provided kind, competent, and compassionate care. While they were tolerant of waits because of extenuating circumstances, being left alone and not told the reasons for delays produced anxiety and powerlessness. In a recent article describing his "experiment" spending the day with his mother-in-law waiting in a clinic for seven hours, a doctor reported a new awareness of what the experience must be like for his own patients: "My appreciation for the aggravation and anxiety my patients endure runs much deeper. They sacrifice so much to see me" (Daberkow, 1999, p. 78).

For participants in the present study, it was an especially frightening experience to wait for a prolonged period in an emergency room. As Reidenbach and Sandifer-Smallwood (1990, p. 50) discovered in a telephone survey, quality of service in the emergency room is evaluated on two key dimensions: the physical appearance of the facility and the quality of treatment. Acknowledging that emergency room patients typically arrive in an agitated state, they suggest that "professionalism and a facility appearance that alleviates this agitation may have a calming effect and heighten perceptions of treatment quality."

Effective communication was reported to be lacking in the outpatient setting and reflected negatively on participants' perceptions of the health care environment. The words of Riikonen (1999) seem applicable to descriptions provided by participants concerning many of their interactions with care providers: "What we have at our hands are 'sickening' or disempowering, noninspiring interactional-linguistic practices we must move away from. . . . I think that the right to good interaction should really be one of the service user's basic rights" (pp. 148–149). According to Gordon and Edwards (1995), health care providers are most comfortable giving information or advice; few want to listen when patients need to express feelings of fear, uncertainty, or depression. In the current study, nurses were seen as essential to good communication between the patient and the physician or nurse practitioner, especially when the patient had been waiting for an extended period of time. Recall how meaningful it was to a participant when a nurse knelt before a patient in the waiting room, making eye contact and giving the patient a brief pat, conveying a caring message not only with words but also with her body.

Participants were keenly aware of encounters when the health care professional was truly listening to them. Gillotti and Applegate (2000) divided communication into two forms: *person-centered* and *position-centered*. In the first of these, the professional relays information to the patient in a sensitive and empathic manner, listens for both cognitive and affective responses, and responds in a kind and caring way. When such communication took place, participants in the present study were more likely to describe the environment as warm and inviting, a place in which they felt cared for. Conversely, in position-centered communication the professional assumes that his/her role is to provide information in an objective, clinical manner that is free from emotion. Study participants interpreted this approach as cold, harsh, and uncaring.

Finally, nurses and other health care professionals need to be ever-vigilant when providing care, whatever the setting may be. No patient should ever feel as if he is being treated more like cattle than a human being. No patient should ever have cause to fear for her well-being because of the lack of individualized care and attention by a health care professional. Brown (1986) found that patients place at the top of their list of caring acts not being considered "just another case," a finding supported by the results of the present study. Additional research is needed to further explore the patient's first-person perspective on receiving care in an outpatient setting. Just as Parimucha, Lussier, and Huelat (2000) advised architects to "think like a patient," we too must learn to see, hear, and feel what our patients are experiencing in order to provide optimal nursing care beyond the hospital walls.

POST-STUDY REFLECTIONS FROM KRISTINA PLAAS

In interviewing individuals about their experiences of receiving health care in an outpatient environment, I found myself repeatedly identifying with them. Re-bracketing was necessary throughout the study, both while interviewing and later while thematizing transcripts, to ensure that my interpretations were solidly based in participant narratives. Their narratives of negative experiences repeatedly kindled a strong empathic response. Even as an experienced nurse and assertive individual, I could relate to participants' feelings of powerlessness and frustration when not being listened to, having to wait for extended periods of time to see the doctor or nurse practitioner, or being treated like just another body on the assembly line. I, too, know of the coldness of the health care environment. Yet, despite these similarities, I have the advantage of understanding how both sides think and operate.

At present, there is a wide gap between what patients want and need and what health care providers offer in the outpatient environment. As technology and treatments have improved, it seems that the gap between patients and providers has grown. Nursing research on the outpatient environment is scarce, yet the environment is one area in which nurses can have a profound influence. This study is but an initial step in increasing our understanding. Further research is needed to isolate specific aspects of the environment which nurses can actively participate in changing in order to provide better care for those who have entrusted their health and well-being to our hands.

Epilogue

We have shared with you, in these pages, the findings of our phenomenological studies at the University of Tennessee. While each study seems to be a "complete" entity, our work is not yet finished. Much remains to be learned about the clinical worlds in which nurses and patients meet one another and establish a connection—or fail to do so. Merleau-Ponty asserted that knowing is never finished because there is no end to the knowable (cited in Kwant, 1963).

Being a descriptive phenomenological researcher has been likened to being a heliograph, a device for sending messages or signaling by flashing the sun's rays from a mirror (Porter, in press). The authors of this book, by sending participants' messages to practicing nurses, have permitted nurses to experience vicariously the life-world of many patients. It is our hope that long after our words are forgotten, the words of our participants will linger in memory. Perhaps somewhere a rehabilitation nurse will recall Rose as she encounters a stroke survivor, providing her patient with the possibility of reopening a closed future. Maybe an emergency room nurse seeing a badly bruised woman, lying in a crumpled heap on a gurney, will ask the husband to leave while she sensitively explores the possibility of abuse. Only when our research makes a difference in the lives of patients such as these will we feel that we have fulfilled our mission.

Reflecting on the invisibility of nurses in many of the studies reported in this book, we are acutely aware that many patients are not getting the nursing care they need and deserve. Particularly poignant was the longing expressed by psychiatric patients for closer connection with their nurses and more intensive individual and group therapies. Some of the chronic patients wistfully recalled the days when they received more substantive treatment while hospitalized—before the days of downsizing RN staffs and substituting medication for interaction. Reflecting upon our research team's previous phenomenological studies of nurses (Brooks et al., 1996; Smith et al., 1996), we are aware that many nurses likewise are longing to do and give more to their patients. But a pervasive sense of powerlessness permeated our interviews of nurses. Over and over again, nurses told our research team that institutional constraints (hospital re-engineering, cutbacks in staffing), uncivil and demeaning treatment (from physicians, supervisors), and lack of collegial support contributed to high levels of frustration, stress, and anger. Contributing to staff nurses' feeling of powerlessness was a belief that no one in management was listening to their concerns. As Benner (2000), has observed, market economics and cost management seem to be dictating contemporary nursing practice.

Elsewhere, we have proposed some solutions to nurses' collective difficulties and private sufferings (Thomas & Droppleman, 1997; Thomas, 1998). While problems at the systems level ultimately require solutions at that level, it is the manager of each nursing unit who embodies higher administration's willingness (or lack, thereof) to seek solutions. If unit managers are not listening to the frustrations of staff nurses, satisfactory solutions are not likely to be discovered. Nurses will continue to feel frustration and patients will continue to feel that no one cares. Management has an obligation to work toward providing adequate resources so that staff can deliver holistic patient care. As Benner noted, "No one can mandate that anyone care or engage in caring practices. But nursing administrators . . . can create working environments and climates that facilitate caring practices" (2001, p. vii).

We remain convinced that there is a moral imperative for each individual practicing nurse to attempt to humanize inhumane treatment settings, clear the debris of his or her own personal and professional life turmoil and pain, and prepare to meet the patient—unencumbered, ready to engage in dialogue. The patient is waiting to be cared for. Even in less-than-ideal circumstances, we must prepare to "meet" him, in the sense that Buber so beautifully described. Swanson (1991) identified *knowing* as one of five dimensions of caring. Knowing is "striving to understand an event as it has meaning in the life of the other" (p. 163). It is precisely this knowing for which phenomenology strives and patients yearn. We believe that phenomenology can be practiced by all nurses as "a manner or style of thinking" (Merleau-Ponty, 1962, p. viii).

Even a "routine" physical assessment can be transformed into a moment of powerful, personal connection. Consider this example. While doing an examination of the various inflamed and deformed joints of an arthritis patient, Claire Hastings made simple statements such as "I can tell that this must be really painful right now" and "It looks like you haven't been able to use this hand for a long time . . ." and concluded her exam by saying, "Rheumatoid arthritis really has not been nice to you." At this point, the patient burst into tears, responding "You know, no one has ever talked about it as a personal thing before, no one's ever talked to me as if this were a thing that mattered, a personal event" (Benner & Wrubel, 1989, pp. 9–11). Eventually, it is our hope that mainstream health care delivery systems will be humanized through the tiny ripples created by such episodes of shared meaning-making between nurse and patient.

We hope that we also said something of interest about a developing style of inquiry in nursing research. Qualitative studies are increasing in number and significance in many different fields, and give participants—patients and nurses alike—a voice that otherwise would remain unspoken and unheard. In dialogic research, the researcher is invariably changed by his or her interaction with participants. The contributors to this book described many new insights in the "Post-Study Reflections" paragraphs at the end of each chapter. As a way to synthesize the changes in perspective they described, we conducted a thematic analysis of these reflections. The following issues became salient to us and to our colleagues as a consequence of the present set of phenomenological studies:

1. Nursing must return to its initial emphasis on holistic care. This means that nurses must not yield to the demands of the profit-driven health care system to emphasize ever-faster performance of tasks and procedures. Patients want to be known, and cared for, in their wholeness, especially when their world is unstable and seems to be falling apart.

2. Illness is never simply a matter of some bodily organ; it always involves the whole person in relation to the major grounds of life. We must be mindful that the ramifications of illness reverberate through families: "When my sister was diagnosed with diabetes, the whole family became diabetic."

3. Nursing education needs to adopt a more open, dialogic style of teaching such that the next generation of nurses will be able to empathize more fully with their patients. A student nurse who does not remember his or her own pain is not likely to be especially caring to someone who now is in pain. Students must be encouraged to reflect on their own prior experiences and on their daily interactions with patients.

4. Technological advances not only have biological implications but also change something about the patient in his or her life world. Much is yet to be learned about patients' lived experiences of organ transplants and mechanical devices.

5. "Being with" a patient is often as significant a role for the nurse as "doing for." Sometimes it may be even more meaningful simply to be with the patient as a person, as one human relating to another. Shotter and Katz (1999, p. 159) remind us that "to be fully 'moved' by an other's suffering, we have . . . to take the trouble to 'enter into' it."

6. The resolution of many situations takes time, and time for our patients in illness (or in the waiting room) is different from time in health. When nurses explain reasons for a prolonged wait and apologize—or "spare a little conversation," as one participant put it—patients report being able to tolerate the slow passage of time.

7. Our patients are spiritual as well as social-biological beings and experiences of spiritual distress can be as disorienting as physical or psychological difficulty.

8. Patients perceive the worlds of the hospital and the clinic to be neither as helpful nor as ameliorative as nurses might hope. Their reports of frightening and dehumanizing experiences bring to mind Nightingale's words in 1859: "It may seem a strange principle to enunciate as the very first requirement in a hospital that it should do the sick no harm."

9. Some of our pre-study assumptions about illness were not always borne out in our interviews. While we never are able to get rid of our prejudgments, we should learn how to hold them in abeyance ("bracket them") in listening to patients. And

we must be open to the serendipitous, the unexpected, as shown in the diametrically opposite meanings of the hospital environment reported by medical and
psychiatric patients.

Although our analysis of researchers' post-study reflections revealed other themes,
some more specific and some more general, the overall conclusion seems to be that
nursing requires an addition to, or even more radically a change in, its philosophical
commitments. To make the fundamental ideas of phenomenology relevant to nurses
we may have to supplant a philosophy useful to biomedical approaches to illness with
one deriving more directly from humanistic concerns. If, and when, we make such a
change, familiar concepts and ideas will appear in a new light and therefore serve to
take us back to why we became nurses in the first place: to care, as best we can, for
suffering people. Although this aspiration most often has been interpreted to mean
"take care of them physically," an existential-phenomenological approach asks us to
see and think about human life in both sickness and health in a quite different way.

Consider, for example, the major existential grounds serving to contextualize human
life: body, time, others, and world. In each domain there is a scientific and an experiential meaning. Body, for example, may mean either the corporeal body of medicine
and physiology or my body as I experience it. While both perspectives may, at times,
provide us with the same meaning—a well-functioning corporeal body does afford
experiences of vitality and activity—sometimes they are curiously disconnected, as the
experience of a phantom limb suggests. Time also provides a clear contrast between
lived and metric time, and human life in the hospital is always experienced in terms of
personal, not clock time. Other people may be experienced as things or Thou, and the
I experiencing the other as Thou is as different as the person being related to. While it
is not reasonable to expect most interactions in crowded clinics and harried hospital
rounds to be I-Thou, it is not too much to expect that we remain open to such possibility. Finally, the world is a world of meanings, of physical structures: from flowers
to personal possessions, from special places to hospitals, the material objects and places
of our world are meaningful. This meaning derives from, and is revealed in, relationships connecting person and world—not from impersonal laws described by physics,
geology, or chemistry.

In the case of either theory, research, pedagogy, or practice, one clear conclusion is
that we are fundamentally beings-in-relations: to one another, to history, to the human
and natural world, to illness, to health, and so on. To recover and describe the nature
of these relationships either as a practitioner or as a researcher it is necessary to adopt
a first-person method in which the perspective of the person is granted an equal value
to that of the researcher. Given these two distinct perspectives, it is clear that we make
contact with one another primarily in conversation. This means that I must hear and
listen to you as you must hear and listen to me. And this is the most important lesson
that each researcher related in his or her post-study reflections: to listen respectfully
to patients and research participants so that we might understand the unique perspectives of their experiences and of their worlds.

Heidegger suggested that the hermeneutic circle is always open, because others always have the possibility of entering into the conversation. Readers are invited to contribute to the ongoing dialogue about the existential phenomena of concern to nurses and their patients. The dialogue transcends this book and its authors, remaining unfinished but nevertheless projecting fascinating possibilities.

References

Abramson, H. S. (1996). A patient's view. In E. D. Baer, C. M. Fagin, & S. Gordon (Eds.), *Abandonment of the patient: The impact of profit-driven health care on the public* (pp. 25–30). New York: Springer.

Ackerman, M., & Stevens, M. (1989). Acute and chronic pain: Pain dimensions and psychological status. *Journal of Clinical Psychology, 45*, 223–228.

Ahern, K. J. (1999). Ten tips for reflexive bracketing. *Qualitative Health Research, 9*, 407–411

Ahlsio, B., Britton, M., Murray, V., & Theorell, T. (1984). Disablement and quality of life after stroke. *Stroke, 15*, 886–890.

Ames, L. B. (1946). The development of the sense of time in the young child. *Journal of Genetic Psychology, 68*, 97–125.

Anderson, D. G. (1996). Homeless women's perceptions about their families of origin. *Western Journal of Nursing Research, 18*(1), 29–42.

Anderson, D. G., & Hatton, D. C. (2000). Accessing vulnerable populations for research. *Western Journal of Nursing Research, 22*(2), 244–251.

ANRED (Anorexia Nervosa and Related Eating Disorders, Inc.) (2000, January 26). *Statistics: How many people have eating and exercise disorders* (available on-line at http://www.anred.com).

Ashurst, P., & Hall, Z. (1989). *Understanding women in distress.* NY: Tavistock/ Routledge.

Ayto, J. (1990). *Dictionary of word origins.* New York: Arcade Publishing (Little Brown).

Bachelard, G. (1969). *The poetics of space* (M. Jones, trans.). Boston: Beacon Press.

Baird, C. L., & Bell, P. A. (1995). Place attachment, isolation, and the power of a window in a hospital environment. *Psychological Reports, 76*, 847–850.

Baker, C. (1992). Discomfort to environmental noise: Heart rate responses of SICU patients. *Critical Care Nursing Quarterly, 15*(2), 75–90.

Ballard, C. G., Davis, R., Cullen, P. C., Mohan, R. N., & Dean, C. (1994). Postnatal depression in mothers and fathers. *British Journal of Psychiatry, 164*, 782–788.

Bates, M., & Rankin-Hill, L. (1994). Control, culture, and chronic pain. *Social Science and Medicine, 39*, 629–645.

Baun, M. M., Oetting, K., & Bergstrom, N. (1991). Health benefits of companion animals in relation to the physiologic indices of relaxation. *Holistic Nursing Practice, 5*(2), 16–23.

Beck, C. T. (1992). The lived experience of postpartum depression: A phenomenological study. *Nursing Research, 41*, 166–170.

Becker, A., Grinspoon, S., Klibanski, A., & Herzog, D. (1999). Eating disorders: Current concepts. *New England Journal of Medicine, 340*(14), 1092–1098.

Becker, C. S. (1992). *Living and relating: An introduction to phenomenology.* Newbury Park, CA: Sage.

Beddoe, S. S. (1999). Reachable moment. *Image: Journal of Nursing Scholarship, 31,* 248.

Beier, B., & Pollio, H. R. (1994). A thematic analysis of the experience of being in a role. *Sociological Spectrum, 14*, 257–272.

Benner, P. (1984). *Stress and satisfaction on the job: Work meanings and coping of mid-career men.* New York: Praeger.

Benner, P. (1994). Introduction. In P. Benner (Ed.), *Interpretive phenomenology: Embodiment, caring, and ethics in health and illness* (pp. xiii–xxvii). Thousand Oaks, CA: Sage.

Benner, P. (1999a). Claiming the wisdom and worth of clinical practice. *Nursing and Health Care Perspectives, 20*(6), 312–319.

Benner, P. (1999b). Quality of life: A phenomenological perspective on explanation, prediction, and understanding in nursing science. In E. C. Polifroni & M. Welch (Eds.), *Perspectives on philosophy of science in nursing* (pp. 303–314). Philadelphia: Lippincott.

Benner, P. (2000). The wisdom of our practice. *American Journal of Nursing, 100*(10), 99–105.

Benner, P. (2001). *From novice to expert: Commemorative edition.* Upper Saddle River, NJ: Prentice Hall Health.

Benner, P., & Wrubel, J. (1989). *The primacy of caring: Stress and coping in health and disease.* Menlo Park, CA: Addison-Wesley.

Bennett, L. (1991). Adolescent girls' experience of witnessing marital violence: A phenomenological study. *Journal of Advanced Nursing, 16*(4), 431–438.

Berger, P., & Luckmann, T. (1966). *The social construction of reality.* New York: Doubleday.

Bevis, E. O. (1993). All in all, it was a pretty good funeral. *Journal of Nursing Education, 32*(3), 101–105.

Bigger, J. T. (1991). Future studies with the implantable cardioverter defibrillator. *PACE, 14*, 883–889.

Biley, F. (1996). *An exploration of the science of unitary human beings and the principle of integrality: The effects of background music on patients and their perception of the environment.* Unpublished Ph.D. thesis, University of Wales, United Kingdom.

Bishop, A. H., & Scudder, J. R. (1999). A philosophical interpretation of nursing. *Scholarly Inquiry for Nursing Practice, 13*(1), 17–27.

Bitner, M. (1990). Evaluating service encounters: The effects of physical surroundings and employee responses. *Journal of Marketing, 54*(2), 69–83.

Bitner, M. (1992). Servicescapes: The impact of physical surroundings on customers and employees. *Journal of Marketing, 56*(2), 57–71.

Bitner, M., Booms, M., & Tetreault, M. (1990). The service encounter: Diagnosing favorable and unfavorable. *Journal of Marketing, 54*(1), 71–85.

Bower, J. (1994). New therapy for ventricular arrhythmias. *AORN Journal, 59*(5), 985–996.

Bowman, J. M. (1991). The meaning of chronic low back pain. *AAOHN Journal, 39*, 381–384.

Boyce, P. (1994). Personality dysfunction, marital problems, and postnatal depression. In J. Cox & J. Holden (Eds.), *Perinatal psychiatry: Use and misuse of the Edinburgh Postnatal Depression Scale* (pp. 90–97). London: Gaskell.

Boyce, W. T., Jensen, E. W., Cassel, J. C., Collier, A. M., Smith, A. H., & Ramey, C. T. (1977). Influence of life events and family routines on childhood respiratory tract illness. *Pediatrics, 60*, 609–615.

Braden, C. J. (1991). Learned response to chronic illness: Disability payments vs. non-recipients. *Rehabilitation Psychology, 36*, 265–277.

Bretall, R. (Ed.) (1946). *A Kierkegaard anthology.* Princeton, NJ: Princeton University Press.

Brooks, A., Thomas, S. P., & Droppleman, P. (1996). From frustration to red fury: A description of work-related anger in male registered nurses. *Nursing Forum, 31*(3), 4–15.

Brown, L. (1986). The experience of care: Patient perspectives. *Topics in Clinical Nursing, 8*(2), 56–62.

Bruch, H. (1985). Four decades of eating disorders. In D. M. Garner & P. E. Garfinkle (Eds.), *Handbook of psychotherapy for anorexia nervosa and bulimia* (pp. 7–18). New York: Garfield Express.

Brumberg, J. (1988). *Fasting girls: The history of anorexia nervosa.* Cambridge, MA: Harvard University Press.

Buber, M. (1924/1970). *I and thou.* (W. Kaufmann, Trans.) New York: Charles Scribner's Sons.

Burkhardt, M. (1991). Exploring understandings of spirituality among women in Appalachia. *Dissertation Abstracts International, 52*, 07B-3523. (University Microfilms No. AAD91–36470).

Burns, J. W., Higdon, L. J., Mullen, J. T., Lansky, D., & Wei, J. M. (1999). Relationships among patient hostility, anger expression, depression, and the working alliance in a work hardening program. *Annals of Behavioral Medicine, 21*(1), 77–82.

Butcher, H. K., Holkup, P. A., & Buckwalter, K. C. (2001). The experience of caring for a family member with Alzheimer's disease. *Western Journal of Nursing Research, 23*, 33–55.

Buytendijk, F. J. J. (1962). *Pain: Its modes and functions.* Chicago: University of Chicago Press.

Cademenos, S. (1981). *A phenomenological approach to pain.* Unpublished doctoral dissertation, Brandeis University.

Caelli, K. (2000). The changing face of phenomenological research: Traditional and American phenomenology in nursing. *Qualitative Health Research, 10*(3), 366–377.

Campbell, J. C. (1986). Nursing assessment for risk of homicide with battered women. *Advances in Nursing Science, 8*(4), 36–51.

Campbell, J. C., Harris, M. J., & Lee, R. K. (1995). Violence research: An overview. *Scholarly Inquiry for Nursing Practice, 9*, 105–126.

Campbell, J. C., & Humphreys, J. (1984). *Nursing care of victims of family violence.* Reston, VA: Reston.

Campbell, J. C., & Humphreys, J. (1993). *Nursing care of survivors of family violence.* St. Louis: C.V. Mosby.

Camus, A. (1970). *Selected essays and notebooks.* (trans. P. Thody.) New York: Marlowe & Company.

Canam, C. (1987). Coping with feelings: Chronically ill children and their families. *Nursing Papers, 19*(3), 9–21.

Cannom, D. S. (1992). Implantable cardioverter defibrillator: The promise and perils of an evolving technology. *PACE, 15*, 1–3.

Cannon, W. B. (1942). "Voodoo" death. *American Anthropologist, 44*, 169–181.

Carpenter, D. R. (1999a). Phenomenology in practice, education, and administration. In H. J. Streubert & D. R. Carpenter (Eds.), *Qualitative research in nursing: Advancing the humanistic imperative* (pp. 65–87). Philadelphia: Lippincott.

Carpenter, D. R. (1999b). Phenomenology as method. In H. J. Streubert & D. R. Carpenter (Eds.) *Qualitative research in nursing: Advancing the humanistic imperative* (pp. 43–63). Philadelphia: Lippincott.

Carpenter, J. S. (1998). Informing participants about the benefits of descriptive research. *Nursing Research, 47*, 63–64.

Carpenter, J. S., Sloan, P., & Andrykowski, M. (1999). Anticipating barriers in pain-management research. *Image: Journal of Nursing Scholarship, 31*, 158.

Carr, D. (1967). Maurice Merleau-Ponty: Incarnate consciousness. In G. A. Schrader (Ed.), *Existential philosophers: Kierkegaard to Merleau-Ponty* (pp. 369–429). New York: McGraw-Hill.

Cash, T. F., & Brown, T. A. (1987). Body image in anorexia nervosa and bulimia nervosa: A review of the literature. *Behavior Modification, 11*, 487–521.

Chernin, K. (1985). *The obsession: Reflections on the tyranny of slenderness.* New York: Harper & Row.

Chesler, M. A., Allswede, J. A., & Barbarin, O. O. (1992). Voices from the margin of the family: Siblings of children with cancer. *Journal of Psychosocial Oncology, 9*(4), 19–42.

Chibnall, J. T., Tait, R. C., & Ross, L. R. (1997). The effects of medical evidence and pain intensity on medical student judgments of chronic pain patients. *Journal of Behavioral Medicine, 20,* 257–271.

Chinn, P. (1983). Nursing theory development: Where we have been and where we are going. In N. L. Chaska (Ed.), *The nursing profession: A time to speak* (pp. 394–405). New York: McGraw-Hill.

Chitty, K. (1996). Clients with eating disorders. In H. S. Wilson & C. R. Kneisl (Eds.), *Psychiatric nursing (5th ed.)* (pp. 420–445). New York: Addison-Wesley.

Churchill, M., Safaoui, J., McCabe, B. W., & Baun, M. M. (1999). Using a therapy dog to alleviate the agitation and desocialization of people with Alzheimer's disease. *Journal of Psychosocial Nursing, 37*(4), 16–22, 42–43.

Cifu, D. X., & Lorish, T. (1994). Stroke rehabilitation. 5. Stroke outcome. *Archives of Physical Medicine and Rehabilitation, 75,* S56–S60.

Cohen, M., & Omery, A. (1994). Schools of phenomenology: Implications for research. In J. M. Morse (Ed.), *Critical issues in qualitative research methods* (pp. 136–156). Thousand Oaks, CA: Sage Publications.

Colaizzi, P. F. (1978). Psychological research as the phenomenologist views it. In R. Valle & M. King (Eds.), *Existential-phenomenological alternatives for psychology* (pp. 48–71). New York: Oxford.

Conn, V. (1999). Nurses as providers of preventive services for relatives of patients with serious mental illnesses. *The Journal of NAMI California, 10*(3), 27–30.

Cooper, D. K., Luceri, R. M., Thurer, R., & Myerburg, R. J. (1986). The impact of the automatic implantable cardioverter defibrillator on quality of life. *Clinical Progress in Electrophysiology and Pacing, 4*(4), 306–309.

Covington, E. C. (1991). Depression and chronic fatigue in the patient with chronic pain. *Primary Care, 18,* 341–358.

Cromer, R. (1968). *The development of temporal reference during the acquisition of language.* Unpublished doctoral dissertation, Harvard University.

Crotty, M. (1996). *Phenomenology and nursing research.* Melbourne, Australia: Churchill Livingstone.

Csikszentmahalyi, M., & Rochberg-Halton, E. (1981). *The meaning of things: Domestic symbols and the self.* Cambridge: Cambridge University Press.

Daberkow, D. (1999, November 22). I finally understand the waiting room ordeal. *Medical Economics, 74*–78.

Dapkus, M. (1985). A thematic analysis of the experience of time. *Journal of Personality and Social Psychology, 49,* 408–419.

Davidson, A. W., & Young, C. (1985). Repatterning of stroke rehabilitation clients following return to life in the community. *Journal of Neurosurgical Nursing, 17,* 123–128.

Davidson, T., VanRiper, S., Harper, P., & Wenk, A. (1994). Implantable cardioverter defibrillators: A guide for clinicians. *Heart and Lung, 23*(3), 205–215.

Davis, G. C. (1998). Nursing's role in pain management across the health care continuum. *Nursing Outlook, 46,* 19–23.

Decker, W. A., & Freeman, M. (1996). The journey challenged by eating disorders. In V. B. Carson & E. N. Arnold (Eds.), *Mental health nursing: The nurse-patient journey* (pp. 909–925). Philadelphia: W.B. Saunders.

DeHaan, R., Horn, J., Limburg, M., Van Der Meulen, J., & Bossuyt, P. (1993). A comparison of five stroke scales with measures of disability, handicap, and quality of life. *Stroke, 24*, 1178–1181.

de Konig, A. J. (1979). The qualitative method of research in the phenomenology of suspicion. In A. Giorgi, R. Knowles, & D. L. Smith (Eds.), *Duquesne studies in phenomenological psychology, vol. 3* (pp. 209–226). Pittsburgh, PA: Duquesne University Press.

DeLuna, A. B., Coumel, P., & Ledercar, J. (1989). Ambulatory sudden cardiac death: Mechanisms of production of fatal arrhythmias on the basis of 157 cases. *American Heart Journal, 117*, 151.

DeSantis, L., & Ugarriza, D. (2000). The concept of theme as used in qualitative nursing research. *Western Journal of Nursing Research, 22*(3), 351–372.

Diekelmann, N. (1992). Learning-as-testing: A Heideggerian hermeneutical analysis of the lived experiences of students and teachers in nursing. *Advances in Nursing Science, 14*(3), 72–83.

Dobash, R. E., & Dobash, R. P. (1988). Research as social action: The struggle for battered women. In K. Yllo & M. Bograd (Eds.), *Feminist perspectives on wife abuse* (pp. 51–74). Newbury Park, CA: Sage.

Doolittle, N. D. (1990). *Life after stroke: Survivors' bodily and practical knowledge of coping during recovery.* Doctoral dissertation, University of California, San Francisco.

Dossey, L. (1984). *Beyond illness.* Boston: Shambhala Publications.

Drew, N. (1999). A return to Husserl and researcher self-awareness. In E. C. Polifroni & M. Welch (Eds.), *Perspectives on philosophy of science in nursing* (pp. 263–272). Philadelphia: Lippincott.

Dromerick, A., & Reding, M. (1994). Medical and neurological complications during inpatient stroke rehabilitation. *Stroke, 25*, 358–361

Drotar, D., & Crawford, P. (1985). Psychological adaptation of siblings of chronically ill children: Research and practice implications. *Journal of Developmental and Behavioral Pediatrics, 6*(6), 355–362.

Dugan, D. (1987/88). Essays on the art of caring in nursing: I. The human spirit in stress management. *Nursing Forum, 23*(3), 108–117.

duMont, P., Droppleman, E., Droppleman, P. G., & Thomas, S. P. (1999). The lived experience of anger among a sample of French women. *The Journal of Multicultural Nursing and Health, 5*(1), 19–26.

duMont, P. (2000, June). *Merleau-Ponty as the lens.* Paper presented at the Conference on Phenomenology and Hermeneutics, Minneapolis, Minnesota.

Dunn, J., & McGuire, S. (1992). Sibling and peer relationships in childhood. *Child Psychology and Psychiatry, 33*(1), 67–105.

duNouy, L. (1936). *Le temps et la vic.* Paris: Gallemord.

Dworkin, S. F., Von Korff, M. R., & Le Resche, L. (1992). Epidemiological studies of chronic pain: A dynamic-ecologic perspective. *Annals of Behavioral Medicine, 14*(1), 3–11.

Easton, K. L., McComish, J. F., & Greenberg, R. (2000). Avoiding common pitfalls in qualitative data collection and transcription. *Qualitative Health Research, 10,* 703–707.

Edwards, R. B. (1989). Pain management and the values of health care providers. In C. S. Hill, Jr., & W. S. Fields (Eds.), *Advances in pain research and therapy, vol. 11* (pp. 101–112). New York: Raven Press.

Eliot, T. S. (1943/1971). *Four quartets.* New York: Harcourt, Brace & World.

Elton, N., Hanna, M., & Treasure, J. (1994). Coping with pain: Some patients suffer more. *British Journal of Psychiatry, 165,* 802–807.

Engelbart, H. J., & Vrancken, M. A. (1984). Chronic pain from the perspective of health: A view based on systems theory. *Social Science and Medicine, 12,* 1383–1392.

Erdmann, B. R. (1987). *Living with chronic pain.* Unpublished doctoral dissertation, University of Tennessee, Knoxville.

Erickson, J. R., & Henderson, A. D. (1992) Witnessing family violence: The children's experience. *Journal of Advanced Nursing, 17,* 1200–1209.

Erikson, E. H. (1980). *Identity and the life cycle.* New York: Norton.

Faux, S. A., Walsh, M., & Deatrick, J. A. (1988). Intensive interviewing with children and adolescents. *Western Journal of Nursing Research, 10*(2), 180–194.

Faberhaugh, S. Y., & Strauss, A. (1977). *Politics of pain management.* Menlo Park, CA: Addison-Wesley.

Fabiszewski, R., & Volosin, K. J. (1992). Refusal of implantable cardioverter defibrillator generator replacement: The nurse's role. *Focus on Critical Care, 19*(2), 97–100.

Fawcett, J. (1995). *Analysis and evaluation of conceptual models of nursing* (3rd ed.). Philadelphia: F. A. Davis.

Fawcett, J. (2000). *Analysis and evaluation of contemporary nursing knowledge: Nursing models and theories.* Philadelphia: F. A. Davis.

Federal Bureau of Investigation (1995). *Uniform crime reports: Crime in the United States, 1994.* Washington, DC: U.S. Department of Justice.

Fehring, R., & Rantz, M. (1991). Spiritual distress. In M. Maas, K. Buckwalter, & M. Hardy (Eds.), *Nursing diagnoses and interventions for the elderly* (pp. 598–609). Redwood City, CA: Addison-Wesley Nursing.

Ferlic, A. (1968). Existential approach in nursing. *Nursing Outlook, 16*(10), 30–33.

Fernandez, L. (1992). *The world of the lupus patient: Phenomenological and psychological perspectives in lupus erythematosus.* Unpublished doctoral dissertation, University of Tennessee.

Ferrari, M. (1984). Chronic illness: Psychosocial effects on siblings. I. Chronically ill boys. *Journal of Child Psychology and Psychiatry and Allied Disciplines, 25*(3), 459–476.

Fields, B., Reesman, K., Robinson, C., Sims, A., Edwards, K., McCall, B., Short, B., & Thomas, S. P. (1998). Anger of African American women in the South. *Issues in Mental Health Nursing, 19*(4), 353–373.

Foucault, M. (1991). The ethic of care for the self as a practice of freedom. In J. Bernauer & D. Rasmussen (Eds.), *The final Foucault* (pp. 1–20). Cambridge: The MIT Press.

Fraisse, P. (1963). *The psychology of time.* New York: Harper & Row.

Frankl, V. (1946/1959). *Man's search for meaning.* Boston: Beacon Press

Friedemann, M-L., & Smith, A. A. (1997). A triangulation approach to testing a family instrument. *Western Journal of Nursing Research, 19*, 364–378.

Frist, T., Jr. (2000, March 8–10). *Facility Management.* Paper presented at the conference of the American Society for Healthcare Engineers and the American Institute of Architecture's Academy of Architecture for Health, Nashville, TN.

Gadamer, H. G. (1966/1977). The universality of the hermeneutic problem. In D. Linge (Ed.), *Philosophical hermeneutics* (pp. 3–17). Berkeley, CA: University of California Press.

Gadamer, H. G. (1960/1975). *Truth and method.* New York: Seabury.

Gadow, S. (1980). Existential advocacy: Philosophical foundation of nursing. In S. Spicker & S. Gadow (Eds.), *Nursing: Images and ideals: Opening dialogue with the humanities* (pp. 79–101). New York: Springer Publishing.

Gadow, S. (1990). The advocacy covenant: Care as clinical subjectivity. In J. S. Stevenson (Ed.), *Knowledge about care and caring: State of the art and future development* (pp. 33–40). Washington, DC: American Nurses Association.

Gallo, A. M. (1988). The special sibling relationship in chronic illness and disability: Parental communication with well siblings. *Holistic Nursing Practice, 2*(2), 28–37.

Gallo, A. M., Breitmayer, B. J., Knafl, K. A., & Zoeller, L. H. (1991). Stigma in childhood chronic illness: A well sibling perspective. *Pediatric Nursing, 17*(1), 21–25.

Gayton, W. F., Friedman, S. B., Tavormina, J. F., & Tucker, F. (1977). Children with cystic fibrosis: I. Psychological test findings of patients, siblings, and parents. *The Journal of Pediatrics, 59*(6), 888–894.

Gelles, R., & Cornell, C. (1990). *Intimate violence in families.* Newbury Park, CA: Sage.

George, J. (1995). *Nursing theories: The base for professional nursing practice.* Norwalk,CT: Appleton & Lange.

George, M. (1996). Postnatal depression, relationships and men. *Mental Health Nursing, 16*(6), 12–15.

Gerace, L. M., Camilleri, D., & Ayres, L. (1993). Sibling perspectives on schizophrenia and the family. *Schizophrenia Bulletin, 19*(3), 637–647.

Gergen, K. (2000, May 2). *The nature of human care.* Paper presented to the Applied Phenomenology Study Group at the University of Tennessee, Knoxville.

Gerteis, M. (1993). Coordinating care and integrating services. In M. Gerteis, S. Edgman-Levitan, J. Daley, & T. L. Delbanco (Eds.), *Through the patient's eyes: Understanding and promoting patient-centered care* (pp. 45–71). San Francisco: Jossey-Bass.

Gerteis, M., Edgman-Levitan, S., Daley, J., & Delbanco, T. L. (Eds.) (1993). *Through the patient's eyes: Understanding and promoting patient-centered care.* San Francisco: Jossey-Bass.

Gillotti, C. M., & Applegate, J. L. (2000). Explaining illness as bad news: Individual differences in explaining illness-related information. In B. B. Whaley (Ed.), *Explaining illness: Research, theories, and strategies* (101–120). Mahwah, NJ: Lawrence Erlbaum Associates.

Giorgi, A. (1975). An application of phenomenological method in psychology. In A. Giorgi, C. T. Fischer, & E. L. Murray (Eds.), *Duquesne studies in phenomenological psychology* (Vol. 2) (pp. 82–103). Pittsburgh: Duquesne University Press.

Goffman, E. (1959). *The presentation of self in everyday life.* Garden City, NY: Doubleday.

Goffman, E. (1961). *Asylums: Essays on the social situation of mental patients and other inmates.* Garden City, NY: Doubleday.

Gogan, J. L., Koocher, G. P., Foster, D. J., & O'Malley, J. E. (1977). Impact of childhood cancer on siblings. *Health and Social Work, 2*(1), 41–57.

Gordon, T., & Edwards, W. S. (1995). *Making the patient your partner: Communication skills for doctors and other caregivers.* Westport, CT: Auburn House.

Granstrom, S. (1985). Spiritual care for oncology patients. *Topics in Clinical Nursing, 7,* 39–45.

Gresham, G. E., Duncan, P. W., Stason, W. B., et al. (1995). *Post-Stroke Rehabilitation.* Clinical Practice Guideline, No. 16. Rockville, MD: U.S. Department of Health and Human Services. Public Health Service, Agency for Health Care Policy and Research. AHCPR Publication No. 95–0062.

Grey, M. (1992). Diabetes mellitus (Type I). In P. L. Jackson & J. A. Vessey (Eds.), *Primary care of a child with a chronic condition* (pp. 229–244). St. Louis: Mosby-Year Book.

Groger, L., Mayberry, P., & Straker, J. (1999). What we didn't learn because of who would not talk to us. *Qualitative Health Research, 9,* 829–835.

Hagan, T. (1986). Interviewing the downtrodden. In P. Ashworth, A. Giorgi, & A. deKonig (Eds.), *Qualitative research in psychology.* Pittsburgh: Duquesne University Press.

Harrell, G., Hutt, M., & Anderson, J. (1980). Path analysis of buyer behavior under conditions of crowding. *Journal of Marketing Research, 17,* 45–51.

Harvey, I., & McGrath, G. (1988). Psychiatric morbidity in spouses of women admitted to a mother and baby unit. *British Journal of Psychiatry, 152,* 506–510.

Hawthorne, M. C. (1988). *The human experience of reparation: A phenomenological investigation.* Unpublished doctoral dissertation, University of Tennessee, Knoxville.

Hatton, D., Bennett, S., Gaffrey, E., & Berends, N. (1995, May). *Staff perceptions of health problems among homeless women shelter residents.* Paper presented at the 28th Annual WSRN Communicating Nursing Research Conference, San Diego, CA.

Hayry, M. (1991). Measuring the quality of life: Why, how and what? *Theoretical Medicine, 12*, 97–116.

Hector, M. (2000, July). *Existential-phenomenological research methodologies: Implications for counseling.* Paper presented at the 27th International Congress of Psychology, Stockholm, Sweden.

Heidegger, M. (1927/1962). *Being and time.* (Trans. J. MacQuarrie). New York: Harper & Row.

Henderson, A. D. (1992). Why is it important for critical care nurses to know anything about wife abuse? *Critical Care Nursing, 12*(2), 27–30.

Henkelman, W. J. (1994). Inadequate pain management: Ethical considerations. *Nursing Management, 25*(1), 48a–48d.

Henriksson, C. M. (1995). Living with continuous muscular pain: Patient perspectives. *Scandinavian Journal of Caring Science, 9*, 77–86.

Hilberman, E. (1980). Overview: The "wife-beater's wife" reconsidered. *American Journal of Psychiatry, 137*, 1336–1346.

Hilbert, R. (1984). The acultural dimension of chronic pain: Flawed reality construction and the problem of meaning. *Social Problems, 31*, 365–378.

Hill, A., & Franklin, J. (1998). Mothers, daughters and dieting: Investigating the transmission of weight control. *British Journal of Clinical Psychology, 37*, 3–13.

Hinkley, B. S., & Jaremko, M. E. (1994). Effects of pain duration in orthopedic patients: The importance of early diagnosis and treatment of pain. *Journal of Pain and Symptom Management, 9*, 175–185.

Hitchcock, L., Ferrell, B., & McCaffery, M. (1994). The experience of chronic non-malignant pain. *Journal of Pain and Symptom Management, 9*, 312–318.

Holden, J. (1994). Can non-psychotic depression be prevented? In J. Cox & J. Holden (Eds.), *Perinatal psychiatry: Use and misuse of the Edinburgh Postnatal Depression Scale* (pp. 90–97). London: Gaskell.

Holm, K., Cohen, F., Dudas, S. Medema, P. G., & Allen, B. L. (1989). Effect of personal pain experience on pain assessment. *Image: Journal of Nursing Scholarship, 21*(2), 72–75.

Holmberg, S., & Coon, S. (1999). Ambient sound levels in a state psychiatric hospital. *Archives of Psychiatric Nursing, 13*(3), 177–126.

Horowitz, L. N. (1992). The automatic implantable cardioverter defibrillator: Review of clinical results, 1980–1990. *PACE, 15*, 604–609.

Hotaling, G., Finkelhor, D., Kirkpatrick, J., & Straus, M. (Eds.) (1988). *Coping with family violence: Research and policy perspectives.* Newbury Park, CA: Sage.

Howell, S. L. (1994). A theoretical model for caring for women with chronic nonmalignant pain. *Qualitative Health Research, 4*, 94–122.

Hurley, M. (Ed.) (1986). *Classification of nursing diagnoses: Proceedings of the sixth national conference.* St. Louis, MO: Mosby.

Husserl, E. (1907/1999). The train of thought in the lectures. In E. C. Polifroni & M. Welch (Eds.), *Perspectives on philosophy of science in nursing* (pp. 247–262). Philadelphia: J.B. Lippincott. (Lectures first delivered in 1907 at Gottingen.)

Husserl, E. (1913/1931). *Ideas: General introduction to pure phenomenology* (W. Gibson, Trans.). New York: Collier Books.

Husserl, E. (1970). *The crisis of European sciences and transcendental phenomenology*. (Trans. D. Carr). Chicago, IL: Northwestern University Press.

Hutchinson, S., Wilson, M., & Wilson, H. (1994). Benefits of participating in research interviews. *Image: Journal of Nursing Scholarship, 26*, 161–164.

Hutton, J., & Richardson, L. (1995). Healthscapes: The role of the facility and physical environment on consumer attitudes, satisfaction, quality assessment, and behaviors. *Health Care Management Review, 20*(2), 48–61.

Ittelson, W., Proshansky, H., & Rivlin, L. (1970). A study of bedroom use on two psychiatric wards. *Hospital and Community Psychology, 21*, 25–28.

Jacob, M. C., Kerns, R. D., Rosenberg, R., & Haythornthwaite, J. (1993). Chronic pain: Intrusion and accommodation. *Behaviour Research and Therapy, 31*, 519–527.

Jacobson, G. (1994). The meaning of stressful life experiences in nine-to eleven-year-old children: A phenomenological study. *Nursing Research, 43*(2), 95–99.

James, W. (1890). *The principles of psychology* (2 volumes). New York: Holt.

Jamieson, E. M., Sewall, M. F., & Suhrie, E. B. (1969). *Trends in nursing history*. Philadelphia: W.B. Saunders.

Janesick, V. J. (1998). The dance of qualitative research design: Metaphor, methodolatry, and meaning. In N. K. Denzin & Y. S. Lincoln (Eds.), *Strategies of qualitative inquiry* (pp. 35–55). Thousand Oaks, CA: Sage Publications.

Janet, P. (1877). Une illusion d'optique interne. *Revue Philosophique, 1*, 497–502.

Jaspers, K. (1955). *Reason and existence*. (Trans. W. Earle). The Noonday Press.

Jaspers, K. (1968). *General psychopathology*. (J. Hoenig & M. W. Hamilton, trans.) Chicago: University of Chicago Press.

Jennings, G. L., Reid, C. M., Christy, I., Jennings, J., Anderson, W. P., & Dart, A. (1998). Animals and cardiovascular health. In C. C. Wilson & D. C. Turner (Eds.), *Companion animals and human health* (pp. 161–171). Thousand Oaks, CA: Sage.

Jennings, J. L. (1986). Husserl revisited: The forgotten distinction between psychology and phenomenology. *American Psychologist, 41*, 1231–1240.

Johnson, C., & Connors, M. (1987). *The etiology and treatment of bulimia nervosa: A biopsychosocial perspective*. New York: Basic Books.

Johnson, M. (2000). Commentary. *Western Journal of Nursing Research, 22*(6), 699–702.

Jourard, S. (1971). *The transparent self*. New York: Van Nostrand.

Jung, C. (1959). *The archetypes of the collective unconscious* (R. Hull, trans.), Vol. 9, part 1 (p. 189). Princeton, NJ: Princeton University Press.

Kainz, H. P. (1988). *Paradox, dialectic and system: A contemporary reconstruction of the Hegelian problematic*. University Park, PA: Pennsylvania State University Press.

Kaldenberg, D. O., & Becker, B. W. (1999). Evaluations of care by ambulatory surgery patients. *Health Care Management Review, 24*(3), 73–83.

Kangas, S., Warren, N. A., & Byrne, M. M. (1998). Metaphor: The language of nursing researchers. *Nursing Research, 47*, 190–193.

Kaplan, H. I., & Sadock, B. J. (1991). *Synopsis of psychiatry (6th ed.)*. Baltimore: Williams & Wilkins.

Kavanaugh, K., & Ayres, L. (1998). "Not as bad as it could have been": Assessing and mitigating harm during research interviews on sensitive topics. *Research in Nursing and Health, 21*, 91–97.

Kaysen, S. (1993). *Girl, Interrupted*. New York: Random House.

Keefe, F. J., & Lefebvre, J. C. (1997). Introduction to the featured section: Pain—From mechanisms to management. *Health Psychology, 16*, 307–309.

Keil, C. P. (1998). Loneliness, stress, and human-animal attachment among older adults. In C. C. Wilson & D. C. Turner (Eds.), *Companion animals in human health*. Thousand Oaks, CA: Sage.

Kendler, K. S. (1991). The genetic epidemiology of bulimia nervosa. *American Journal of Psychiatry, 148*, 1627.

Kenemore, E., & Spira, M. (1996). Mothers and their adolescent daughters: Transitions and transformations. *Child and Adolescent Social Work Journal, 13*(3), 225–240.

Keren, R., Aarons, D., & Velti, E. (1991). Anxiety and depression in patients with life-threatening ventricular arrhythmias: Impact of the implantable cardioverter defibrillator. *PACE, 14*, 841–843.

Kesselring, A. (1990). *The experienced body: When taken-for-grantedness fails*. Unpublished doctoral dissertation. University of California, San Francisco.

Kim, M., McFarland, G., & McLane, A. (Eds.) (1984). *Classification of nursing diagnoses: Proceedings of the fifth national conference*. St. Louis, MO: Mosby.

King, M. C., & Ryan, J. (1989). Abused women: Dispelling myths and encouraging intervention. *Nurse Practitioner, 14*(5), 47–57.

King, R. B. (1990). *Quality of life after stroke*. Doctoral dissertation, University of Illinois at Chicago.

King, S., & de Sales, T. (2000). Caring for adolescent females with anorexia nervosa: Registered nurses' perspective. *Journal of Advanced Nursing, 32*(1), 139–147.

Kirkevold, M. (1997). The role of nursing in the rehabilitation of acute stroke patients: Toward a unified theoretical perspective. *Advances in Nursing Science, 19*, 55–64.

Kluckhon, F. R. (1953). Dominant and variant value orientations. In C. Kluckhon, H. A. Murray & D. M. Schneider (Eds.), *Personality in nature, culture, and society* (pp. 342–357). New York: Knopf.

Kobasa, S. (1984). The hardy personality: Toward a social psychology of stress and health. In W. D. Gentry, H. Benson, & C. J. de Wolff (Eds.), *Behavioral medicine, work and stress*. The Hague: Martinus Nijhoff.

Koch, T. (1995). Interpretive approaches in nursing research: The influence of Husserl and Heidegger. *Journal of Advanced Nursing, 21*, 827–836.

Kolcaba, K. Y. (1995). The art of comfort care. *Image: Journal of Nursing Scholarship, 27*, 287–289.

Kotler, P. (1973). Atmospherics as a marketing tool. *Journal of Retailing, 49*(4), 48–64.

Kramer, R. F. (1984). Living with childhood cancer: Impact on the healthy siblings. *Oncology Nursing Forum, 11*(1), 44–51.

Krauss, J. (2000). Protecting the legacy: The nurse-patient relationship and the therapeutic alliance. *Archives of Psychiatric Nursing, 14*(2), 49–50.

Kuhlemeier, K. V., & Stiens, S. A. (1994). Racial disparities in severity of cardiovascular events. *Stroke, 25,* 2126–2131.

Kvale, S. (1996). *InterViews: An introduction to qualitative research interviewing.* Thousand Oaks, CA: Sage.

Kwant, R. C. (1963). *The phenomenological philosophy of Merleau-Ponty.* Pittsburgh, PA: Duquesne University Press.

Lai, Y. (1999). Effects of music listening on depressed women in Taiwan. *Issues in Mental Health Nursing, 20*(3), 229–246.

Lakoff, G., & Johnson, M. (1980). *Metaphors we live by.* Chicago, IL: The University of Chicago Press.

Lakoff, G., & Johnson, M. (1999). *Philosophy in the flesh: The embodied mind and its challenge to western thought.* New York: Basic Books.

Landenburger, K. (1989). A process of entrapment in and recovery from an abusive relationship. *Issues in Mental Health Nursing, 10,* 209–226.

Langer, M. K. (1989). *Merleau-Ponty's "Phenomenology of Perception": A Guide and Commentary.* London: Macmillan.

LaSorsa, V., & Fodor, I. (1990). Adolescent daughter and midlife mother dyad. *Psychology of Women Quarterly, 14,* 593–606.

Latham, J., & Davis, B. D. (1994). The socioeconomic impact of chronic pain. *Disability and Rehabilitation, 16,* 39–44.

Lazarus, R. S., & Folkman, S. (1984). *Stress, appraisal and coping.* New York: Springer.

LeFort, S. M. (2000). A test of Braden's Self-Help Model in adults with chronic pain. *Journal of Nursing Scholarship, 32,* 153–160.

Leininger, M. (1991). *Culture care diversity and universality: A theory of nursing.* New York: National League for Nursing Press.

Leonard, V. (1999). A Heideggerian phenomenologic perspective on the concept of the person. In E. C. Polifroni & M. Welch (Eds.), *Perspectives on philosophy of science in nursing* (pp. 315–327). Philadelphia: Lippincott.

Levine, M. E. (1969). The pursuit of wholeness. *American Journal of Nursing, 69*(1), 93–98.

Levine, M. E. (1971). Holistic nursing. *Nursing Clinics of North America, 6,* 253–264.

Lincoln, Y. S., & Guba, E. G. (1987). But is it rigorous? Trustworthiness and authenticity in naturalistic evaluation. *Evaluation Studies Review Annual, Vol. 12*(pp. 425–436). Newbury Park, CA: Sage.

Lindeke, L. L., Hauck, M. R., & Tanner, M. (1998). Creating spaces that enhance nurse practitioner practice. *Journal of Pediatric Health Care, 12*(3), 125–129.

Lively, S., Friedrich, R. M., & Buckwalter, K. C. (1995). Sibling perception of schizophrenia: Impact on relationships, roles, and health. *Issues in Mental Health Nursing, 16*, 225–238.

Loose, V. (1994). Lydia E. Hall: Rehabilitation nursing pioneer in the ANA Hall of Fame. *Rehabilitation Nursing, 19*, 174–176.

Love, C., & Seaton, H. (1991). Eating disorders: Highlights of nursing assessment and therapeutics. *Nursing Clinics of North America, 26*(3), 677–680.

Lovestone, S., & Kumar, R. (1993). Postnatal psychiatric illness: Impact on partners. *British Journal of Psychiatry, 163*, 210–216.

Ludwig, A. M. (1966). Altered states of consciousness. *Archives of General Psychiatry, 15*, 225–234.

Luft, J. (1970). *Group processes: An introduction to group dynamics.* Palo Alto, CA: Mayfield.

Macann, C. (1993). *Four phenomenological philosophers.* London: Routledge.

MacGillivray, W. (1986). *Ambiguity and embodiment: A phenomenological analysis of the lived body.* Unpublished doctoral dissertation, University of Tennessee, Knoxville.

MacQuarrie, J. (1973). *Existentialism.* London: Penguin Books.

Main, M. C., Gerace, L. M., & Camilleri, D. (1993). Information sharing concerning schizophrenia in a family member: Adult siblings' perspectives. *Archives of Psychiatric Nursing, 7*(3), 147–153.

Marck, P. (2000). Nursing in a technological world: Searching for healing communities. *Advances in Nursing Science, 23*(2), 62–81.

Markenson, J. A. (1996). Mechanisms of chronic pain. *American Journal of Medicine, 101*, Suppl. 1A, pp. 7–17.

Martell, L. K. (1990). Postpartum depression as a family problem. *MCN, The American Journal of Maternal Child Nursing, 15*, 90–93.

Martin, D. (1988). *Battered wives.* San Francisco: Volcano Press.

Martinson, I. M., & Campos, R. G. (1991). Adolescent bereavement: Long-term responses to a sibling's death from cancer. *Journal of Adolescent Research, 6*(1), 54–69.

Matas, K. E. (1997). Human patterning and chronic pain. *Nursing Science Quarterly, 10*(2), 88–95.

McCaffery, M., & Thorpe, D. (1989). Differences in perception of pain and the development of adversarial relationships among health care providers. In C. S. Hill & W. S. Fields (Eds.), *Advances in pain research and therapy, vol.11*(pp. 113–125). New York: Raven Press.

McCollum, A. T. (1971). Cystic fibrosis: Economic impact upon the family. *American Journal of Public Health, 61*, 1335–1340.

McHolm, F. (1991). A nursing diagnosis validation study: Defining characteristics of spiritual distress. In R. Carroll-Johnson (Ed.), *Classification of nursing diagnoses* (pp. 112–119). Philadelphia: J. B. Lippincott.

McKeever, P. (1983). Siblings of chronically ill children: A literature review with implications for research and practice. *American Journal of Orthopsychiatry, 53*(2), 209–217.

McMahon, M. (1995). *Engendering motherhood: Identity and self-transformation in women's lives*. New York: Guilford Press.

McWilliam, C. L., Stewart, M., Brown, J. B., Desai, K., & Coderre, P. (1996). Creating health with chronic illness. *Advances in Nursing Science, 18*, 1–15.

Meighan, M. M. (1998). *Testing a nursing intervention to enhance parental-infant interaction and promote paternal role attainment*. Unpublished doctoral dissertation, University of Tennessee, Knoxville.

Menke, E. M. (1987). The impact of a child's chronic illness on school-aged siblings. *Children's Health Care, 15*(3), 132–140.

Merleau-Ponty, M. (1945/1962). *The phenomenology of perception* (C. Smith, trans.). London: Routledge and Kegan Paul.

Merleau-Ponty, M. (1970). *Themes from the lectures at the College of France 1952–1960*. (J. O'Neill, trans.). Evanston, IL: Northwestern University Press.

Merleau-Ponty, M. (1973). *The prose of the world* (J. O'Neill trans., C. Lefort ed.). Evanston, IL: Northwestern University Press.

Merritt-Gray, M., & Wuest, J. (1995). Counteracting abuse and breaking free: The process of learning revealed through women's voices. *Health Care for Women International, 16*, 399–412.

Mertz, M. G. (1999). What does Walt Disney know about patient satisfaction? *Family Practice Management, 6*(10), 33–35.

Miller, W. L., & Crabtree, B. F. (1998). Clinical research. In N. K. Denzin & Y. S. Lincoln (Eds.), *Strategies of qualitative inquiry* (pp. 292–314). Thousand Oaks, CA: Sage.

Miller, W. L., Yanoshik, M. K., Crabtree, B. F., & Reymond, W. K. (1994). Patients, family physicians, and pain: Visions from interview narratives. *Clinical Research and Methods, 26*, 179–184.

Mills, T. (1985). The assault on the self: Stages in coping with battering husbands. *Qualitative Sociology, 8*(2), 103–123.

Minkowski, E. (1970). *Lived time: Phenomenological and pathological studies* (N. Metzel, trans.). Evanston, IL: Northwestern University Press.

Minuchin, S. (1974). *Families and family therapy*. Cambridge, MA: Harvard University Press.

Minuchin, S., Rosman, B. L., & Baker, L. (1979). *Psychosomatic families*. Cambridge, MA: Harvard University Press.

Moore, T. (1992). *Care of the soul*. New York: HarperCollins.

Moran, D. (2000). *Introduction to phenomenology*. London: Routledge.

Morris, D. (1998). Illness and health in the postmodern age. *Advances in Mind-Body Medicine, 14*, 237–251.

Morse, J. (1991). Strategies for sampling. In J. Morse (Ed.), *Qualitative nursing research* (pp. 127–145). Newbury Park, CA: Sage.

Morse, J. (1994). Designing funded qualitative research. In N. K. Denzin & Y. S. Lincoln (Eds.), *Handbook of qualitative research* (pp. 220–235). Thousand Oaks, CA: Sage.

Morse, J. (2000). On comfort and comforting. *American Journal of Nursing, 100*(9), 34–37.

Morse, J., & Doberneck, B. (1995). Delineating the concept of hope. *Image: Journal of Nursing Scholarship, 27,* 277–285.

Morse, J., Penrod, J., & Hupcey, J. (2000). Qualitative outcome analysis: Evaluating nursing interventions for complex clinical phenomena. *Journal of Nursing Scholarship, 32,* 125–130.

Moser, S. A., Crawford, D., & Thomas, A. (1993). Updated care guidelines for patients with automatic implantable cardioverter defibrillators. *Critical Care Nurse, 13*(2), 62–71.

Moss, D. M. (1989). Brain, body and world: Body image and the psychology of the body. In R. S. Valle & S. Halling (Eds.), *Existential-phenomenological perspectives in psychology* (pp. 63–81). New York: Plenum.

Munhall, P. L. (1994). *Revisioning phenomenology: Nursing and health sciences research.* New York: National League for Nursing Press.

Muscari, M. E. (1998). Walking a thin line: Managing care for adolescents with anorexia and bulimia. *MCN, the American Journal of Maternal Child Nursing, 23*(3), 130–141.

Newman, K. D. (1993). Giving up: Shelter experiences of battered women. *Public Health Nursing, 10*(2), 108–113.

Newman, M. A. (1994). *Health as expanding consciousness*(2nd ed.). New York: National League for Nursing Press.

Newshan, G. T. (1996). *Is anybody listening? A phenomenological study of pain in hospitalized persons with AIDS.* Unpublished doctoral dissertation, New York University.

Nichols, S. K., & Wolverton, C. L. (1991). Outcome criteria for patients with implantable defibrillators. *Dimensions of Critical Care Nursing, 10*(5), 294–304.

Niemi, M., Laaksonen, R., Kotila, M., & Waltimo, O. (1988). Quality of life four years after stroke. *Stroke, 19,* 1101–1107.

Nightingale, F. (1860/1969). *Notes on nursing: What it is and what it is not.* New York: Dover.

Noll, S. F., & Roth, E. J. (1994). Stroke rehabilitation. 1. Epidemiologic aspects and acute management. *Archives Physical Medicine and Rehabilitation, 75,* S38–S41.

North American Nursing Diagnosis Association (1996). *Nursing diagnoses: Definitions and classification 1997–1998.* Philadelphia: Author.

Oakden, E. C., & Sturt, M. (1922). The development of knowledge of time in children. *British Journal of Psychology, 12,* 309–337.

O'Hara, M. W. (1995). *Postpartum depression: Causes and consequences.* New York: Springer-Verlag.

O'Loughlin, A. (1999). On living with chronic pain. In I. Madjar & J. Walton (Eds.), *Nursing and the experience of illness: Phenomenology in practice* (pp. 123–144). London: Routledge.

Oiler, C. (1982). The phenomenological approach in nursing research. *Nursing Research, 31*(3), 178–181.

Omery, A. (1983). Phenomenology: A method for nursing research. *Advances in Nursing Science, 5*(2), 49–63.

Palazolli, S. (1978). *Self starvation: From the intrapsychic to the transpersonal approach*. New York: Jason Aronson.

Paley, J. (1997). Husserl, phenomenology, and nursing. *Journal of Advanced Nursing, 26*(1), 193–197.

Paley, J. (1998). Misinterpretive phenomenology: Heidegger, ontology, and nursing research. *Journal of Advanced Nursing, 27*(4), 817–824.

Parimucha, J. P., Lussier, J., & Huelat, B. J. (2000, March 8–10). *Facility management: It costs how much? Bottom line reality*. Paper presented at the conference of the American Society for Healthcare Engineers and the American Institute of Architecture's Academy of Architecture for Health, Nashville, TN.

Parse, R. R. (1981). *Man-living-health: A theory of nursing*. New York: Wiley.

Parse, R. R. (1992). Human becoming: Parse's theory of nursing. *Nursing Science Quarterly, 5*, 35–42.

Parse, R. R. (1995). *Illuminations: The human becoming theory in practice and research*. New York: National League for Nursing Press.

Paterson, J. G., & Zderad, L. T. (1976). *Humanistic nursing*. New York: Wiley.

Peacher, R. (1996). The experience of place. *Dissertation Abstracts International: Section B: The Sciences and Engineering, 57*(2–B), 1450.

Peplau, H. E. (1952). *Interpersonal relations in nursing*. New York: Putnam.

Pfettscher, S., de Graff, K., Tomey, M., Mossman, C., & Slebodnik, M. (1998). Florence Nightingale: Modern Nursing. In A. M. Tomey and M. R. Alligood (Eds.), *Nursing theorists and their work* (pp. 69–85). New York: Mosby.

Phillips, K. (1994). *Testing biobehavioral adaptation in persons living with AIDS using Roy's theory of the person as an adaptive system*. Unpublished doctoral dissertation, University of Tennessee, Knoxville.

Pieranunzi, V. R. (1997). The lived experience of power and powerlessness in psychiatric nursing: A Heideggerian hermeneutical analysis. *Archives of Psychiatric Nursing, 11*, 155–162.

Pike, K., & Rodin, J. (1991). Mothers, daughters and eating disorders. *Journal of Abnormal Psychology, 100*, 198–204.

Piles, C. (1990). Providing spiritual care. *Nurse Educator, 15*(1), 36–41.

Plessner, H. (1961/1970). *Laughing and crying* (J. Churchill & M. Grene, trans.). Evanston, IL: Northwestern University Press.

Plugge, H. (1967). *Der Mensch und sein Leib*. Tubingen: Max Neimeyer.

Polkinghorne, D. (1989). Phenomenological research methods. In R. S. Valle & S.

Halling (Eds.), *Existential-phenomenological perspectives in psychology* (pp. 41–62). New York: Plenum.

Pollio, H. R. (1982). *Behavior and existence: An introduction to empirical humanistic psychology*. Monterey, CA: Brooks/Cole.

Pollio, H. R., Barlow, J., Fine, H., & Pollio, M. R. (1977). *The poetics of growth: Figurative language in psychology, psychotherapy, and education*. Hillsdale, NJ: Erlbaum.

Pollio, H. R., Henley, T. B., & Thompson, C. J. (1997). *The phenomenology of everyday life*. New York: Cambridge University Press.

Pollio, H. R., Levasseur, P., Anderson, J., & Thweatt, M. (2001, March). *Current cultural meanings of nature: An analysis of contemporary motion pictures*. Paper presented at the Southeastern Psychological Association, Atlanta, GA.

Pollio, H. R., & Thweatt, M. (2000). Experiencing the landscape in landscape painting. *Soundings, 83*, 147–168.

Porter, E. (1998). On "being inspired" by Husserl's phenomenology: Reflections on Omery's exposition of phenomenology as a method of nursing research. *Advances in Nursing Science, 21*, 16–28.

Porter, E. (1999a). 'Getting up from here': Frail older women's experiences after falling. *Rehabilitation Nursing, 24*, 201–206, 211, 226.

Porter, E. (1999b). Defining the eligible, accessible population for a phenomenological study. *Western Journal of Nursing Research, 21*, 796–804.

Porter, E. (in press). Sparking students' interest in the clinical relevance of qualitative research. *Journal of Nursing Education*.

Porter, E., & Lanes, T. (2000). Targeting intermediaries to recruit older women for qualitative, longitudinal research. *Journal of Women and Aging, 12*, 63–75.

Powell, T. H., & Gallagher, P. A. (1993). *Brothers and sisters: A special part of exceptional families*. Baltimore: Paul H. Brookes.

Quill, T. E., Barold, S. S., & Sussman, B. L. (1994). Discontinuing an implantable cardioverter defibrillator as a life-sustaining treatment. *The American Journal of Cardiology, 74*, 205–207.

Radner, G. (1989). *It's always something*. New York: Avon.

Ramacharandan, V. S., & Hirstein, W. (1998). The perception of phantom limbs. *Brain, 121*, 1603–1630.

Rampling, D. (1980). Abnormal mothering in the genesis of anorexia nervosa. *Journal of Nervous and Mental Disease, 168*, 501–504.

Ray, M. A. (1994). The richness of phenomenology: Philosophic, theoretic, and methodologic concerns. In J. M. Morse (Ed.), *Critical issues in qualitative research methods* (pp. 117–133). Thousand Oaks, CA: Sage.

Redeker, N. (2000). Sleep in acute care settings: An integrative review. *Journal of Nursing Scholarship, 32*(1), 31–38.

Reed, P. G. (2000). Nursing reformation: Historical reflections and philosophic foundations. *Nursing Science Quarterly, 13*(2), 129–136.

Reeder, F. (1987). The phenomenological movement. *Image: Journal of Nursing Scholarship, 19*(3), 150–152.

Reidenbach, R., & Sandifer-Smallwood, B. (1990). Exploring perceptions of hospital operations by a modified SERVQUAL approach. *Journal of Health Care Marketing, 10*(4), 47–55.

Reinharz, S. (1992). *Feminist methods in social research.* New York: Oxford University Press.

Remen, R. (1988, Autumn). Spirit: Resource for healing. *Noetic Sciences Review,* 61–65.

Richardson, J. (1986). *Existential epistemology: A Heideggerian critique of the Cartesian project.* Oxford, England: Oxford University Press.

Riddoch, G. (1941). Phantom limbs and body shape. *Brain, 64,* 197–222.

Riemen, D. J. (1998). The essential structure of a caring interaction. In J. W. Creswell (Ed.), *Qualitative inquiry and research design: Choosing among five traditions.* Thousand Oaks, CA: Sage Publications.

Riikonen, E. (1999). Inspiring dialogues and relational responsibility. In S. McNamee & K. Gergen (Eds.), *Relational responsibility* (pp. 139–149). Thousand Oaks, CA: Sage.

Risse, G. B. (1999). *Mending bodies, saving souls: A history of hospitals.* Oxford, UK: Oxford University Press.

Roberts, S. J. (2000). Development of a positive professional identity: Liberating oneself from the oppressor within. *Advances in Nursing Science, 22*(4), 71–82.

Robinson, D. N. (1995). The logic of reductionistic models. *New Ideas in Psychology, 13,* 1–8

Robley, L. R. (1995). The ethics of qualitative nursing research. *Journal of Professional Nursing, 11*(1), 45–48.

Rodgers, B. L. (1991). Deconstructing the dogma in nursing knowledge and practice. *Image: Journal of Nursing Scholarship, 23,* 177–181.

Rodin, J. (1993). Cultural and psychosocial determinants of weight concerns. *Annals of Internal Medicine, 119*(7 part 2), Suppl., 643–645.

Rogers, M. E. (1970). *An introduction to the theoretical basis of nursing.* Philadelphia: F. A. Davis.

Ronco, P. (1972). Human factors applied to hospital patient care. *Human Factors, 14,* 461–470.

Rondeau, K. V. (1998). Managing the clinic wait: An important quality of care challenge. *Journal of Nursing Care Quality, 13*(2), 11–20.

Rorty, M., Yager, J., Rossotto, E., & Buckwalter, G. (2000). Parental intrusiveness in adolescence recalled by women with a history of bulimia nervosa and comparison women. *International Journal of Eating Disorders, 28*(2), 202–208.

Rosen, J. C. (1992). Body image disorder: Definition, development, and contribution to eating disorders. In J. H. Crowther, D. L. Tennenbaum, S. E. Hobfoll, & M. A. P. Stephens (Eds.), *The etiology of bulimia: The individual and family context* (pp. 157–177). Washington, DC: Hemisphere.

Rosen, J. C. (1996). Body dysmorphic disorder: Assessment and treatment. In J. K. Thompson (Ed.), *Body image, eating disorders, and obesity: An integrative guide for assessment and treatment* (pp. 149–170). Washington, DC: American Psychological Association.

Roth, J. A. (1963). *Timetables.* New York: Bobbs-Merrill.

Rubin, E. (1921). *Visuell wahregenommene figuren.* Copenhagen: Glydendalske.

Sacco, R. L. (1995). Risk factors and outcomes for ischemic stroke. *Neurology, 45*(suppl.), S10–S14.

Sampselle, C., Bernhard, L., Kerr, R., Opie, N., Perley, M., & Pitzer, M. (1992). Violence against women: The scope and significance of the problem. In C. Sampselle (Ed.), *Violence against women: Nursing research, education, and practice issues* (pp. 3–16). New York: Hemisphere Publishing.

Sandelowski, M. (1986). The problem of rigor in qualitative research. *Advances in Nursing Science, 8*(3), 27–37.

Sandelowski, M. (1993). Rigor or rigor mortis: The problem of rigor in qualitative research revisited. *Advances in Nursing Science, 16*(2), 1–8.

Sandelowski, M. (1997). "To be of use": Enhancing the utility of qualitative research. *Nursing Outlook, 45,* 125–132.

Sandin, K. J., Cifu, D. X., & Noll, S. F. (1994). Stroke rehabilitation. 4. Psychologic and social implications. *Archives of Physical Medicine Rehabilitation, 75,* S52–S55.

Sartre, J. P. (1956). *Being and nothingness.* (Hazel Barnes, trans.). New York: Philosophical Press.

Schorr, J., & Schroeder, C. (1989). Consciousness as a dissipative structure: An extension of the Newman model. *Nursing Science Quarterly, 2*(4), 183–192.

Schroeder, C. (1992). The process of inflicting pain in nursing: Caring relationship or torture? In D. Gaut (Ed.), *The presence of caring in nursing* (pp. 211–220). New York: National League for Nursing.

Schwarz, N. (1999). Self-reports: How the questions shape the answers. *American Psychologist, 54*(2), 93–105.

Secrest, J. (1997). *Quality of life following stroke: The survivors' perspective.* Unpublished doctoral dissertation, University of Tennessee, Knoxville.

Seers, K., & Friedli, K. (1996). The patients' experiences of their chronic non-malignant pain. *Journal of Advanced Nursing, 24,* 1160–1168.

Seidner, B. (1987). *A phenomenological analysis of the experience of falling apart.* Unpublished doctoral dissertation, University of Tennessee, Knoxville.

Seitz, F. C. (1993). The evaluation and understanding of pain: Clinical and legal/forensic perspectives. *Psychological Reports, 72,* 643–657.

Sexton, A. (1981). *The complete poems.* Boston, MA: Houghton Mifflin.

Seymour, E., Fuller, B. F., Pederson-Gallegos, L., & Schwaninger, J. E. (1997). Modes of thought, feeling, and action in infant pain assessment by pediatric nurses. *Journal of Pediatric Nursing, 12*(1), 32–50.

Shoebridge, P., & Gowers, S. (2000). Parental high concern and adolescent-onset anorexia nervosa: A case control study to investigate direction of causality. *British Journal of Psychiatry, 176*, 132–137.

Shotter, J., & Katz, A. M. (1999). Creating relational realities: Responsible responding to poetic 'movements' and 'moments.' In S. McNamee & K. J. Gergen (Eds.), *Relational responsibility* (pp. 151–161). Thousand Oaks, CA: Sage.

Shupe, A., Stacey, W., & Hazelwood, L. (1987). *Violent men, violent couples: The dynamics of domestic violence.* Toronto: D.C. Heath.

Silva, M. C. (1995). *Ethical guidelines in the conduct, dissemination, and implementation of nursing research.* Washington, DC: American Nurses Association.

Simmel, M. (1962). Phantom experiences following amputation in childhood. *Journal of Neurology and Neurological Psychiatry, 25*, 69–78.

Skevington, S. M. (1983). Chronic pain and depression: Universal or personal helplessness? *Pain, 15*, 309–317

Sloane, R., & Sloane, B. (1992). *A guide to health care facilities: Personnel and management* (3rd ed.). Ann Arbor, MI: Health Administration Press.

Smith, B. A. (1999). Ethical and methodologic benefits of using a reflexive journal in hermeneutic-phenomenologic research. *Image: Journal of Nursing Scholarship, 31*, 359–363.

Smith, G. C., Smith, M. F., & Toseland, R. W. (1991). Problems identified by family caregivers in counseling. *The Gerontologist, 31*(1), 15–22.

Smith, M., Droppleman, P., & Thomas, S. P. (1996). Under assault: The experience of work-related anger in female registered nurses. *Nursing Forum, 31*(1), 22–33.

Smolak, L., Murnen, S., & Ruble, A. (2000). Female athletes and eating problems: A meta-analysis. *International Journal of Eating Disorders, 27*(4), 371–380.

Souhrada, L. (1990, February 20). A-1 renovations: Planning for the future. *Hospitals*, 58–66.

Sourkes, B. M. (1987). Siblings of the child with a life-threatening illness. *Journal of Children in Contemporary Society, 19*, 3–4.

Spiegelberg, H. (1981). *The context of the phenomenological movement.* The Hague: Martinus-Nijhoff.

Springer, D. V. (1951). Development of concepts related to the clock as shown in young children's drawings. *Journal of Genetic Psychology, 79*, 47–54.

Springer, D. V. (1952). Development in young children of an understanding of time and the clock. *Journal of Genetic Psychology, 80*, 83–96.

Stark, F. (1948). *Perseus in the wind.* London: John Murray.

Steeves, R., & Kahn, D. (1987). Experience of meaning in suffering. *Image, 19*(3), 114–116.

Stern, D. (1995). *The motherhood constellation: A unified view of parent-infant psychotherapy.* Cambridge, MA: Harvard University Press.

Storr, J. (1996). A nurse's view. In E. D. Baer, C. M. Fagin, & S. Gordon (Eds.), *Abandonment of the patient* (pp. 31–36). New York: Springer.

Stranahan, S. (2001). Spiritual perception, attitudes about spiritual care, and spiritual practices among nurse practitioners. *Western Journal of Nursing Research, 23,* 90–104.

Straus, E. (1947). Disorders of personal time in depressive states. *Southern Medical Journal, 40,* 254–259.

Straus, E. (1964). Chronognosy and chronopathy. In E. Strais (Ed.), *Phenomenology: Pure and applied. The First Lexington Conference.* Pittsburgh: Duquesne University Press.

Straus, M. (1976). Sexual inequality, cultural norms, and wife beating. *Victimology: An International Journal, 1,* 54–76.

Sunderland, S. (1978). *Nerves and nerve injuries, 2nd ed.* Edinburgh: Churchill-Livingston.

Swanson, K. M. (1991). Empirical development of a middle range theory of caring. *Nursing Research, 40,* 161–166.

Swanson, K. M. (1993). Nursing as informed caring for the well-being of others. *Image: Journal of Nursing Scholarship, 25*(4), 352–357.

Tait, R. C., & Chibnall, J. T. (1997). Physician judgments of chronic pain patients. *Social Science and Medicine, 45,* 1199–1205.

Tanner, C., Benner, P., Chesla, C., & Gordon, D. (1993). The phenomenology of knowing the patient. *Image: Journal of Nursing Scholarship, 25,* 273–280.

Taylor, A. G., Skelton, J. A., & Butcher, J. (1984). Duration of pain condition and physical pathology as determinants of nurses' assessments of patients in pain. *Nursing Research, 33,* 4–8.

Taylor, E., Highfield, M., & Amenta, M. (1994). Attitudes and beliefs regarding spiritual care. *Cancer Nursing, 17*(6), 479–487.

Taylor, S., & Epstein, R. (1999). *Living well with a hidden disability.* Oakland, CA: New Harbinger Publications.

Taylor, S. C. (1980). The effect of chronic childhood illnesses upon well siblings. *Maternal-Child Nursing, 9*(2), 109–116.

Teplitz, L., Egenes, K. J., & Brask, L. (1990). Life after sudden death: The development of a support group for automatic implantable cardioverter defibrillator patients. *Journal of Cardiovascular Nursing, 4*(2), 20–32.

Thomas, S. P. (1998). *Transforming nurses' anger and pain: Steps toward healing.* New York: Springer Publishing.

Thomas, S. P. (2000). Response by Thomas. *Western Journal of Nursing Research, 22*(6), 702–705.

Thomas, S. P., & Donnellan, M. M. (1993). Stress, role responsibilities, social support, and anger. In S. P. Thomas (Ed.), *Women and anger* (pp. 112–128). New York: Springer.

Thomas, S. P., & Droppleman, P. G. Channeling nurses' anger into positive interventions. *Nursing Forum, 32*(2), 13–21.

Thomas, S. P., McCoy, J. D., & Martin, R. (2000, August). *Men's anger: A phenome-*

nological exploration of its meaning. Poster presented at the annual meeting of the American Psychological Association, Washington, DC.

Thomas, S. P., Shattell, M., & Martin, T. (2001, February). *The phenomenal world of the hospitalized psychiatric patient*. Paper presented at the Second International Interdisciplinary Conference "Advances in Qualitative Methods," Edmonton, Alberta, Canada.

Thomas, S. P., Smucker, C., & Droppleman, P. (1998). It hurts most around the heart: A phenomenological exploration of women's anger. *Journal of Advanced Nursing, 28*(2), 311–322.

Thompson, C., Locander, W., & Pollio, H. R. (1989). Putting consumer experience back into consumer research: The philosophy and method of existential-phenomenology. *Journal of Consumer Research, 16*, 133–146.

Thompson, J. K., Heinberg, L. J., Altabe, M., & Tartleff-Dunn (1999). *Exacting beauty*. Washington, DC: American Psychological Association Press.

Thorne, S., & Paterson, B. (1998). Shifting images of chronic illness. *Image: Journal of Nursing Scholarship, 30*(2), 173–178.

Thweatt, M. (2000). *The experience of being lost*. Unpublished doctoral dissertation, the University of Tennessee, Knoxville.

Travelbee, J. (1971). *Interpersonal aspects of nursing* (2nd ed.). Philadelphia: Davis.

Trice, L. (1990). Meaningful life experiences to the elderly. *Image, 22*(4), 248–251.

Tuan, Y. (1977). *Space and place: The perspective of experience*. Minneapolis, MN: University of Minnesota.

Ulrich, R. (1984). View through a window may influence recovery from surgery. *Science, 224*, 420–421.

Ulrich, Y. C. (1991). Women's reasons for leaving abusive spouses. *Health Care for Women International, 12*, 465–473.

Vaillot, Sr. M. C. (1966). Existentialism: A philosophy of commitment. *American Journal of Nursing, 66*, 500–505.

Valle, R. S., & King, M. (1978). An introduction to existential-phenomenological thought in psychology. In R. S. Valle & M. King (Eds.), *Existential-phenomenological alternatives for psychology*. New York: Oxford University Press.

Valle, R. S., King, M., & Halling, S. (1989). An introduction to existential-phenomenological thought in psychology. In R. S. Valle & S. Halling (Eds.), *Existential phenomenological perspectives in psychology* (pp. 3–16). New York: Plenum.

Van den Berg, J. H. (1961). *The changing nature of man*. New York: Dell.

van Kaam, A. L. (1966). *Existential foundations of psychology*. Pittsburgh, PA: Duquesne University Press.

Van Maanen, J. (1982). Introduction. In J. Van Maanen, J. M. Dabbs, & R. R. Faulkner (Eds.), *Varieties of qualitative research* (pp. 11–29). Beverly Hills, CA: Sage.

van Manen, M. (1990). *Researching lived experience*. London, Ontario: Althouse.

van Manen, M. (1998). Modalities of body experience in illness and health. *Qualitative Health Research, 8*(1), 7–24.

Vavaro, F. F. (1989). Treatment of the battered woman: Effective response of the emergency department. *American College of Emergency Physicians, 11*, 8–13.

Verdeber, S. (1986). Dimensions of person-window transactions in the hospital environment. *Environment and Behavior, 18*, 450–466.

Viney, L. L. (1989). *Images of illness.* Malabar, FL: Robert E. Krieger Publishing.

Vlay, S. C., Olson, L. C., Fricchione, G. L., & Friedman, R. (1989). Anxiety and anger in patients with ventricular tachyarrhythmias: Responses after automatic internal cardioverter implantation. *PACE, 12*, 366–373.

Von Fiandt, K. (1952/1966). *The world of perception.* Homewood, IL: Dorsey Press.

Wade, T. D., Bulik, C. M., Neale, M., & Kendler, K. S. (2000). Anorexia nervosa and major depression: Shared genetic and environmental risk factors. *The American Journal of Psychiatry, 157*(3), 469–471.

Walker, C. L. (1988). Stress and coping in siblings of childhood cancer patients. *Nursing Research, 37*(4), 208–212.

Walker, J. D. (1993). Enhancing physical comfort. In M. Gerteis, S. Edgman-Levitan, J. Daley, & T. L. Delbanco (Eds.), *Through the patient's eyes: Understanding and promoting patient-centered care* (pp. 119–153). San Franscisco: Jossey-Bass.

Walker, L. E. (1979). *The battered woman.* New York: Harper & Row.

Wallace, T., Roberton, E., Millar, C., & Frisch, S. (1999). Perceptions of care and services by the clients and families: A personal experience. *Journal of Advanced Nursing, 29*, 1144–1153.

Walsh, B. T., & Devlin, M. J. (1998). Eating disorders: Progress and problems. *Science, 280*(5368), 1387–1390.

Watson, J. (1985). *Nursing: Human science and human care.* Norwalk, CT: Appleton-Century-Crofts.

Watson, J. (1999). *Postmodern nursing and beyond.* London: Churchill Livingstone.

Watson, J. (2001). Postmodern nursing and beyond. In N. L. Chaska (Ed.), *The nursing profession: Tomorrow and beyond* (pp. 299–309). Thousand Oaks, CA: Sage.

Weatherall, J., & Creason, N. (1987). Validation of the nursing diagnosis, spiritual distress. In A. McLane (Ed.), *Classification of nursing diagnoses: Proceedings of the seventh conference* (pp. 182–185). St. Louis, MO: Mosby.

Werner, H. (1948). *Comparative psychology of mental development.* Chicago: Follett.

Wertz, F. J. (1983). From everyday to psychological description: Analyzing the moments of a qualitative data analysis. *Journal of Phenomenological Psychology, 14*, 197–242.

Wertz, F. J. (1989). Approaches to perception in phenomenological psychology: The alienation and recovery of perception in modern culture. In R. S. Valle & S. Halling (Eds.), *Existential-phenomenological perspectives in psychology* (pp. 83–97). New York: Plenum.

White, J. (2000). The prevention of eating disorders: A review of research on risk factors with implications for practice. *Journal of Child and Adolescent Nursing, 13*(2), 76–88.

Whorf, B. L. (1956). *Language, thought and reality*. Cambridge, MA: MIT Press.

Wilde, M. H. (1999). Why embodiment now? *Advances in Nursing Science, 22*(2), 25–38.

Wolf, B. (1977). *Living with pain*. New York: Seabury.

Wolf, Z. (1988). *Nurses work: The sacred and the profane*. Philadelphia: University of Pennsylvania Press.

Wood, A., Meighan, M., Thomas, S. P., & Droppleman, P. G. (1997). The downward spiral of postpartum depression. *MCN, The American Journal of Maternal Child Nursing, 22*, 308–317.

Woodside, A., Nielsen, R., Walters, F., Muller, G. (1988). Preference segmentation of health care services: The old-fashioneds, value conscious, affluents, and professional want-it-alls. *Journal of Health Care Marketing, 8*(2), 14–24.

Wuest, J., & Merritt-Gray, M. (1999). Not going back: Sustaining the separation in the process of leaving abusive relationships. *Violence Against Women, 5*(2), 110–133.

Yalom, I. (1980). *Existential psychotherapy*. New York: Basic Books.

Zalon, M. L. (1997). Pain in frail, elderly women after surgery. *Image: Journal of Nursing Scholarship, 29*(1), 21–26.

Zipfel, S., Lowe, B., Reas, D. L., Deter, H., & Herzog, W. (2000). Long-term prognosis in anorexia nervosa: Lessons from a 21–year follow-up study. *The Lancet, 355*(9205), 721–722.

Index